ROUTLEDGE LIBRARY EDITIONS:
SCIENCE AND TECHNOLOGY IN THE
NINETEENTH CENTURY

Volume 1

MEDICAL FRINGE AND
MEDICAL ORTHODOXY
1750–1850

MEDICAL FRINGE AND MEDICAL ORTHODOXY 1750–1850

Edited by
W. F. BYNUM AND ROY PORTER

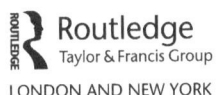

LONDON AND NEW YORK

First published in 1987 by Croom Helm Ltd
This edition first published in 2019
by Routledge
2 Park Square, Milton Park, Abingdon, Oxon OX14 4RN
and by Routledge
52 Vanderbilt Avenue, New York, NY 10017

Routledge is an imprint of the Taylor & Francis Group, an informa business

© 1987 W. F. Bynum and Roy Porter

All rights reserved. No part of this book may be reprinted or reproduced or utilised in any form or by any electronic, mechanical, or other means, now known or hereafter invented, including photocopying and recording, or in any information storage or retrieval system, without permission in writing from the publishers.

Trademark notice: Product or corporate names may be trademarks or registered trademarks, and are used only for identification and explanation without intent to infringe.

British Library Cataloguing in Publication Data
A catalogue record for this book is available from the British Library

ISBN: 978-1-138-39006-5 (Set)
ISBN: 978-0-429-02175-6 (Set) (ebk)
ISBN: 978-1-138-39128-4 (Volume 1) (hbk)
ISBN: 978-1-138-39136-9 (Volume 1) (pbk)
ISBN: 978-0-429-42274-4 (Volume 1) (ebk)

Publisher's Note
The publisher has gone to great lengths to ensure the quality of this reprint but points out that some imperfections in the original copies may be apparent.

Disclaimer
The publisher has made every effort to trace copyright holders and would welcome correspondence from those they have been unable to trace.

MEDICAL FRINGE & MEDICAL ORTHODOXY 1750-1850

Edited by W.F. Bynum and Roy Porter

CROOM HELM
London • Sydney • Wolfeboro, New Hampshire

© 1987 W.F. Bynum and Roy Porter
Croom Helm Ltd, Provident House, Burrell Row,
Beckenham, Kent BR3 1AT
Croom Helm Australia Pty Ltd, Suite 4, 6th Floor,
64-76 Kippax Street, Surry Hills, NSW 2010, Australia

British Library Cataloguing in Publication Data

Medical fringe and medical orthodoxy 1750-1850.
 (Wellcome Institute series in the history
 of medicine)
 1. Medicine — History — 18th century
 2. Medicine — History — 19th century
 I. Bynum, W.F. II. Porter, Roy, 1946-
 III. Series
 610'.9'033   R148

ISBN 0-7099-3959-0

Croom Helm US, 27 South Main Street,
Wolfeboro, New Hampshire 03894-2069

Library of Congress Cataloging-in-Publication Data
Medical fringe and medical orthodoxy.
 (The Wellcome Institute series in the history of
medicine)
 "Many of the papers in this volume were first presented at a one-day Symposium on Medical Orthodoxy and Medical Fringe held at the Wellcome Institute for the History of Medicine on 15 February 1985" —
Acknowledgements.
 1. Quacks and quackery — Social aspects — History —
18th century — Congresses. 2. Quacks and quackery —
Social aspects — History — 19th century — Congresses.
3. Social medicine — History — 18th century — Congresses.
4. Social medicine — History — 19th century — Congresses.
5. Medicine — History — 18th century — Congresses.
6. Medicine — History — 19th century — Congresses.
I. Bynum, W.F. (William F.), 1943-
II. Porter, Roy, 1946- . III. Symposium on Medical
Orthodoxy and Medical Fringe (1985: Wellcome Institute
for the History of Medicine) IV. Series. [DNLM:
1. History of Medicine, Modern — congresses. 2. Quackery
— history — congresses. 3. Therapeutic Cults — history —
congresses. WB 900 M489]
R730.M46 1987   362.1'09'033   86-19641
ISBN 0-7099-3959-0

Printed and bound in Great Britain by Mackays of Chatham Ltd, Kent

CONTENTS

Acknowledgements	vi
Introduction	1
1. Treating the Wages of Sin: Venereal Disease and Specialism in Eighteenth-century Britain *W.F. Bynum*	5
2. Publicity and the Public Good: Presenting Medicine in Eighteenth-century Bristol *Jonathan Barry*	29
3. Orthodoxy and Fringe: Medicine in Late Georgian Bristol *Michael Neve*	40
4. 'I Think Ye Both Quacks': The Controversy between Dr Theodor Myersbach and Dr John Coakley Lettsom *Roy Porter*	56
5. Property Rights and the Right to Health: The Regulation of Secret Remedies in France, 1789-1815 *Matthew Ramsey*	79
6. 'The Vile Race of Quacks with which this Country is Infested' *Irvine Loudon*	106
7. The Orthodox Fringe: The Origins of the Pharmaceutical Society of Great Britain *S.W.F. Holloway*	129
8. Bones of Contention? Orthodox Medicine and the Mystery of the Bone-setter's Craft *Roger Cooter*	158
9. Physical Puritanism and Sanitary Science: Material and Immaterial Beliefs in Popular Physiology, 1650-1840 *Virginia Smith*	174
10. Early Victorian Radicals and the Medical Fringe *J.F.C. Harrison*	198
11. Social Context and Medical Theory in the Demarcation of Nineteenth-century Boundaries *P.S. Brown*	216
12. Medical Sectarianism, Therapeutic Conflict, and the Shaping of Orthodox Professional Identity in Antebellum American Medicine *John Harley Warner*	234
Index	261

ACKNOWLEDGEMENTS

Many of the papers in this volume were first presented at a one-day symposium on 'Medical Orthodoxy and Medical Fringe' held at the Wellcome Institute for the History of Medicine on 15 February 1985. The generous support of the Wellcome Trustees made possible that symposium and, in a very real sense, this book as well.

INTRODUCTION

Few medical historians today would argue that regular medicine and fringe medicine have had their own autonomous histories, developing as completely distinct separate species, the one (in the eyes of its friends) scientific, professional, effective, or (in the eyes of its opponents) monopolistic and authoritarian; the other (according to some) vulgar, cranky and dangerous, or (to others) natural, democratic, harmless. The days of such 'saints and sinners' histories are over. Scholars of all stripes agree nowadays that — to a greater or lesser degree — the frontiers between orthodox and unorthodox medicine have been flexible; indeed, the very distinction between the two is one that has been socially constructed. So mobile have been their boundaries, that one age's quackery has often become another's orthodoxy, or vice versa. Thus, plotting the territorial shifts, gains and losses for 'proper' and 'improper' medicine, is acknowledged to be a task requiring the social historian.

But if it is generally accepted that regular and irregular medicine have dialectically interacted within the larger social whole, it is curious how each continues to be studied on its own. Most of the best social history or historical sociology of medical developments since the Industrial Revolution has looked at the operation of professionalisation and modernisation *within* orthodox medicine; and so we now have admirable studies, for example, of the tensions between physicians and apothecaries or the relations between the profession and Parliament. At the same time the medical sects have also found their historians, especially amongst scholars concerned with working-class and labour history. These two genres of research have established themselves, but very little has been published which links and straddles them.

To do that is the aim of this book. In it the dozen contributors have provided a series of studies examining how the relations between regular and irregular medicine have been constituted in particular fields at particular times. In some cases, they complement each other, and their relations are amicable; in others, there is deep conflict. Sometimes we see the isomorphisms, in others the differences between 'insider' and 'outsider' medicine stand out most. Examining how 'high' and 'low' medicine came to adopt their own identities through conflict and competition with each other is a particularly important feature of these analyses. For arguably, it was the hundred years covered by this book (the mid-eighteenth to the mid-nineteenth centuries) that saw the emergence of the familiar distinction between regular and fringe medicine which we nowadays feel comfortable enough in making. If a historian speaks of a distinction before the nineteenth century between 'proper' medical practitioners and the rest, his distinction is not one which was to any great degree based upon a contemporary formal, legal, or statutory basis. Certainly, the medical historian surveying the eighteenth-century scene can point to certain practitioners who had society's approval stamped on to pieces of paper: these were university graduates, or members or licentiates of the various medical colleges. But such men (and all of them, with the exception of a number of licensed midwives, were *men*) amounted to only a relatively small percentage even of those who would have popularly been regarded as regular practitioners, let alone of all the people who (men or women, on a full-time or part-time, commercial or amateur basis) were engaged in healing the sick. Most practising surgeons and apothecaries held no public certificate.

The beginning of the end of this 'unregulated' situation — very different from what commonly obtained on the continent — came with the Apothecaries Act of 1815, the terms of which envisaged a time in the future when all 'general practitioners' would have to be licensed by one of numerous licensing bodies. The end came in 1858 with the Medical Act which established the *Medical Register*. From then on, the official public divide between the regular practitioners and the fringe healer was (at one level at least) clearly fixed: did a man's name (and still it was men only) appear on the register or not?

So in an important way the essays in this book are not just about the positioning and nature of the divide between medical orthodoxy and medical fringe, but are about its very creation, or at least the crystallisation of it as part of the public domain of medicine. Before, there was more of a continuity; after, more of a polar division. It is appropriate, therefore, that several of the contributors deal at some length with the various sectarian and professional groupings leading to, or created by, these landmarks of legislation. Thus Irvine Loudon and S.W.F. Holloway both look at the tussles towards the lower end of orthodox medicine between the apothecaries and the druggists and chemists. Apothecaries, who might have expected to find their place in the sun a little more secure after the 1815 Act, in fact found themselves being grossly undermined, professionally and economically, by the rise of the retail druggist; druggists, for their part, were anxious to turn their commercial success into professional consolidation. Or, looking further towards the fringe, P.S. Brown and J.F.C. Harrison examine how a newly self-conscious, self-defining, radical 'fringe' came to emerge in the early Victorian years, aggressively repudiating medical orthodoxy on high moral grounds (pure medicine would follow nature, trust the people, adopt a democratic epistemology, scorn monopoly and oligarchy). There had been 'irregular practitioners' aplenty before Victoria. But most of these were individuals, performing their healing practices, selling patent medicines: men like Theodor von Myersbach, examined in Roy Porter's essay. On the whole such itinerants, advertisers or empirics were not peddling ideologies or '-isms'. They weren't sectaries by choice: they were the classic 'quacks'. This changed in the nineteenth century, with the importation (often from America, as John Harley Warner's essay suggests) of medical sects which were heterodox by choice. To this degree, the growing nineteenth-century rupture between orthodox and fringe medicine was as much a creation of sect groups from below as it was of professional and controlling strategies from above.

In France (as Matthew Ramsey's discussion shows) the state, the law, and the medical corporations played important parts from early times in determining the fate of irregular medicine. In England, the state never outlawed fringe medical practices, and the ultimate arbiter remained to a much larger degree the public. How would the public vote with its feet? Some of the attempts in the late eighteenth century by a quack and a scion of the profession to convince the public of their respective claims to medical authority are examined in Porter's article. But what actually happened in practice? Which sectors of the public resorted to official or unofficial medicine, and why? Bynum's study of treatments for venereal disease in the eighteenth century indicates that regular surgeons and 'quack' practitioners presented themselves and their cures to the public in ways more remarkable for their similarities than for their differences. This is a conclusion confirmed to some extent by the two local studies in this volume, Michael Neve's and Jonathan Barry's examinations of Bristol. For as Neve suggests, even a regular physician such as Thomas Beddoes could actually appear a 'quack' to certain sectors of the public, worried about his radicalism and mystified by his Pneumatic Institute for the treatment of consumption by gases. Barry in turn shows how we must not automatically assume that 'quacks' were popular: there was a good deal of public scepticism about 'charlatans' and many of them must have led a precarious and marginal existence.

The subject thus proves complex. Not least, it is important to remember that at no point did there emerge a single 'orthodoxy' confronted by a single 'fringe'. Yet it is important not to create the impression that orthodox and fringe medicine were poles apart and fundamentally unalike in theory, therapeutics and general rhetoric. Roger Cooter's essay on that neglected figure, the bone-setter, to a large degree traces the historical complementary and peaceful coexistence between the bone-setter and the surgeon. In a similar way, Virginia Smith argues that medicine on all rungs of the ladder has been preoccupied with shared concerns: with cleanliness, temperance, moderation, hygiene, dietetics, bathing and so forth. In some ages, in some health-care systems, these have been seen mainly as 'fringe' specialities; in others, they have been true-blue orthodoxy. There are no automatic affinities between the social position of the fringe and its intellectual affiliations.

Above all, this book enters a plea against historical fragmentation. It could make for bad history if all orthodox medical historians studied orthodox medicine, while social, radical and labour historians studied the history of the 'fringe'. All schools of medicine took on their identities — shifting all the time — in relation to perceived rivals, above, below and all around. They must be studied in their mutual, dynamic relations, as a whole. This book aims to make a start on this necessary work.

1 TREATING THE WAGES OF SIN: VENEREAL DISEASE AND SPECIALISM IN EIGHTEENTH-CENTURY BRITAIN

W.F. Bynum

Introduction

If desperate diseases may require desperate remedies, do secret diseases elicit secret remedies?

The history of venereal disease, particularly since the eighteenth century, suggests that this may be so. The acquisition of a disorder generally contracted outside the socially sanctioned bounds of matrimony — the consequence of *coitus impurus* — has often left its victim the prey of remorse, guilt and desperation. These emotions may in turn disrupt the ordinary commercial dimensions of medical practice, and the moral neutrality which is supposed to attend the mundane encounter of sufferer and healer. Shame and guilt may heighten the possibilities for exploitation, for the desperation may arise as much from the fear of discovery as from any perceived threat to health or life. It can create a ripe field for subtle or not-so-subtle advertising, for promises in excess of the evidence, and for fees over the odds: rich pickings for quacks, charlatans and disreputable frauds.

Much of the traditional historical literature on quackery tacitly or implicitly assumes that venereal disease has been a quack's paradise. C.J.S. Thompson's *Quacks of Old London* details several venereological entrepreneurs among his galaxy of mountebanks and quacks, and Alex Comfort's *The Anxiety Makers* includes venereal disease along with reproduction, masturbation and constipation as highly charged areas of the body economy, prone to exploitation.[1] The essays by Barry and Loudon in this volume (pp. 29-39 and 106-28) demonstrate how the use of local newspapers, handbills and other sources — many of them ephemeral in character — can uncover a vigorous trade in venereal disease in eighteenth- and early-nineteenth-century provincial Britain. Sorting out the sheep from the goats may not be so easy, however, since, as Porter has argued, the boundaries between 'regular' and 'irregular' practice are difficult to draw in the individualistic and unregulated medical world prior to the parliamentary Acts of the nineteenth century.[2] Further, there exists a historiography which stresses the sexual openness

5

6   *Treating the Wages of Sin*

of Enlightenment values in those days of directories of prostitutes and public mistresses. In a society where sexual intercourse could be depicted as a relatively uncomplicated physical act, without the psychological overtones it was later to acquire, and where young men were expected to sow a few oats, it might be expected that venereal disease would be viewed as a nuisance but not a stigma, perhaps even as the 'cavalier's disease'.[3] When we add to this the fact that syphilis was one of the few diseases for which orthodox medicine could claim a specific remedy (mercury), the flourishing of a quack venereology might seem more appropriate to Victoria's century, when hypocrisy abounded, euphemism was the order of the day, and the Contagious Diseases Acts (themselves euphemistically titled) could be debated repeatedly in Parliament for twenty years without anyone uttering the word 'syphilis'.[4]

It is not necessary to deny the existence of 'quackery' before the 1858 Medical Act finally and statutorily identified the 'regulars'. We can even accept the eighteenth century as quackery's 'golden age' — indeed, Porter has marshalled convincing evidence why this should be so, particularly in the growth of new forms of commercialism and consumerism.[5] My own work is based primarily on printed books and pamphlets, and so would tend to be biased in favour of literate elites. Even within this literature, however, we can find behaviour which is often difficult to characterise neatly: on the one hand, books published with title pages proclaiming the author as orthodox and 'regular' which are no more than puffs for secret remedies; and on the other hand, pamphlets which at first blush seem to be 'quackish', since coming from outside medical circles, but which are open, honest and humane.[6]

One feature of the venereal world was touted at the time, and has been repeated since, as a tellingly suspicious feature of shady behaviour: specialisation. Those who treated a single disease, whether venereal disease or gout, or those who performed a single task, like bone-setting, stone-cutting or cataract-couching, were branded as quacks or individuals of limited capacities, who failed to participate in the liberal aspirations of the orthodox occupation of medicine.[7] George Rosen argued that such marginal specialisms were common precursors of the formation of modern medical specialties like ophthalmology and urology, and that at least some of the opposition and even hostility which was accorded to the early specialties within medicine resulted from the traditional association of specialism and quackery.[8] The case for venereology has even further credibility within Rosen's classic framework, for the founding of specialised hospitals within the orthodox medical community provided a field of observation and a concentration of clinical cases similar to those offered by eye hospitals and dispensaries, or institutions devoted to treating bladder stones. Indeed, in the instance of venereal disease, lock hospitals had existed in London since the late Middle Ages, and although these medieval establishments had all disappeared by the mid-eighteenth century, the foundation of a new lock hospital in 1747 (part of the wave of specialist institutions which were to complement the early general voluntary hospitals) might, according to Rosen's model, have given a nucleus for a 'modern' specialty.[9] At least as early as 1802, George Rees was delivering a private course of lectures on venereal disease at his house in Soho Square, further evidence of the early perception of the coherence of the subject. If, as one recent commentator would have it, venereology did not emerge as a specialty until the present century, in this case Rosen's preconditions might be necessary but they are hardly sufficient, since they existed for a century or more before the specialty actually developed.[10]

We should not push his model too far, however, in identifying premodern occupational confinement as 'quackery'. There were, after all, the traditional divisions of labour accorded to physicians, surgeons and apothecaries (even if these were not always observed in practice) and further refinements which, though not overtly deemed quackish, were also part of the medical world we have lost. Male midwives, for instance, could hope to 'specialise' in their practice by the mid-eighteenth century, and the trade in lunacy encouraged a number of medical men to devote themselves to that branch of the occupation.[11] Psychiatry and obstetrics both became ultimately relatively unprestigious medical specialties, although the relationship between their antiquity and their present status is not a simple one, and both orthopaedic surgery and ophthalmology would rank well on a hierarchy of modern specialisms, despite their ancestry among the bone-setters and couchers.

Recent research has suggested that the tripartite model for medical practice in the eighteenth century is far too simple, particularly in the provinces, where many practitioners were generalists (prescribing, selling, advising, cutting and delivering), and even in London the divisions, despite the existence of three medical corporations, were not all that precise.[12] In the section that follows, I shall look at that division, as it related to the treatment of venereal disease. In the third section, I examine some of the general characteristics in this literature before, finally, looking at some examples of the professional behaviour which it reflects, especially those kinds of behaviour which are normally associated with the fringe, and the changing norms as the century wore on. I shall suggest that the venereological literature implies that, by the early nineteenth century, it is much easier to identify aberrant behaviour among 'ordinary' practitioners and briefly outline how the formation of a more unified medical orthodoxy might be important for understanding the emergence of a more highly structured 'fringe'.

Venereal Disease and the Medical Division of Labour

A parent in Georgian London concerned about his son's future occupation might well have consulted R. Campbell's *London Tradesman* (1747), with its descriptions of both 'liberal and mechanical' professions and trades, information on length and costs of apprenticeships, and often trenchant remarks on the skills and character traits needed for success. Campbell had a relatively low opinion of physicians, suggesting that too many of them placed too much emphasis on the trappings of the profession (the wig, chariot and cane), and too little on common sense and careful observation. Surgeons fared better, requiring (Campbell believed) just as liberal an education and capable of doing much good and of earning suitable rewards. 'An ingenious Surgeon, let him be cast on any Corner of the Earth, with but his Case of Instruments in his Pocket, he may live where most other professions would starve,' he observed.[13]

For the most part, Campbell was content with the traditional division of labour: although the 'Physician should know something of the Surgeon's Business, and he of the Doctor's, and the Apothecary of both,' in reality the more 'each confines himself to his own particular Branch, the greater success he may expect in his practice'.[14] Better a master of one trade than Jack of all, a sentiment echoed some seventy years later by Leonard Stewart, who lamented the extent to which the coming of the 'general practitioner' (a term he used) threatened to retard the advance of medical knowledge.[15] One condition, however, straddled the three branches of medicine — venereal disease. Campbell made no mention of it under 'Physician', and commented of apothecaries only that 'they all of them cure the Venereal Disease; I mean, they have their Patients upon whom they practise in that Distemper, who often find their Mistresses have only clapped them, but Doctor Apothecary has poxed them'.

Campbell was equally scathing when it came to surgical claims about curing venereal disease:[16]

> But there is one Branch belonging to the Doctor, [i.e. physician] which the Town Surgeon has almost monopolized to himself; that is, the

Cure of the Venereal Disease; upon which alone the Subsistance of three Parts in four of all the Surgeons in Town depends; and three Parts in four of their Practice depend upon their Ignorance in this very Distemper, which they pretend to cure: I mean, that if all knew as much as they pretend, they would not have half so many Patients, nor those half so long under their Cure. Before the Discovery of Mercury as a Specific against his Disorder, the Venereal Disease was always the Province of the Physician, as much as any other acute Distemper; the Surgeon was never called but when Amputations or outward Applications were necessary: But when the Virtues of prepared Mercury became generally known, the Surgeon usurped the Place of the Doctor, and monopolized this odious Distemper to himself. For this Reason the *London* Surgeon must study this Disease more than any other, as it is not only the most frequent but the most profitable Branch of his Profession; though I would advise him in all difficult Cases to take a Physician to his Assistance.

As a historical thesis, Campbell's remarks are wide of the mark. In the first place, the sixteenth-century literature on syphilis was not the exclusive product of physicians' pens, and in any case the relations between physic and surgery were rather different on the continent than in Britain. The most influential native pre-eighteenth-century works on the subject were probably those of William Clowes (1540?-1604) and Richard Wiseman (1622?-76), both surgeons, but Gideon Harvey (1640?-1700?), a physician, published two treatises on venereal disease, and Thomas Sydenham's (1623-88) comments on its diagnosis and treatment were afterwards much cited.[17] Furthermore, there is not much to suggest that 'prepared' mercury in itself encouraged the surgeons to poach venereal disease from the physicians, since mercurial compounds and salves were already in use during the late-fifteenth-century outburst of syphilis. Indeed, Owsei Temkin has outlined an alternative sixteenth-century scenario, in which the introduction of guaiac for the treatment of syphilis helped to 'individualise' the management of the condition and so made it more interesting to physicians, as opposed to the surgeons and barbers who upheld the universal specificity of mercury.[18]

Be that as it may, venereal disease is commonly cited as a surgical prerogative: gonorrhoea, after all, often led to urethral obstruction requiring manipulation, and the genital and skin manifestations of syphilis placed it 'naturally' within the purview of surgeons, who liked to see what they were treating. But was Campbell justified in giving such attention to the surgical importance of venereal disease, even if recommending that difficult cases should also involve a physician colleague? And did its treatment really preoccupy 75 per cent of eighteenth-century London surgeons? So large a group could hardly be called marginal to the medical establishment as a whole, but were these venereologists pillars of the community or despised and untrusted exploiters of fear and shame? In order to examine these issues, I have compiled a bio-bibliography of works on venereal disease published in Britain between 1700 and 1800, drawn principally from the Wellcome Institute's own catalogue, from that of the National Library of Medicine in Washington (Surgeon General's Library), and from Proksch's monumental *Die Litteratur über die venerischen Krankheiten*.[19] It is not complete, since I have excluded references to books which I have been unable to consult; it includes no medical theses (of which there were probably more than two dozen) or articles in medical or general periodicals; nor does it incorporate the thirty or more translations into English of foreign-language monographs on venereal disease, or the systematic considerations of venereal disease within larger, more general medical or surgical works. The absence of unbound ephemera, advertisements, broadsheets, etc., biases the sample in favour of more established practitioners; even so, this material still reflects a wide variety of standards of professional behaviour or conduct.

Even with the exclusions mentioned above, 100 separate publications on venereal disease have been identified, ranging from pamphlets of a few pages to substantial quartos. While by no means complete, it does give a good social, occupational and educational cross-section of individuals with a serious interest in the condition. They were produced by seventy-four separate named authors (several authors writing more than one work) and include half a dozen anonymous pamphlets and tracts. A couple of the authors do not appear to have been engaged in any form of medical practice, several were irregular or clearly fringe practitioners, and occasionally it has not been possible to place orthodox-sounding individuals within the conventional tripartite occupational division. Surprisingly, perhaps, apothecaries are virtually absent.

This leaves sixty-four 'regular' authors, of whom surgeons outnumbered physicians by a ratio of about two to one. Forty-five surgeons and nineteen physicians wrote on venereal disease during the century, figures which suggest that there is only a grain of truth in the general picture of venereal disease as a surgical monopoly. The rate of publication increased perceptibly, fifty-five of the items appearing in the last third of the period, but the physician/surgeon ratio does not vary significantly at any point. The raw figures thus support the popular

Treating the Wages of Sin 11

stereotype, but they also remind us that it is no more than a stereotype. The professional standing of the authors varied wildly, from individuals (physicians and surgeons) with no other publication and about whom there is little evidence of education, career or even birth and death dates, to some of the most eminent practitioners of the period. In the latter group may be included Nicholas Robinson (1697-1775), Daniel Turner (1667-1741), Thomas Beddoes (1760-1808), John Armstrong (1709-79), and John Hunter (1728-93), a nice mixture of physicians and surgeons, symbolised perhaps by the fact that Turner was a surgeon-turned-physician.[20] At the other end of the scale, men like Henry Saffory, Charles Swift and John Warren left behind little for posterity apart from their publications on venereal disease.[21] At the very least, however, the liberal sprinkling of professional elites (a trend which continued throughout the nineteenth century) gives the lie to the idea of a fringe monopoly in the treatment of what one anonymous pamphleteer actually called the 'secret disease'.[22] Certainly, there was money to be made by 'regulars' and 'irregulars' alike. For instance, when in 1748 the *Gentleman's Magazine* provided a listing of available nostrums and patent medicines, those for venereal complaints (and impotence) regularly cost a good deal more than those for coughs, colds, the 'itch' or 'pain'.[23]

The literature itself further clouds the notion that physicians were theory-prone speculators, and surgeons practical-minded operators. To be sure, there was some awareness of the medical division of labour, and a certain amount of inter-occupational sniping. One surgeon remarked that he would let physicians get on with the vain task of speculating on the precise cause of venereal disease, while he himself was busy simply curing it. One physician noted in his case histories his consultations with a surgeon with whom he was working in concert. But for the most part, it is impossible to predict attitudes or preoccupations among physicians and surgeons. Some surgeons, for instance, were deeply interested in issues like the New or Old World origin of syphilis, and many physicians were concerned principally with the simple practicalities of therapy, including, it might be added, the nature of the solutions for irrigating the bladder in cases of gleet or gonorrhoea. Another physician implied that he himself sometimes applied a mercurial ointment to his patients.[24]

It is significant that in the course of James Boswell's long and complicated affair with what he called 'Signor Gonorrhea', he consulted and was treated by both physicians and surgeons: surgeons such as Alexander Douglas, Duncan Forbes and Percival Pott, but also physicians such as John Gregory and Sir John Pringle.[25] That these were all worthy, or even eminent representatives of their respective callings suggests that Boswell at least did not feel compelled to take himself off to some backstreet irregular. The surgeons appear always to have performed the urethral dilatations and injections (although in one or two instances the operator is not made clear) but the attitudes and advice of his doctors routinely cut across medical and surgical divisions. The surgeon Douglas treated Boswell with a low diet, rest and internal medicine, and the physician Pringle was one of a group of consultants who at one stage advised a surgical procedure on the bladder of the long-suffering patient. Apparently only once in his long, licentious history (nineteen attacks of venereal disease) did Boswell try a nostrum which might be called a quack remedy. His doctors attempted to dissuade him from this step, but with his marriage imminent, he was determined to try to clear himself once and for all of his venereal taint. Accordingly, he bought and used a nostrum called Kennedy's Lisbon Diet Drink. At half a guinea a bottle and a bottle a day, it was expensive, but a friend testified that a course of the drink had cured him after he had already spent £300 on more conventional treatment. Unfortunately, it did not work for Boswell, who ended up calling it 'nonsense' and its vendor 'a gaping babbler'. The nostrum was well advertised, much was claimed for it, and it came with a long list of grateful testimonials: all the hallmarks, we might say, of a quack remedy. However, its inventor and proprietor, Gilbert Kennedy (c 1680-1780), had studied at the universities of Glasgow and Edinburgh, was a pupil of Boerhaave in Leyden, had an MD from Rheims and obtained another (by diploma in 1749) from Oxford. In 1737 he was elected a Fellow of the Royal Society.[26] Quack is as quack does.

All this does not mean, of course, that there was no eighteenth-century medical division of labour, no group consciousness among physicians, surgeons and apothecaries. Physicians generally placed their medical degree after their names on the title page and surgeons more often than not identified themselves as such. Nevertheless, it is individualism rather than collectivism, commercialism rather than enquiry, which shine through most of the eighteenth-century venereal disease literature; characteristics which make exceptions such as John Hunter's *Treatise on the Venereal Disease* (1786) all the more striking.[27] In the sections that follow, I shall examine some of the ramifications of this individualism and the range of values and varieties of professional behaviour which venereal disease elicited from those who wrote about it.

Themes from the Literature

Two important factors bore directly on most eighteenth-century writing on venereal disease: its sexual dimension and the availability of a widely respected treatment.

That the condition was routinely spread through sexual contact was a commonplace, although the nature of the *modus operandi* left plenty of room for observation, comment and speculation. Simple theories were patently inadequate, since there were too many instances of individuals with known sexual exposure to someone with active venereal disease failing to contract it, and others coming down with the symptoms while denying unclean intercourse. That permanent immunity did not result from a flagrant episode of the disease, as in smallpox, further complicated the matter. So did presumed non-venereal sources of infection, especially diseased nurses passing the 'virus' (as it was usually called) to their sucklings. These and other ambiguities convinced John Andree in 1779 that the disease must ultimately be generated *de novo* within the body.[28] These issues also made it easy to provide moral readings of its aetiology and spread. Chaste kissing, for instance, was assumed to be safe, but lascivious kissing could spread venereal disease.[29] Moderate copulation between undiseased partners was not dangerous, but if indulged in too frequently, one or both of the partners might come down with a venereal complaint. Since the 'gleet' (a whitish urethral discharge), the 'whites' (whitish vaginal discharge), gonorrhoea and syphilis were often assumed to be either stages in, or varieties of, what was the same category of disease, it is easy to see how these interpretations made perfectly logical (as well as moral) sense. Most writing in the period referred simply to 'the venereal disease' as a blanket category to describe all of these conditions.

The sexual aspect of the topic had other implications, however, particularly in the audience to which treatises were addressed. Surprisingly, the standard eighteenth-century 'sex manuals' — such as Nicolas Venette's *Mysteries of Conjugal Love Reveal'd*, or the perennial bestseller *Aristotle's MasterPiece* — contain virtually nothing about venereal disease.[30] Nor, with a few exceptions, do the spate of popular medical advice books which throughout the century were a regular feature of the publishing scene. Venereal disease was discreetly omitted, for instance, from the two most successful examples of the genre, John Wesley's *Primitive Physic* (1st edn 1747) and William Buchan's *Domestic Medicine* (1st edn 1769). The clergyman Wesley's reticence might have been predicted, but not so Buchan's (for reasons, as he later explained, of 'delicacy'). Buchan eventually made amends, not by adding a section to his original work, but by writing a whole separate treatise on the subject. Although not so popular as the wildly successful *Domestic Medicine*, his *Observations Concerning the Prevention and Cure of the Venereal Disease* (1st edn 1796) did reach its fourth edition by 1808.[31]

It is probable that the relative paucity of information about venereal disease from the advice literature was related to the targeted market — usually, it would seem, the respectable middle-class family. It could also be argued that the concerned layman was also being reached by the 'specialised' venereal literature, and certainly a high percentage of the books and pamphlets seem to have been written with at least one eye on the consumer rather than fellow 'professionals'. Entrepreneurialism and the relatively fluid 'professional' boundaries meant that almost any publication — particularly on a practical topic — could be seen as a form of advertising. A large number of venereologists, for instance, gave their addresses at the end of the preface, or on the title page, where it may also have been announced that both the treatise itself, and the various preparations mentioned within it, could be purchased. Examples include John Martin, whose *Treatise . . . of the Venereal Disease in both Sexes* (6th edn 1708) was available (so the title page has it) at six London booksellers, and 'at the Author's House, the further End of *Hatton Garden*, on the Left-hand beyond the *Chappell*, *John Marten* Surgeon writ over the Door'.[32] Vincent Brest saw fit to inform the reader that he was '*Surgeon, and Cupper to His Royal Highness* Frederick *Prince of Wales*', also mentioning that he himself lived in Panton Street.[33] This practice, it should be said, became less common towards the end of the century, but George Rees in 1802 announced on the title page of his book the specific address in Soho Square where he delivered his lectures.[34] The line between disseminating useful information and advertising may be a fine one, but there can be no doubt that many authors believed that potential clients might buy and read their books.

The lay readership can also be inferred in the raciness of a good deal of this literature. The subject lent itself to a fair amount of sexual explicitness, of course, but a good deal of amorous and semi-erotic material occasionally got thrown in. Although professing himself horrified at having to go into details, Marten provided explicit descriptions of buggery ('an abominable, beastly sodomitical and shameful Action') and of fellatio ('so very Beastly and so much to be abhorr'd, as to cause at the mentioning, or but thinking of it, the utmost detestation and loathing'). Letters from victims of venereal disease (whether genuine or composed by Marten is unclear) often linger on how the infection was acquired. The stories, of course, generally have a happy ending, since Marten is able to effect a cure, and the titillation seems almost as central as the warnings.

There was a perceptible refinement as the century progressed. Tales of sexual heroics were less common and the writing generally becomes tamer. What changes less, however, is the overwhelming therapeutic orientation and the individual doctor's claims to therapeutic power. In that sense, practitioners were still telling clients what they wished to hear.

Given the diversity of the symptoms and conditions grouped under the rubric of 'the venereal disease', the therapeutic discussions were, not surprisingly, complicated. The gleet, the whites and gonorrhoea each commanded its own cluster of remedies, as did the 'pox', or syphilis. This latter, as the gravest illness of the group, naturally attracted the most attention. Despite the lumping together of syphilis and gonorrhoea, few claimed for mercury any efficacy in the latter. Rather, it was for syphilis that mercurial preparations were generally reserved, many believing that mercury alone offered the chance of a radical (or specific) cure, a fact summarised by the sober Buchan:[35]

> I have taken much pains to find any well-authenticated case where the lues venerea had been cured without the use of mercury; but all my inquiries have proved unsuccessful. It is of no avail to say that symptoms will disappear under the use of other medicines, which seemed to resist the powers of mercury. This I meet with every day under the use of the bark, or of butter-milk: but it does not follow that either bark or butter-milk will cure the lues venerea.

As Buchan went on shrewdly to observe, both doctors and their patients generally attributed the 'cure' to the last medicine given.

Despite mercury's reputation, it was central to much therapeutic discussion. Eighteenth-century established 'regular' doctors accepted the traditional assertion that quacks who were out to capture the venereal market often covered themselves by selling preparations which actually contained mercury. How common this was can of course never be known with certainty, for even those 'quacks' who have left behind tangible historical traces routinely chose not to divulge the composition of their nostrums. But in so far as the accusation was correct, these selfsame 'quacks' were guilty only of the relatively minor deception of not telling the client what he was taking, and were innocent of the more serious ones (in eighteenth-century terms) of selling a worthless preparation, and denying the patient the 'proven' therapy of orthodoxy.

It was, of course, not so simple, for mercury was far from an innocuous substance, and writers routinely accused their colleagues — quack, fringe or regular — of failing to pay sufficient attention to the potential dangers of this dangerous remedy, and of ruining for ever the constitutions of their unhappy patients. Temkin's suggestion that a sixteenth-century doctor believed mercury to be less problematical, or requiring less management, than guaiac, certainly does not hold two centuries later. Indeed, it was asserted, precisely because of its danger and its power, mercury needed more caution in management than almost any other drug.[36]

Balancing the two required a skilful combination of the right preparation, correct administration and delicate titration. There was plenty of room for argument about these matters, and since mercury could be prepared in a variety of ways (or used in its elemental form), and further combined with a number of other medicaments, it was easy to claim that one's own preparation (stated or secret) was best. Despite lack of unanimity about dosage or preparation or management, there was fairly good agreement from the core of elite practitioners that mercury was a powerful and potent drug, and possibly even a specific, for cases of syphilis.

There was also a shared sense — towards the end of the century — of progress in its application. Taking mercury to the point of salivation, sore gums and loose teeth was the traditional recommendation. This had unfortunate consequences for the patient, for not only was it uncomfortable and dangerous, it also was impossible to accomplish without being obvious to those who came in contact with the patient, since it left a metallic smell to the breath, to say nothing of the constant salivation (as much as three or four pints in a day), which could last for several weeks. This in itself announced to anyone who knew the clues that the individual was under treatment for syphilis, even if the chancre, buboes, rash or other physical manifestations could be hidden from public view. Scurrilous literary references to 'stinking breath' had other connotations than simply the lack of oral hygiene. The mercurial salivation made contracting syphilis doubly awkward and virtually impossible to conceal from one's family, friends and servants. Small wonder that Andree remarked in 1779 that 'the method practised in Hospitals, of salivating for the cure of most venereal disorders, cannot be adopted in private, as very few patients would submit to so severe a mercurial course, unless for the cure of the worst state of the disease'.[37] Like most of his regular colleagues, Andree continued to put stock in mercury (even for private patients), hallowed as it was by more than three centuries of use. But by the closing decades of the century, most commentators believed that the violent salivations of the age of Turner had been unnecessarily harsh and dangerous, and that the newer preparations, whether applied by friction or taken internally, were altogether milder and safer, but equally effective against the disease — perhaps more effective, since not undermining the patient's constitution. Some authors throughout the century attacked salivation but not mercury and, indeed, because the popular mind equated the two, were able to offer seemingly radical new treatments while in fact staying within the bounds of mercurial orthodoxy.[38]

The precise mechanism whereby mercury acted as a specific was, of course, the subject of considerable enquiry, although these debates cannot be discussed here. One consequence of mercury's dramatic effects was the common assumption that the syphilitic virus was being literally driven out of the victim's body, and suggested to many that preparations with analogous physiological effects might work just as effectively, but without the side-effects. A good many of the alternatives or adjuncts prepared during the century possessed some physiological property which recommended them as capable of doing what mercury did. Antimony was occasionally flirted with, but the botanical world produced most of the alternative *pharmacopoeia syphilitica*.[39]

Of these, guaiac was the most time-honoured and carried with it almost as long a tradition as mercury. That the guaiacum tree was native to the Americas had initially seemed to provide some evidence favouring the American origin of syphilis (the tacit assumption being that God placed remedies near to diseases, to make them a bit easier to discover). Once a remedy gets rooted in both professional and public consciousness, it is difficult to abandon it, although guaiac's reputation declined in the century. 'It was formerly supposed that the decoction of guaiacum alone was a remedy for the venereal disease. Although this opinion is now abandoned, it is still by many supposed to co-operate with mercury,' wrote Alexander Buchan (William's son) in 1803.[40] That it produced a sweating still gave it some rational claims as an adjunct, however.

Of the other three most popular herbal remedies (mezereon, sassafras, sarsparilla) it may be significant that two of them were obtained from plants native to the New World, and of the twenty botanical remedies listed in William Meyrick's *New Family Herbal* (1790) as being useful against various forms of the venereal disease, almost half were not native to Britain. The exotic continued to attract itself for what was always seen as originally an imported disease. With its sudorific properties, for instance, juniper was 'supposed by many to be equally efficacious in the French disease with those of guaiacum and sassafras.'[41] Although there were dozens of preparations on the market by the turn of the century, most 'regular' ones turn out to be versions of only a handful of core ingredients, and despite the amount of ink spilled on the subject, there was fairly good professional agreement about the five front-line drugs of choice: mercury, guaiac, sarsparilla, sassafras and mezereon. Radical deviations from that can with some confidence be placed beyond the professional pale, and it seems not unreasonable to assume that a good many secret remedies contained one or more of the above ingredients.

Despite the profusion of therapeutic possibilities, mercury and remedies with analogous actions still set the orthodox standard, and therapy itself dominated the literature. Within those boundaries, however, there was much room for manoeuvre, for style, for presentation. In the section that follows, I shall look in a little more detail at five authors, selected at intervals through the century.

Some Contributors to the Genre

With a literature so diverse in production and intent, it is impossible to discern any clearly demarcated thread during the course of the century. Indeed, by carefully selecting the examples, it would probably be possible to support any number of mutually exclusive hypotheses about diagnostic criteria, treatments of choice, or standards of professional behaviour. Nevertheless, if there are no precise strands, there are, I think, at least some general trends, and there can be no doubt that by the century's end, informal codes of conduct were better defined, and better adhered to, than they had been at the beginning of our period. I shall choose my examples for more detailed consideration to illustrate this, realising of course that exceptions could be found which might support an alternative gloss. My individuals wrote at roughly generational intervals.

In 1708, a small one-shilling pamphlet appeared. Appealingly entitled *The Charitable Surgeon*, its author was identified only as 'T.C., Surgeon'. In the preface he promised other treatises on 'divers other parts of the Physical and Chirurgical Practice', but I can find no evidence that these ever appeared. If books were advertisements, why publish quasi-anonymously? One answer was provided in the preface: 'T.C.' had retired from practice and was living in the country, so had no direct need of publicity. What of the title? It appears that 'T.C.' believed himself 'charitable' because his pamphlet offered fourteen non-mercurial preparations which, he was confident, would cure a whole variety of signs and symptoms of venereal complaints, together with a 'yard-syringe' and a 'womb-syringe' to administer some of them. With this information, the sufferer would not need the 'help of any Physician, Surgeon or Apothecary', or be 'expos'd to the hazardous attempts of Quacks and Pretenders'. The poor would also be aided, since only a short course of his medicines (priced at between 2s. 6d. and 7s. 6d.) would cure. Although the absence of the name on the title page precluded selling his 'discoveries' himself, they were all available from the bookseller who published his pamphlet, 'Edmund Curle, at the Peacock without Temple Bar'.[42] And what of his medicines, with names like 'the Anodyne Injection', 'the Grand Preservative', 'the Specifick Electuary'? Some details were given for each of them, but as 'T.C.' explained,[43]

> The mimicking of Medicines also, by almost every Apothecary's Boy, Quack, Physick-Vendor, etc. who knows not a good Ingredient or Drug from a bad one, nay, scarcely knows one from another, or at leastwise their Nature or Principles so, as to compound them Artfully or Aright, was the next Inducement for my concealing one, even the principal Ingredient in every particular Medicine, (as will be observ'd in the Book) because as I had undertook to accommodate the People both with Method and Medicine, I was willing for their Good, that nothing should be wanting to render it effectually Serviceable, which could not be, were the Medicines wrongly compounded or not prepar'd with the best Ingredients.

Besides, 'T.C.' insisted, by keeping things secret but available, he could hope to put a stop to and restrain 'the Quacks and ignorant Professors'.

Was 'Mr C'. a quack himself? Certainly not in his own mind, although his defensiveness in explaining his anonymity, and insisting that his secret ingredient was never mercury, suggests that he was conscious that he might be taken for one. His pamphlet is also thin on evidence of clinical knowledge and is squarely addressed to the public, not to any medical or surgical colleagues. In the end, I think, we must accept 'T.C.' exactly as he represents himself: as a surgeon, for he did nothing more than named medical men, like Gideon Harvey just before, or John Marten, just after, had done.

Of somewhat different mettle was Daniel Turner who in 1711 disfranchised himself from the Barber-Surgeons Company and turned physician, practising that branch of the profession until his death thirty years later. Turner had already published some surgical treatises, and although as a physician he wrote on fevers, most of his subsequent output concerned the no-man's land between physician and surgeon, skin diseases (on which he wrote the first monograph in English) and venereal disorders.[44] He was also particularly active in campaigning against superstition and against quacks and shady behaviour among his colleagues in all three branches of medicine. That he felt that venereology was an especially vulnerable area for exploitation may be seen from the fact that almost half of his *The Modern Quack* (1718) was devoted to the subject.[45] Fear of exposure was the prime ingredient which allowed fortunes to be made from venereal disease by uneducated fringe practitioners. The unwitting victim might end up paying 'twenty five Guineas, of which fifteen were paid for *Secrecy*, and ten for a pretended cure'. Four behavioural characteristics set quacks apart: the claim to secret remedies (with instructions where these might be purchased); advertising and the use of testimonials; resort to uroscopy; and the use of public display and what we would call crowd psychology. Turner was aware that some of his professional brethren sometimes resorted to these methods, but in so far as they did, they too were simply acting as 'quacks'.

Turner's attitudes to quacks extended to his two monographs on venereal disease, one on gleet and another (which went through four editions) on syphilis.[46] In both productions, he remained essentially true to his sense of professionalism. In both, to be sure, we can discern a certain condescension to practitioners of his former calling, surgery: *Syphilis* was dedicated to a surgeon, Samuel Palmer, and its preface addressed to the Barber-Surgeons Company. Palmer was chosen, Turner informed his readers, because he regarded secret remedies as anathema, the surgeons preached at because venereal disease so often came their way. Turner's seriousness of intent expressed itself in several ways: not simply in openness of his remedies, nor his traditional use of Latin for especially intimate details, nor his readiness to speculate about mechanisms of aetiology and pathogenesis, but in the sheer poignancy of some of his case histories. These latter carry a ring of authenticity, and while there were the inevitable cures effected by Turner from the ruins of quackish maltreatment, not all his patients ended their encounters with venereal disease in the 'happily ever after' camp. There was, for instance, the man who believed that his nose had been rotted away by the distemper; Turner convinced him rationally (though perhaps not emotionally) that this had not happened, but the man was a broken reed, fit only to retire to a country village,

> Employing himself in a Garden, saying nothing to any Body, or sitting in a Chimney-Corner, where he will sometimes weep, especially

when they are unmindful to keep him to his Meals, or when he has been long empty; then feeling of his Nose, he will run to the Glass, that he may have both Senses to ascertain he has not lost it.

Another man, having been infected through an encounter with a prostitute, found his relationship with his wife much affected. Turner reported curing the man and although the wife escaped infection, the episode left them cold towards each other: 'tho' they lie under one Roof, they have bedded separately'.[47] Throughout, Turner gives the impression that he cared for his patients and even if the failures are mostly attributed to the prior ministrations of quacks, he did occasionally include cases for which only palliative treatment was possible. For syphilis itself, mercury was the drug of choice, generally to the point of salivation.

After Daniel Turner turned to physic, he acquired a medical degree, the first to be awarded by Yale University.[48] We do not know where John Profily MD got his. His only apparent publication, *An Easy and Exact Method of Curing the Venereal Disease* (1748), suggests that he had practised in Dublin, although it was published in London and has a Latin dedication to the President and Fellows of the College of Physicians in London. A stout octavo, with several nicely produced engravings, it has the physical appearance of a learned treatise. It is not, being aimed squarely at the medical consumer ('My design is to make every patient become his own Physician in common Cases'). Rather engagingly written as a series of dialogues between patient and physician, it uses the immediacy of this quasi-Socratic form to instil in the reader an overwhelmingly favourable impression of Profily's therapeutic expertise. The world it evokes is a doctor's paradise: the patients are invariably docile and tractable, ask only questions for which the physician has an answer, take their medicines properly, are cured and gratefully pay their bills. The following are typical patient responses: 'Sir, I have observed all your Directions, and I find myself a great deal better.' 'Sir, I have the pleasure to tell you, I find myself almost well.' 'My Wife is perfectly recovered as I am, and full of Gratitude to you for your Directions.' 'I shall take care to observe your Directions.'[49]

Profily littered his narrative with instructions for a number of remedies, and his range of ingredients was unexceptional: guaiac and sarsparilla, as well as mercury — but the thrust of his narrative towards the non-mercurial cure of venereal complaints without salivating, is most clearly borne out by the volume's climax, a thirty-page description of a public experiment which Profily carried out in Dublin in 1746, advertised in the local papers and offering to cure, without charge, the first nine patients (three females and six males) who presented themselves 'in the Worst Stage of the Venereal Disease'. For this he asked two or more physicians and surgeons to examine the patient before and after treatment. Confinement was not necessary, although the patient was required to sleep at Profily's house and agree to be discharged on failure to conform to his instructions. Preliminary examination of the patients (whose names and occupations were revealed) was thorough by the standards of the time (an overall inspection plus a brief history) and, needless to say, the only 'failure' was a patient dismissed for failing to follow instructions. One hesitates to call it quackish (particularly since Profily admitted using crude mercury as the basic therapeutic ingredient), but it was blatantly commercial.

The constraints on professional behaviour grew tighter during the second half of the century. What this meant was that those who wished to align themselves with the 'regulars' were less free to engage in some of the activities — secret remedies, blatant advertising, etc. — which, though perhaps frowned upon by some, were more common in the earlier period. Since the legal status of the profession had not changed, this process was informal and of course subject to abuse and exception. But that does not make it less real, and certainly the literature on venereal disease reflects this tightening and growth of professional consciousness.

A good example may be found in the case of J. Smyth MD. Smyth apparently wrote only two small pamphlets, both on venereal disease, and eventually published together as a single work. If the title page is to be believed, his *A New Treatise on the Venereal Disease* was a wildly successful production, passing through twenty-eight editions in about as many years. Like so many relatively obscure works of the period, however, its publishing history is murky. The Wellcome Institute, British Library and National Library of Medicine possess a total of eight editions, the earliest called the sixth (1771), the last called the twenty-eighth (1798). The eighteenth (1781) is the most common. All were printed 'for the author', who, at least from 1781, lived in Great Suffolk-Street, Charing Cross, London. Curiously, the four Wellcome editions are all dedicated to Charles Lucas MD, an Irish apothecary-turned-physician and politician, despite the fact that by the last edition, Lucas had been dead for twenty-seven years. Although Smyth was consistently described as possessing the MD, and practising also as a man-midwife, I have been unable to discover where his medical degree came from and he cannot be identified from J.F. Simmons' 1783 *Medical Register*.

The earliest editions were rather typical productions of what might be called the professional fringe: professional in his parading of credentials and apparent respectability, but fringe (particularly by the 1770s) in what his privately published pamphlet attempted to do, which is to sell his Specific Drops for Venereal Complaints, and his Restorative Medicine for a variety of sexual disorders, including impotency and barrenness. The intended readership was clearly the potential consumer, and despite an occasional sideways glance at other venereologists such as Jean Astruc (1684-1766), his discussion quickly turned from the signs and symptoms of venereal disease to a series of remarkable cures effected by his medicine. The testimonials were glowing: 'I think it my duty to inform you, that after taking nine bottles of your Restorative Drugs, I am perfectly recovered from a debilitated state, the course of which I unfortunately brought on myself, by a practice I am ashamed to mention,' wrote Mr Nicholson, of Twickenham, who had presumably spent nine guineas with Smyth, since the concoction cost a guinea a bottle. Both the drops and the medicine could be obtained from him, or from any one of thirty or so agents listed in the back of the volume.[50]

The purpose of the 1798 (twenty-eighth) edition (which is almost certainly an unaltered reprint of the 1792 edition, called the twenty-sixth) was identical: to sell his remedies. But the tone was more defensive. Gone were the testimonials (although Smyth told the reader that many could be read at his own home), and the preliminary 'Advertisement' contained a short biographical apologia, explaining that he had served 'a legal apprenticeship to one of the first Chymists in London', had been appointed 'Surgeon to a Regiment in his Majesty's Service', and then attended 'with some advantage a [unspecified] celebrated University' where he had taken his degree. A list of the suppliers of both the book and the medicine was still appended, but the price was no longer stated and an offer of postal service no longer made. The writing, too, was less florid. All in all, it seems that Smyth had had to make a decision on whether or not to use the weight and authority of the medical profession, and having decided in the affirmative, had toned down his message to conform to the expectations of his readers. He was still an individualist. The public had, he was certain, bought his medicines over the years because they worked, not simply because of his superior education, but by the end of his life he was an entrepreneur working within more clearly defined constraints. In fact, by the time the last edition appeared, he may well have been dead, since he was no longer listed as a supplier of his medicines.[51]

I am not, of course, suggesting that medicine had by 1800 become a coherent, unified occupation, simply that the boundaries were sharper then they had been a century before, and that behaviour which would have been tolerated, or even admired, in earlier generations, was not so in the more 'refined' circumstances of the late eighteenth and early nineteenth centuries. One last brief example from the turn of the century will serve: John Pearson's *Observations on the . . . Lues Venerea* (1800).

Although Pearson (1758-1826) was a pupil of John Hunter, his monograph on venereal disease was hardly touched by the theoretical issues which Hunter had earlier raised regarding the aetiology and pathogenesis of the condition. Rather, it was a practical exercise, aimed, like the other productions we have examined, at improving treatment and management. It possesses, however, three characteristics which set it apart from a good deal of the earlier literature. First, it was aimed directly at colleagues rather than the general public. His case histories have been shorn of spicy details and concentrate tersely on the evolving medical nuances of pathology. Second, his therapeutic evaluations were much more tentative and critical. He offered no wholesale condemnation of various remedies in favour of a particular favourite (although mercury in moderate doses remained his standby); rather, he was prepared to evaluate the strengths and weaknesses of the whole of the venereal pharmacopoeia. The principal innovation in his work concerned the evaluation of acids, especially nitrous, in the treatment of syphilis. His series of twenty-one cases in which nitrous acid had been employed included instances in which he judged it as a useful adjunct to mercury, and cases in which 'the Nitrous Acid was given without Success'. A third significant feature of Pearson's work was that it was based on his experience as senior surgeon to the lock hospital rather than simply his private practice.[52]

Venereal disease, of course, continued to attract much medical attention, and to be a condition with considerable commercial potential for both medical orthodoxy and medical fringe. But it becomes, I suggest, easier to identify the 'regulars' from the 'irregulars' long before the legal establishment of the *Medical Register* in 1858. If, as Porter has argued, eighteenth-century 'irregulars' mirrored many aspects of more orthodox Georgian medical practice — through display, individualism and even cultivated eccentricity — is it too much to suggest that the dialectic continued in the nineteenth? As the medical profession began to close ranks, so too did the fringe with its alternative cosmologies of homeopathy, herbalism, spiritualism or Coffinism. Within this newer framework, venereal disease continued to occupy a special place, and its nineteenth-century history would provide an instructive lesson in the mirroring of orthodoxy by fringe, and in the wider social relations of all healers and sufferers.[53]

Notes

1. C.J.S. Thompson, *The Quacks of Old London* (London, Brentano's, 1928); Alex Comfort, *The Anxiety Makers* (London, Nelson, 1967); Eric Jameson, *The Natural History of Quackery* (London, Michael Joseph, 1961).

2. Roy Porter, 'Before the Fringe', in R. Cooter (ed.), *Alternatives: Essays in the Social History of Irregular Medicine* (London, Macmillan, forthcoming); idem, 'The Language of Quackery in England, 1660-1800', in P. Burke and R. Porter (eds), *Language and Society* (Cambridge, Cambridge University Press, 1987).

3. Paul-Gabriel Boucé (ed.), *Sexuality in Eighteenth-century Britain* (Manchester, Manchester University Press, 1983); idem, 'Aspects of Sexual Tolerance and Intolerance in XVIIIth-century England', *British Journal of Eighteenth-century Studies*, 3 (1980), 173-91; Roy Porter, 'Spreading Carnal Knowledge or Selling Dirt Cheap? Nicolas Venette's *Tableau de l'Amour Conjugal* in Eighteenth-century England', *Journal of European Studies*, 14 (1984), 233-55; Owsei Temkin, 'On the History of " Morality and Syphilis" ', in his *The Double Face of Janus* (Baltimore and London, Johns Hopkins University Press, 1977), 472-84.

4. F.B. Smith, 'Ethics and Disease in the Late Nineteenth Century: the Contagious Diseases Acts', *Historical Studies*, 15 (1971), 118-35; Paul McHugh, *Prostitution and Victorian Social Reform* (London, Croom Helm, 1980); Judith Walkowitz, *Prostitution and Victorian Society* (Cambridge, Cambridge University Press, 1980); Edward J. Bristow, *Vice and Vigilance* (Dublin, Gill & Macmillan, 1977).

5. Porter (note 2); N. McKendrick, J. Brewer and J.H. Plumb, *The Birth of a Consumer Society* (London, Europa, 1982); R. Hambridge, 'Empiricomany, or an Infatuation in Favour of *Empiricism* or *Quackery*. The Socio-economics of Eighteenth-century Quackery', in S. Soupel and R. Hambridge, *Literature and Science and Medicine* (Los Angeles, Clark Memorial Library, 1982).

6. For instance, H. Deacon, *A Compendious Treatise on the Venereal Disease, Gleets, etc.* (London, The Author, 1789), is a work which never reveals the occupation of its author, yet makes no claims to secret remedies or commercialism.

7. Jameson (note 1), ch. 3, addresses fringe 'specialisms'.

8. George Rosen, *The Specialization of Medicine with Particular Reference to Ophthalmology* (New York, Froben Press, 1944).

9. For the lock hospitals, cf. James Bettley, 'Post Voluptatem Misericordia: The Rise and Fall of the London Lock Hospitals', *London Journal*, 10 (1984), 167-75. For the social setting in London, cf. M. Dorothy George, *London Life in the Eighteenth Century* (Harmondsworth, Penguin, 1965). On hospitals more generally, cf. John Woodward, *To Do the Sick No Harm* (London, Routledge & Kegan Paul, 1974).

10. G. Rees, *A Treatise on the Primary Symptoms of Lues Venerea* (London, M. Allen, 1802); E.D. Cotterall, 'The Emergence of a Specialty', *Sexually Transmitted Diseases*, 10 (1983), 85-92.

11. Jean Donnison, *Midwives and Medical Men* (London, Heinemann, 1977); A. Wilson, 'William Hunter and the Varieties of Man-midwifery', in W.F. Bynum and Roy Porter (eds), *William Hunter and the Eighteenth-century Medical World* (Cambridge, Cambridge University Press, 1985); William Ll. Parry-Jones, *The Trade in Lunacy* (London, Routledge & Kegan Paul, 1972); Ida Macalpine and Richard Hunter, *George III and the Mad-business* (London, Allen Lane, 1969).

12. The classic formulation of the tripartite division in the period is Bernice Hamilton,

26 Treating the Wages of Sin

'The Medical Professions in the Eighteenth Century', *Economic History Review* (2nd series), 4 (1951), 141-69. More recent revisionist work includes Irvine Loudon, 'The Nature of Provincial Medical Practice in Eighteenth-century England', *Medical History*, 29 (1985), 1-32; Joan Lane, 'The Role of Apprenticeship in Eighteenth-century Medical Education in England', in Bynum and Porter (note 11); *idem*, 'The Medical Practitioners of Provincial England in 1783', *Medical History*, 28 (1984), 353-71.

13. R. Campbell, *The London Tradesman* (London, T. Gardner, 1747), 57; cf. Geoffrey Holmes, *Augustan England: Professions, State and Society, 1680-1730* (London, George Allen) Unwin, 1982).

14. Campbell (note 13), 52.

15. Leonard Stewart, *Remarks on the Present State of the Medical Profession* (London, John Hatchard, 1826), 17.

16. Campbell, (note 13), 52-3.

17. William Clowes, *A Briefe and Necessarie Treatise, Touching the Cure of the Disease called Morbus Gallicus* (London, T. Cadman, 1585); Richard Wiseman, *Severall Chirurgicall Treatises* (London, Flesher, 1676); Gideon Harvey, *Great Venus Unmasked* (London, N. Brook, 1672); *idem*, *Little Venus Unmask'd* (London, W. Thackeray, 1670).

18. Owsei Temkin, 'Therapeutic Trends and the Treatment of Syphilis Before 1900', in Temkin (note 3.).

19. J.K. Proksch, *Die Litteratur über die venerischen Krankheiten*, 3 vols. in 5 (Bonn, Hanstein, 1889-1900); *idem*, *Die Geschichte der venerischen Krankheiten*, 2 pts (Bonn, Hanstein, 1895). Ben Barkow has been of great help in compiling the bio-bibliography.

20. Nicholas Robinson, *A New Treatise of the Venereal Disease* (London, Knapton, 1736); John Armstrong, *A Synopsis of the History and Cure of Venereal Diseases* (London, A. Millar, 1737); Daniel Turner, *Syphilis. A Practical Dissertation on the Venereal Disease* (London, R. Bonwicke, 1717); *idem*, *A Discourse Concerning Gleets* (London, J. Clarke, 1729); John Hunter, *A Treatise on the Venereal Disease* (London, The Author, 1786); Thomas Beddoes, *Reports Principally Concerning the Effects of the Nitrous Acid in the Venereal Disease* (Bristol, N. Biggs, 1797).

21. Henry Saffory, *The Inefficacy of all Mercurial Preparations in the Cure of Venereal and Scorbutic Disorders, Proved* (London, The Author, 1773); Charles Swift, *Salivation Exploded* (Lambeth, T. Romney, 1812); John Warren, *A New Method of Curing and Preventing the Virulent Gonorrhea* (London, W. Flexney, 1771).

22. *A Plain and Practical Discovery of the Nature and Cause of the Secret Disease* (London, 18th Century). Eminent nineteenth-century British practitioners who wrote on venereal disease include Benjamin Bell, Jonathan Hutchinson, and Erasmus Wilson. For a discussion, including the continental venereologists, cf. J.T. Crissey and L.C. Parish, *The Dermatology and Syphilology of the Nineteenth Century* (New York, Praeger, 1981).

23. Roy Porter, 'Lay Medical Knowledge in the Eighteenth Century: The Evidence of the *Gentleman's Magazine*', *Medical History*, 29 (1985), 138-68; *idem*, 'Laymen, Doctors and Medical Knowledge in the Eighteenth Century: The Evidence of the *Gentleman's Magazine*', in R. Porter (ed.), *Patients and Practitioners* (Cambridge, Cambridge University Press, 1985), 283-314.

24. Some representative treatises not otherwise cited include, J. Becket, *A New Essay on the Venereal Disease* (London, The Author, 1765); William Rowley, *The Most Cogent Reasons Why Astringent Injections; Caustic Bougies and Violent Salivations Should Be Banished* . . . (London, The Author, 1800); N.D. Falck, *A Treatise on the Venereal Disease* (London, The Author, 1772); S.F. Simmons, *Observations on the Cure of the Gonorrhoea* (London, J. Murray, 1780).

25. For a good discussion of Boswell's bouts of venereal disease, see William B. Ober, 'Boswell's Clap', in his *Boswell's Clap and Other Essays* (Carbondale, Southern Illinois University Press, 1979).

26. For Kennedy, see E.A. Underwood, *Boerhaave's Men at Leyden and After* (Edinburgh, Edinburgh University Press, 1977). One of the most enthusiastic advocates of the

Lisbon Diet Drink was John Leake (1729-92), the founder of the Westminster Lying-in Hospital. Leake's *Dissertation on the Properties and Efficacy of the Lisbon Diet-drink and its Extract* reputedly went through at least eight editions between 1767 and 1787. It is not clear whether Leake's Diet Drink was the same as Kennedy's, but ironically, the sale of Leake's was complicated, since a journeyman bookbinder named Walter Leake took out a patent for a pill which came to be called Leake's Pill. It was reputed to have the same effect as the Diet Drink and so hurt the sales of the latter (cf. 'Leake', in *Dictionary of National Biography*). Lisbon had a reputation in the mid-eighteenth century for possessing a climate which was beneficial to venereal disease sufferers.

27. The standard discussion of Hunter's work on venereal disease is still Proksch (note 19, *Die Geschichte* . . .). See also, Kenneth M. Flegal, 'Changing concepts of the Nosology of Gonorrhea and Syphilis', *Bulletin of the History of Medicine*, 48 (1974), 571-88.

28. John Andree, *Observations on the Theory and Cure of the Venereal Disease* (London, W. Davis, 1779), 2.

29. For instance, John Atkins, *The Navy-surgeon* (London, Caesar Ward, 1734), 209ff.

30. Porter (note 3); *idem*, ' "The Secrets of Generation Display'd"': Aristotle's Masterpiece in Eighteenth-century England', *Eighteenth Century Life*, 9 (1985), 1-21. Curiously, it became more common for nineteenth-century editions of *Aristotle's Masterpiece* to include a short section on the treatment of venereal disease.

31. For Buchan, cf. C.J. Lawrence, 'William Buchan: Medicine Laid Open', *Medical History*, 19 (1975), 20-35; Charles Rosenberg,'Medical Text and Social Context: Explaining William Buchan's "Domestic Medicine",' *Bulletin of the History of Medicine*, 57 (1983), 22-42. Although none of the editions of *Domestic Medicine* appearing in Buchan's lifetime apparently include venereal disease, some at least of the later ones did, e.g. one of my own copies, not dated but published *c* 1870 by Milner & Company, in London, pp. 331-51.

32. John Marten, *A Treatise of All the Degrees and Symptoms of the Venereal Disease in Both Sexes*, 6th edn (London, S. Crouch, 1708). I have used the facsimile reprint by Garland Publishing (New York, 1985).

33. Vincent Brest, *An Analytical Inquiry into the Specifick Property of Mercury, Relating to the Cure of Venereal Diseases* (London, J. Nourse, 1732).

34. Rees (note 10).

35. William Buchan, *Observations Concerning the Prevention and Cure of the Venereal Disease*, 3rd edn (London, J. Cadell, 1803), iii-iv.

36. Temkin (note 18), 523; cf. Buchan (note 35), 284: 'Though some inconveniences may attend the administration of mercury, yet I know no medicine of equal value.'

37. Andree (note 28), v.

38. For instance, George Key. *A Dissertation on the Effects of Mercury on Human Bodies* (London, T. Osbourne, 1747); and Charles Hales, *Salivation Not Necessary for the Cure of the Venereal Disease*, 3rd edn (London, J. Almon, 1764).

39. For a brief discussion of antimony, see R. James, *A Medicinal Dictionary* 3 vols (London, T. Osbourne, 1743-5), 2, art, 'Lues venerea'.

40. Alexander Buchan, in Buchan (note 35), 'Supplement', lxxiii.

41. William Meyrick, *The New Family Herbal* (Birmingham, J. Pearson, 1790). Buchan (note 35); and John Pearson, *Observations on the Effects of Various Articles of the Materia Medica in the Cure of Lues Venerea*, (London, J. Callow, 1800), contain full, systematic discussions. For guaiac, see R.S. Munger, 'Guaiacum, the Holy Wood for the New World', *Journal of the History of Medicine*, 4 (1949), 196-229.

42. Edmund Curll (Curle) (1675-1747) was one of the most flamboyant publishers, booksellers and men of letters of his time: cf. Ralph Straus, *The Unspeakable Curll* (London, Chapman & Hall, 1927), 26ff., for a discussion of the polemic surrounding the publication of T.C.'s volume: it was suggested, though denied by Curll, that John Marten was its author. Mrs Christine English has suggested to me that the author and title are actually

playfully the same, i.e. 'T.C., Surgeon,' actually simply abbreviates 'The Charitable Surgeon'.

43. T.C., *The Charitable Surgeon: Or, the Best Remedies for the Worst Maladies, Reveal'd* (London, E. Curle, 1708), v and *passim*.

44. For Turner's dermatology, cf. Crissey and Parish (note 22), 8ff.

45. [Daniel Turner], *The Modern Quack; or the Physical Impostor, Detected* (London, J. Roberts, 1718). This edition and the second (1724) were published anonymously, but the third edition (1739) appeared over Turner's name.

46. Daniel Turner, *Syphillis, A Practical Dissertation on the Venereal Disease . . . to Which . . . Is Added, the Author's Discourse, of Gleets*, 4th edn (London, J. Walthoe, 1732). In addition, Turner republished an English edition of Ulrich von Hutten's *De morbo Gallico* (London, J. Clarke, 1730), and wrote the preface to the English edition of Aloysius Luisinus's *Aphrodisiacus, Containing a Summary of the Ancient Writers on the Venereal Disease* (London, John Clarke, 1736).

47. Turner, *Syphillis* (sic), 3rd edn (London, J. Walthoe, 1727), quotations from pp. 102 and 212.

48. John E. Lane, 'Daniel Turner and the First Degree of Doctor of Medicine Conferred in the English Colonies of North America by Yale College in 1723', *Annals of Medical History*, 2 (1919), 367-80.

49. John Profily, *An Easy and Exact Method of Curing the Venereal Disease* (London, J. Robinson, 1748), *passim*. Except for a second edition of this book, Profily appears to have published nothing else.

50. J. Smyth, *A New Treatise on the Venereal Disease; Gleets, Seminal Weaknesses etc..*, 18th edn (London, The Author, 1781), 47.

51. J. Smyth, *A Practical Essay on the Venereal Disease*, 28th edn (London, The Author, 1798). Heading the list of suppliers on p. 48 was 'Mr. William Moore, Druggist, No. 80, Fleet-street, London'.

52. Pearson (note 41). Significantly, perhaps, Pearson was a pious man who wrote the life of his teacher, the evangelical Leeds surgeon William Hey (1736-1819). One of Pearson's sons became an Anglican clergyman.

53. Two recent works which deal with aspects of the later history of syphilis are D.B. Perett, 'Ethics and Error: The Dispute between Ricord and Auzias-Turenne over Syphilization, 1845-70', (unpublished PhD thesis, Stanford University, 1977); J.H. Jones, *Bad Blood. The Tuskegee Syphilis Experiment* (New York, Free Press, 1981).

2 PUBLICITY AND THE PUBLIC GOOD: PRESENTING MEDICINE IN EIGHTEENTH-CENTURY BRISTOL

Jonathan Barry

Roy Porter has recently suggested that the term 'quackery' is best used heuristically to designate those 'at the leading edge of advertising . . . who actively and energetically peddled their services in the medical market place,' helping in the 'creation of widespread impersonal medical markets', which combined 'the healing and the performing arts'.[1] In this brief sketch of medical publicity in eighteenth-century Bristol I shall consider whether a firm definition of provincial quackery can be established on these grounds, and also whether, as Porter assumes, the use of publicity was a sign of success, or whether it was both a symptom, and possibly a cause, of weakness. To establish this final point it is necessary to place medical publicity in a wider context — namely, recurring discussions of the relationship between public good, private interest, and publicity, especially in the press. I shall concentrate on the efforts of practitioners to attract personal custom, rather than the subject of patent medicines, since Dr Brown's excellent study of the neighbouring town of Bath has already illuminated an experience essentially similar to that of Bristol.[2]

Before challenging some of Porter's work, I should make it clear that the Bristol evidence supports the great majority of the points he has made about eighteenth-century quackery. No hard and fast lines are evident between fringe and orthodoxy in the areas of therapeutic efficacy, choice of remedial methods, or involvement in trade and the marketplace. The complexity of the medical scene, and the importance of lay patronage, within a generally agreed framework of medical ideas, barred the establishment of a clear distinction between an orthodox profession and fringe practitioners. There is no evidence that the commercial quacks offered any coherent alternative to the medical cosmology of ordinary practitioners, and every sign that they sought to imitate those elements of orthodox practice which attracted lay respect.

It is therefore very tempting to look to the nature of their publicity to discover the essential difference between quack and regular practitioner. In quacks' advertisements we find all those features which Porter has identified, such as the use of jargon, of classical and oriental names, of royal and cosmopolitan associations, of slick packaging and measures intended to reassure the wary, and of dramatic presentation. Their own claims to infallibility, secret methods and other exclusive talents were matched by subtle denigration of other practitioners. In 1715, for example, Dr Clark, 'sworn physician and oculist' to Charles II, James II and Queen Anne, offered his secret of 'the lamp of light' to cure the blind, stressing his patronage by royalty and others of the highest rank and quality. He promised success where others had failed, and not merely for blindness but through his 'infallible' secret for the king's evil, cancers and stone, 'without the dreadful way of cutting'.[3] In addition to such famous national figures as the Chevalier Taylor and James Graham,[4] Bristol's leading quacks included: Dr Benjamin Thornhill, of the 'orthodox city of Wells', who cured the lame, blind, dumb, deaf and diseased, claimed 4,789 cures of the king's evil, and offered help to those 'lately sporting in the garden of Venus' and now tasting 'the bitter grapes';[5] Bartholomew di Dominiceti, nobleman and physician from Venice;[6] Dr Georgslanger Benevenuti, Saxon physician and oculist;[7] Joseph Grimaldi, surgeon, dentist and clown (father of *the* Grimaldi);[8] and Peter de Pustule, surgeon, apotehcary, 'pollincter and botanist' from Havana.[9]

But two notes of caution are necessary. First, one can easily focus, as I have just done, on the more ostentatious quacks, who were generally seeking to displace the physician in public esteem, and overlook the humbler quacks, who peddled simpler cures for ruptures, eye and teeth disorders or venereal diseases. The humbler quacks, competing with surgeons and apothecaries rather than physicians, were therefore more businesslike in their rhetoric, and less concerned to establish their Enlightenment credentials.[10] Not only did they outnumber the Taylors and the Grahams, to judge purely from newspaper advertisements, but they were much more likely not to advertise in such an expensive medium; instead, they tended to rely on the cheaper publicity of handbills and public display. Second, the protests against quacks at this period also tended to be against the outrageous quacks who threatened the physicians, both because their pretensions were greater and because their orthodox rivals had the leisure and opportunity to respond in print. There was a typically laconic warning in 1763 against the quack doctors and strollers, 'with whom the kingdom swarms', after one tried to rape a 12-year-old epileptic who applied for relief,[11] whereas the Chevalier Taylor warranted a full-scale satirical advertisement in 1730, denouncing the famous 'no mountebank, no quack, no doctor T . . . sole master of all the Arcanums, Nostrums and specifics in Nature . . . The only oculist for the teeth in the universe'. This picked out for ridicule his use of long words, his claim to cure all diseases, 'whether curable or incurable', his monstrous wigs, ornamental sword, velvet sleeves, fashionable greatcloak, and his 'promised, though unintended, editions of Books'.[12]

How far, moreover, did their methods of publicity distinguish even the outrageous quacks like Taylor? As Porter notes, many of their tricks were merely extensions of the publicity devices of regular practitioners, particularly physicians. They were regularly burlesqued for the literary pretension and use of learned language by which they distinguished themselves.[13] As the surgeons bettered themselves they advanced their claims to merit by using science. The split in the 1740s between surgeons and barber-surgeons was both hastened and legitimised by the greater scientific pretensions of the pure surgeons, several of whom used the Surgeons' Hall to give public anatomy lectures, and in 1741 an epitome of theses was published in Latin.[14] The surgeon Townsend, who was 'no classic', filled his surgery with surgical apparatus 'to influence the minds of the vulgar'.[15] It is hard to distinguish this from Taylor's lectures on the eye, or Dominiceti's impressive collection of anatomy specimens and steam baths.[16] Each of the professional groups had distinctive trade symbols, from the physician's carriage and the gild regalia of the barber-surgeons to the humble barber's pole. The elaborate packaging of patent preparations was matched by the splendid bottles and jars of the apothecaries' shops, carefully painted by local artists in gilt.[17]

Certainly the itinerant life led by many quacks meant that they needed to establish their presence, and their particular claim to distinction, as soon and as noticeably as possible. This in turn made them take to exaggerated lengths the methods common to the profession — indeed, to any trade of the period. Their temporary status also meant that they had to improvise the space needed for practice out of inn chambers and public stages.[18] But if the public nature of these settings strikes us as unprofessional, we should not forget that the barber-surgeon's shop was a similar mixture of surgery, shop, public haunt and often public house. Quack oculists were not unique in operating before audiences, to judge by Claver Morris's reference to 'many spectators' at a lithotomy performed in 1723 by Bristol's leading surgeons.[19] If, as Adrian Wilson has suggested, childbirth was also a public ceremony,[20] as were bathing cures at the Hotwells, then we need to re-examine our assumptions about the private character of medical care. In one important respect, furthermore, the itinerant was less public than other practitioners: he was not part of the community and would depart with the secrets entrusted to him, and this may explain his attractiveness to those with venereal problems. Bristol-settled specialists in this practice — such as Dr Speakman and his family — stressed the preservation of secrecy.[21]

The element in quack advertisements that most strikes us is the long listing of cures. Many of these were probably bogus, and contemporaries singled out quacks by unacceptably grandiose claims to success. But the *need* to list successful cures arose from the fundamental *problem* faced by the quack: the lack of the personal ties of reputation and neighbourhood which brought business to the medical practitioner, particularly as most quacks lacked a distinctive form of treatment. Practitioners of all kinds used the listing of cures whenever they ventured into new areas of treatment.[22] The literature of the Bristol Hotwells, for example, is replete with cases of cures. John Underhill's treatise of 1703 is little more than a compendium based on the register of cures kept at the Hotwells and told largely in lay words, although the author underlined his own status as a physician by using pompous and Latinate phraseology, even calling himself Johannus Subtermontanus![23] Later Hotwells physician denounced Underhill's uncritical use of lay testimony, but they provided many case studies of their own.[24]

Such practices were encouraged by the theoretical confusion besetting eighteenth-century English medicine, in which Galenic, Hippocratic, chemical and iatro-mechanical systems all jostled for acceptance and were combined eclectically by each physician, then deployed in a mixture of theoretical discussion and empirical narrative. The physician was no more certain of impressing the public with a theoretical account of his principles than was the quack. Both knew that the layman was impressed by theory, but that the bottom line was always practice. In his highly influential *Essay upon Nursing*, the Bristol physician William Cadogan sought to reconstruct childcare from first principles. But in doing so he claimed to avoid 'all terms of art and vain language' in favour of 'the open observations of nature', and he denounced quacks who preyed on the credulous by pretence to great knowledge of 'occult qualities'. After his medical account, he concluded with the clinching comment that 'I am a Father and have already practised [my method] with most desirable success.'[25] Physicians could exploit the confused therapeutic position by arguing that they alone could judge the correct blend of remedies in a specific case, so undermining the specific or universal panaceas of the quack,[26] but when the physician was arguing the advantages of a specific therapy he often shared many of the aims and techniques of the quack. Dr Sutherland, for example, in his discussion of the Bristol waters, vacillated uneasily between arguments from theoretical principles and empirical evidence, before concluding that the water was 'of such efficacy . . . as in the highest degree to exceed all shop remedies and approach nearest in nature to what has been searched after — an universal medicine'.[27] Although the Hotwells practice was unusual in its seasonal clientele and mixture of local and visiting practitioners, the same pattern can be traced in other therapies such as the use of electricity or the establishment of inoculation houses.[28]

Regular practitioners also seized the opportunity to publicise their successes through the growth in hospitals. As soon as the city workhouse, St Peter's Hospital, opened in 1697 with medical facilities, that inveterate self-publicist Thomas Dover offered his services as physician free.[29] But it was the surgeons, first at St Peter's and after 1737 also at the infirmary, who achieved the greatest prestige. The hospitals' daring operations on cataracts, stones, cancerous breasts, harelips, dropsy, even the delivery of triplets, were widely covered in the papers, and written up in pamphlets or in the *Philosophical Transactions of the Royal Society*.[30] These established a tradition of heroic medicine equal to the most dangerous methods of the quacks, and often treating similar ailments. Increasingly fierce competition to hold honorary hospital posts suggests a growing awareness of the career benefits of such public positions. Questions began to be asked about whether the doctors were serving the hospitals or vice versa; to excluded doctors, it seemed that private monopolies were being created out of public services. In 1759 the apparent efforts of one surgeon to monopolise lithotomies became a focus of press censure on these grounds,[31] while in 1767 a discussion about the choice of physicians began with the query; 'Does the Infirmary want a physician — or a physician an Infirmary?'[32] Of course, the increasingly bitter disputes on this theme, replete with the language of honorary posts and medical advance through hospital experience, itself generated publicity for the medical disputants.[33]

The establishment of a medical reputation through service to local charity carried further advantages. It enabled the practitioner to seem generous and benevolent, serving the poor gratis. In 1770 the St Peter's doctors announced that, despite their boycott of the hospital during a dispute, they would still visit the poor free of charge. They scorned any suggestion that they be turned into 'hirelings' by the establishment of salaried hospital posts.[34] Such a tradition was hardly new. The barber-surgeons' ordinances of 1652 provided for regulation of fees for treating the poor and free treatment of the poorest.[35] Local practitioners, especially young men seeking to establish a reputation, advertised that they were open to the poor, at least for a few hours a week. In 1757 the surgeon and man midwife Hands proposed to see the poor gratis on Sunday morning and to hasten to the delivery of poor pregnant women as if they gave a fee.[36]

Quacks felt obliged to emulate these practitioners in establishing their credentials as benevolent men, and stressed the point in their advertising,[37] while their opponents pounced on any shortcomings in this respect. In 1766 the same paper carried both Dr Benevenuti's claim to be remaining in Bristol longer than intended 'from solicitude of the poor', and a report by 'Benevolus' that the Italian gentleman 'who lately honoured the populace on the quay with his orations and advertised to cure almost all disorders,' had initially dismissed a poor man who applied to him for three days. Apparently the Italian then insisted on payment of three crowns, refusing to continue treatment when only one was paid.[38] On the other hand, even quacks tried to distinguish genuine paupers from pretenders by demanding certificates from parishes or clergymen before giving free care, like other doctors.[39] Even amongst the better-off, the physician was expected to display liberality. Smollett portrays Ferdinand Fathom attracting Hotwells clients by providing prescriptions free, although his sense of affront when offered payment did not extend to voluntary presents![40] All medical men were operating within a market economy; nevertheless, it was one where the traditions of *noblesse oblige* were firmly embedded in public expectations of medical practice.

Printed claims of efficacy and good intentions also had to be supplemented, particularly in the opening years of the century, by more traditional testimonies. Early advertisers spent much of their *printed* publicity establishing that they had been approved by sources of authority *outside* the marketplace. Apart from the stress on aristocratic support or scientific pedigree which Porter has highlighted, they also claimed, like the oculist Fairclough in 1701,[41] to be 'known to the Corporation and the Merchants at the Tolzey' or, like Dr Clark in 1715, to be 'sworn' surgeons or physicians, which presumably refers to the holding of an episcopal licence.[42] In 1761 a surgeon claimed to travel by Act of Parliament,[43] while Dominiceti produced a certificate to his integrity and judgement signed by clergy, churchwardens, surgeons, apothecaries, chemists, druggists, attorneys, merchants and tradesmen.[44] Rhetorically at least, quacks welcomed the scrutiny of local medical men, and Dr Hillman, counsellor to the court of the King of Prussia, claimed that 'many of the faculty as well as divers other spectators' saw him restore sight at an inn.[45] Dominiceti stressed his friendly relations with the

Bath and Bristol faculty and invited them to visit his house.[46]

Underlying the hyperbole of quack advertisements was surely an awareness of public scepticism, increasing the need to have the quack's claims validated by external authority, particularly the testimony of established local figures. The quack concentrated on local examples of cures because these could be confirmed by sight and conversation. It was equally essential that the cured patient should be seen to testify voluntarily, from a sense of gratitude and to further the public good.[47]

In this account I have stressed the *problems* faced by the quacks, rather than the *opportunities* offered by publicity, in explaining their characteristic forms of self-advertisement. In part, this is intended to suggest that the quack's lot may not have been as happy as some accounts tend to suggest. The absence of serious attacks on quackery by local practitioners suggests that the quack was not a major threat to the prosperity of regular doctors at this period: this situation was to change by the early nineteenth century. Porter and Loudon have both suggested that this lack of concern was the result of a 'sellers' market', as demand for medical relief outpaced supply, especially after 1740.[48] But even if this was true for the profession as a whole, the individual practitioner might still be expected to have felt endangered at a time when no single group of practitioners held a theoretical or therapeutic dominance.

I believe it more likely that the lack of concern about quackery arose from the fact that, in the struggle to be noticed and gain a reputation in provincial communities, the advantage lay with those who could exploit local associations and 'regular' practice. An exception may have to be made for those itinerants who specialised in eye, ear and tooth complaints while gifted individuals with a regular practice in one area sometimes found it worthwhile to travel elsewhere to take full advantage of their particular expertise. The two Thomas Mountjoys, father and son, regularly left their apothecary practice at Wootton to visit Bristol each summer to treat children for rickets and ruptures.[49] Otherwise, it is legitimate to doubt whether the high-pressure world of the quack was actually a better formula for success than the cautious cultivation of a local reputation, especially as the regular practitioner could make subtle use of many of the same publicity devices as the quack, and develop his own specialism in some modish disease or therapy. This might lead to publication of a small pamphlet, possibly reinforced, in cases of initial apprenticeship to a surgeon or apothecary, by a Scottish degree and a hospital post. Bristol examples from mid-century include the surgeons Abel Dagge[50] and James Norman,[51] who published locally on the treatments of fevers and gonorrhoea, and Daniel Smith, who developed a remedy for gout, published pamphlets attacking Cadogan and Williams on this subject and then took an MD, publishing *An Apology to the Public for Commencing the Practice of Physick*.[52] Perhaps the most successful, if also dangerous, method of extending a reputation and gaining practice was to enter midwifery, as most of Bristol's surgeons and surgeon-apothecaries began to do from about the 1720s.[53]

Finally, I would like to suggest that the medical scene illustrates a more general point about eighteenth-century publicity. In their enthusiasm for attending the 'birth of the consumer society' historians have tended to over-emphasise the instrumental intervention of the press, neglecting the traditional forms of delivery more natural to small provincial communities. The rise of the provincial press offers a plethora of new sources, but we should not exaggerate their effect or be misled by their character. The elite appeal of the newspaper publicity is hardly surprising, given the likely readership of the papers, and matches the nature of other goods advertised, which were primarily luxury items, trade and property notices and the like. It would be invaluable to compare the style of handbills to newspaper advertisements, but almost none of the former survive, at least for Bristol. The greater survival of handbills and the growth of a more popular press in the early nineteenth century may do much to account for an apparent change in the style and appeal of later fringe medicine.

Above all, it should be stressed that advertising through the press was not necessarily more effective than more traditional methods. Reliance on printed publicity carried penalties as well as advantages. The press was distrusted as a source of false information, as well as praised as a potential benefactor. Its use, at least for news, was normally restricted by conventions and expectations about impartiality, often breached in practice but never overtly flouted. Local partisans used the papers carefully as a means of propaganda, inserting short items with veiled references to controversial issues. Personal disputes, when they erupted, were widely deplored, and though they were often vigorously prosecuted this was generally done by means of pseudonyms and satirical generalisations which were intended to evade the charge of personal aggrandisement.[54] Often press items merely reported, very briefly, other forms of publicity which carried more impressive local connotations, such as civic and other rituals. Both the practitioners and subscribers to the infirmary, for example, achieved their greatest publicity on the annual march through the town to a sermon and dinner, with the faculty in their finery and civic dignitaries to grace the occasion.[55]

Generally the quacks would turn to newspaper publicity only after they had already exhausted other ways of attracting attention and were settled in the town, either to drum up more trade or publicise an established record of success. In presenting himself to the public, the quack risked flouting the general conventions governing the use of the press and so being branded as untrustworthy by general readers as well as by the medical community. He had to attempt to establish his own uniqueness, while simultaneously concealing his private interest by a claim to serve the public good. A minority adopted the most dramatic mode of achieving this, employing a rhetoric in which they conflated their personal triumphs with the public good. The majority limited their press publicity to brief and modest notices, preferring to bury their personalities, in print if not in practice, under the testimonies of others. If we restrict the term 'quacks' to those who exploited without reservation the possibilities of press publicity, then we will still have to continue the elusive, if heuristically fruitful, hunt for a term to describe the majority of 'irregular practitioners' who operated on the fringe of eighteenth-century medical practice.

Notes

I should like to thank David Harley and Irvine Loudon for their assistance in the preparation of this paper.

1. R. Porter, 'The Language of Quackery in England 1660-1800', in P. Burke and R. Porter (eds), *Language and Society* (Cambridge, Cambridge University Press, 1986).
2. P.S. Brown, 'The Vendors of Medicines Advertised in Eighteenth-century Bath Newspapers', *Medical History*, 19 (1975), 352-69; *idem*, 'Medicines Advertised in Eighteenth-century Bath Newspapers', *Medical History*, 20 (1976), 152-68; a bibliography of medical sources for Bristol is given in J. Barry, 'Guide to Sources and Writings on the History of Medicine in Bristol 1600-1900', *Bulletin of the Society for the Social History of Medicine*, 35 (December 1984), 48-52.
3. *Bristol PostBoy*, 16 April 1715.
4. Taylor: *Bristol Oracle and Country Advertiser*, 8 October 1743; *Bristol Oracle* 17 September 1748; *Felix Farley's Bristol Journal*, 16 December 1758, 30 May 1761, 24 December 1763 and see note 12. Graham: *Felix Farley's Bristol Journal*, 3 May, 18 June 1774; *Bristol Journal* 13 August, 12-19 November 1774.
5. *Farley's Bristol Newspaper*, 1 July 1727 and on, e.g. 15 July 1727, 5 July 1728.
6. *Felix Farley's Bristol Newspaper*, 8 January, 23 April 1757, 3 May 1760, 22 August 1761, 27 February 1762, 12 May 1764; B. de Dominiceti, *A Short and Calm Apology* (Bristol, S. Farley, 1762); *idem*, *Medical Anecdotes of the Last Thirty Years* (London, L. Davis, 1781).
7. *Felix Farley's Bristol Journal*, 5 April 1766 and see note 38.
8. *Bristol Journal*, 28 August 1773, 11 June 1774.
9. *Felix Farley's Bristol Journal*, 26 February 1763.
10. For example, Mary Beck of Bedminster in *Bristol Journal*, 25 December 1771. Generally, female quacks advertised much less flamboyantly than men.

11. *Felix Farley's Bristol Journal*, 25 July, 13 August 1763.
12. *Farley's Bristol Newspaper*, 4 April 1730.
13. Richard Smith's potted biographies of Bristol medical men in his 'Biographical Memoirs of the Infirmary', now in Bristol Archives Office, generally note the literary and classical leanings of practitioners, as well as marking the few exceptions. For a typical satire see the comments on the fiercely disputatious Dr Rigge in J. Thistlethwaite, *The Consultation* (Bristol, W. Pine, 1774), 22-4.
14. G. Parker, 'Early Bristol Medical Institutions', *Transactions of the Bristol and Gloucestershire Archaeological Society*, 44 (1922), 155-78; J. Page, *Compendium Anatomicum* (Bristol, 1741); *Bristol Oracle and Country Advertiser* 20 October, 3 November 1744; *Oracle and Country Advertiser*, 25 October 1746; *Bristol Oracle*, 1 November 1746; R. Smith, 'Biographical Memoirs', I, 50-5, 118; and ibid., II, 210.
15. *Ibid.*, I, 95, 159.
16. Taylor: *Bristol Oracle and Country Intelligencer*, 5 October 1743; Dominiceti, *Apology* (note 6), 12.
17. G. Munro Smith, *A History of Bristol Royal Infirmary* (Bristol, J.W. Arrowsmith, 1917) prints many colourful items on trade practices from Richard Smith's notes. Probate inventories in Bristol Archives Office include references to barbers' poles (e.g. M. Lewis in 1717) and Company gowns (e.g. S. Noade in 1742, where the gown is valued at £3!). The coach company records in Public Record Office (C/104/139) show doctors paying up to £100 a year for a chariot, horses and drivers, while the ledger of Michael Edkins, painter (Bristol Central Library, Bristol Collection no. 20196) includes work gilding for apothecaries.
18. Bristol Quarter Sessions Minutes in Bristol Archives Office, for January 1670; *Bristol PostBoy*, 25 September 1714, 25 August 1715.
19. H. Hobhouse (ed.), *Diary of a West Country Physician* (London, Simpkin, Marshall, 1933), 99.
20. A. Wilson, 'Participant or Patient?' in R. Porter (ed.), *Patients and Practitioners* (Cambridge, Cambridge University Press 1985), 129-44.
21. *Felix Farley's Bristol Journal*, 28 September 1754, 8-22 May 1762; *Bristol Chronicle*, 27 September 1760.
22. For example, the advertisements for his treatment for gout and rheumatism of Bristol apothecary Thomas Hayward in *Bristol Oracle and Country Intelligencer*, 23 July 1743 and on.
23. J. Underhill, *A Short Account of the Bristol Hotwell-Water* (Bristol, W. Bonny, 1703)
24. G. Randolph, *An Inquiry into the Medicinal Virtues of Bristol-Water* (Oxford, J. Fletcher, 1745), 21-3; A. Sutherland, *The Nature and Qualities of Bristol Water* (Bristol, E. Farley & Son, 1758), 22-3.
25. W. Cadogan, *An Essay upon Nursing* (London, J. Roberts, 1748), 4, 34.
26. Sutherland (note 24), 110-12, 122.
27. *Ibid.* 153.
28. See references in J. Barry, 'Piety and Patient: Medicine and Religion in Eighteenth-century Bristol', in Porter (note 20), 153-5.
29. J. Johnson, *Transactions of the Corporation of the Poor* (Bristol, P. Rose, 1826), 108ff.; E.E. Butcher (ed.), *Bristol Corporation of the Poor* (Bristol Record Society III, 1932), 10-12, 111-12; T. Dover, *An Ancient Physician's Legacy*, 2nd edn (London, For the Author, 1732), 98-9; Smith (note 17).
30. *Farley's Bristol Newspaper*, 28 January 1727; *Bristol Oracle and Country Advertiser*, 8 October 1743; *Felix Farley's Bristol Journal*, 22 March 1755, 21 February 1756, 23 February 1760, 14 February 1761 and on (surgical dispute); *Philosophical Transactions*, 21 (1720), 44-6; *ibid.*, 49 (1755), 93-5, 264-5; S. Pye, *Some observations on . . . Lithotomy* (London, J. & W. Innys, 1724); J. Middleton, *A Short Essay on . . . Lithotomy* (London, G. Strahan, 1727).
31. *Felix Farley's Bristol Journal*, 22 September 1759 and on.

32. *Ibid*, 10 January 1767. Cf. *ibid.*, 28 December 1754; *Bristol Oracle*, 28 November 1747; *The Bristol Infirmary Contest* (Bristol, E. Farley, 1755).

33. See *Felix Farley's Bristol Journal* and *Bristol Journal*, 22 October 1768 and on, e.g. 14 January 1769 and 16 June 1770; Smith (note 17), 419ff.

34. See 1770 reference in note 33; Butcher (note 29), 111-16.

35. Bristol Archives Office, 04369(1), ordinance no. 7.

36. Hands: *Felix Farley's Bristol Journal*, 22 October 1757, 18 October 1760. In 1750 James Grace, surgeon-apothecary, explicitly compared his offer of free service to that of the hospitals (*Bristol Journal*, 19 May 1750). The inoculation houses made the same offer (*ibid*, 22 October 1768, 20 January 1770).

37. *Felix Farley's Bristol Journal*, 29 September 1759, 19 January 1760.

38. *Ibid.* 10 May 1766.

39. *Bristol PostBoy*, 25 September 1714; *Felix Farley's Bristol Journal*, 26 June 1752.

40. T. Smollett, *The Adventures of Ferdinand, Count Fathom* (Oxford, Oxford University Press, 1971), 166f., 247-50.

41. *The PostMan*, 18-20 September 1701 (I owe this reference to David Harley).

42. *Bristol PostBoy*, 16 April 1715; cf. *ibid.* 25 September 1714.

43. *Felix Farley's Bristol Journal*, 2 May 1761.

44. Dominiceti, *Apology* (note 6), 30.

45. *Felix Farley's Bristol Journal*, 17 September 1757.

46. Dominiceti, *Apology* (note 6), 15-17, 22.

47. *Farley's Bristol Newspaper*, 16 July 1726, 5 July 1728; *Bristol PostBoy*, 13 March 1714.

48. Porter (note 1); I. Loudon, 'The Nature of Provincial Medical Practice in Eighteenth-century England', *Medical History*, 29 (1985), 1-32. See also their contributions to this volume.

49. *Felix Farley's Bristol Journal*, 21 April 1759; *Bristol Journal*, 26 April 1760, 15 July 1766, 29 April 1775.

50. *Ibid.*, 31 January, 27 December 1767, 3 November 1770, 4 April, 12 December 1772.

51. Smith (note 13), I, 106-7; *Felix Farley's Bristol Journal*, 24 January 1756.

52. *Bristol Journal*, 6 June 1772, 9 April 1774; *Bonner and Middleton's Bristol Journal*, 17 June 1775; D. Smith, *An Apology to the Public* (London, Carnan and Newbury, c. 1775).

53. S. Stone, *The Complete Practice of Midwifery* (London, T. Cooper, 1737), x.

54. These general points cannot be substantiated here. See J. Barry, 'The Cultural Life of Bristol, 1640-1775' (unpublished D.Phil thesis, University of Oxford, 1985), 123-8.

55. Smith (note 17), 24; *Felix Farley's Bristol Journal*, 16 July 1757.

3 ORTHODOXY AND FRINGE: MEDICINE IN LATE GEORGIAN BRISTOL

Michael Neve

> QUACKERY. The extension of it remains to be proved. There may be an increase of advertised medicines, but when I consider the immense number of herbs mentioned in our old herbals, and recollect how busy were our old women, I see that they very much exceed the quack medicines, and I venture to believe that medicine, in proportion to the population of the country, is less frequently administered by unprofessional hands than at any former period.
>
> *Thomas Beddoes*

To examine provincial medical culture such as that of Bristol at the end of the eighteenth century is to uncover a world of considerable confusion. As other contributors to this volume make clear, the various distinctions introduced into the medical profession in the nineteenth century, including the increased fear of 'quackery' itself, can seem to have very little explanatory value for the earlier period. The medical world of the eighteenth century is almost defined by the absence of demarcation that was one of the trade marks of professional struggle in the period after 1790. Not even the radical chemist Thomas Beddoes, who was virulent in his attacks on irregular practice, could fully decide how extensive that practice actually was.

Certain doubts may therefore be cast on the idea of an extensive 'fringe', as against a large body of locally based practitioners who, in many cases, do not even appear in any known archive, let alone express the nature of their remedies. The 'fringe' should then be divided between stylish itinerants, such as Chevalier Taylor MD, one of whose specialities seems to have been his ability not to have been present when consulted, and local medical dealers whose profile in the commercial sector was maintained by a mixture of local reputation and advertisement.[1] It certainly seems important to distinguish sharply between itinerant showmen and local medical men, whether one is attempting to examine the dispensing of medicine in Bristol or the protecting of the reputation of the Bath waters by practitioners determined for obvious commercial reasons to maintain their efficacy.[2]

An admirable desire to investigate 'irregular practice' and the scale of public desire for commercially marketed medicine in the late eighteenth and early nineteenth centuries should not lead medical historians to over-estimate the strength of the 'irregulars', as against the orthodox, at least in provincial centres such as Bristol. Local medical archives, including the now much quoted memoirs of the Bristol surgeon Richard Smith, do not provide a vast amount of materials on the activities of 'quacks', and it is not clear that this is simply because an infirmary-based collector of medical information and anecdote would be ideologically averse to collecting parallel information about the 'fringe'.[3] Apart from some fleeting references in the early volumes, the Smith memoirs are an overwhelming testament to the existence of a large body of what can only be called regular practitioners.

This does not mean that quacks were not present, especially in the treatment of sexually transmitted disease, or that a local figure such as George Winter — author of *Elements of Agriculture* and a history of animal magnetism — might not, as shown by Loudon, dispense medicine to the local poor later in the century.[4] It may indeed be the case that the absence of major campaigns to vilify quacks beteen 1740 and 1790 sprang from the prosperity of apothecaries, and indeed surgeons, who would be untouched by the activities of medicinally minded Anglican clergy or chariot-borne oculists. As was said of Taylor in the *Gloucester Journal* for 18 September 1733: 'From the shortness of his stay in each place he gives no personal attendance in his manner of removing the Disorders of Sight and Hearing'.[5] If this is the case, then the build-up of a large number of 'regular practitioners', or men who stayed put, as well as the eclectic mixture of medical techniques that might be employed by them, would provide the background to the beginning of the attack on the 'fringe' from the 1790s onwards. It is certainly puzzling, for example, that so few of the local collections of broadsides — at least in the Bristol material — give evidence of any kind of routine stage-setting, let alone performance, that might allow the quacks to be clearly identified. In some important sense, both archivally and perhaps in historical reality, 'quackery' does not seem to have been a major eighteenth-century problem.

One speculation that will be hinted at in this short essay is that the fate of barber-surgeons after 1745 is not historically certain, and a reasonable guess is that many such figures continued to exist after the mid-century, even if they chose not to appear in the pages of local directories. The problem again, a problem with some modest historical implications, is that of the records themselves. Loudon has followed certain hints by G. Munro Smith on the rise of the dispensing druggist as the adversary of the apothecary medicine of the 'golden age'.[6] And, at least in the Bristol case, the basis for researching into this is once again the Richard Smith memoirs. Certain clues suggest that, at least up to the end of the eighteenth century, barber-surgeons continued to exist perhaps to the annoyance of surgeons and surgeon-apothecaries, and may even have formed a 'quack' target for that group of practitioners. Newspaper evidence shows that in 1752, on 28 September, a young woman who had been bled at a barber's shop in March Street 'fainted away and died'. In March 1754, 'Henry Haines, barber, Redcliff Pitt' advertised himself as shaving 'for twopence, cuts hair for three halfpence, and bleeds for sixpence. All customers who are bled he treats with two quarts of good ale, and those whom he shaves or cuts their hair with a pint each.' In the 1774 list of medical practitioners for Bristol (included in volume 1 of the Smith memoirs) one of the barber-surgeons is also a publican.[7]

As Mary Fissell has suggested in her study of eighteenth-century Bristol medical culture, the possibility certainly exists that a proper examination of the apprentice-records, however inadequate (bearing in mind that only freemen would be listed, along with legitimate apprentice-takers), might well reveal a continuity of barber-surgeon practice. This would add weight to the view that there were large numbers of *local* medical practitioners, opposed to barber-surgeons, whose practice was distinct from that of itinerants. They would be the servants of medical consumers, and calling them 'quacks' is not historically appropriate.[8]

As late as 1807, even sources other than the apprentice records indicate the continued existence of barber-surgeons. Richard Smith writes:

> I just mention en passant that the last remnant of barber surgery dropped with Old Parsley, who lived next door to the Guildhall so lately as 1807 — this man dressed more wigs, drew more teeth, and spilled more blood than any man in Bristol — at his window, and by the side of his door hung immense and double strings of teeth, drawn by one terrible jerk, having never used a gum lancet in his life — thousands of people yet alive can testify by this, for he regularly brought his patients to the door, either for the sake of a good light or for notoriety.

The acknowledged presence of barber-surgeons in the late 1740s might now be extended, indeed might be a feature of medical practice throughout the 'long eighteenth century'.[9]

The drug consumption of medical customers undoubtedly benefited, and was met by, the apothecaries, of whom Bristol produced some strikingly wealthy examples. The apothecaries had their own fringe, the now 'marginalised' barber-surgeon, and were also able to benefit from what can only be called an urban population with a major, opium-based drug habit. Any population-based view of medical remedies must, after all, presuppose such a habit along with a public able to purchase patent medicines through known local vendors and through newspaper advertisement.

In late-eighteenth-century Bristol patent medicines, if newspaper advertisements are anything to go by, were widely available. They range from the universally popular James's Fever Powder, or Dr Ward's extensive list of cheap medicines, to Hill's medicine for mad-dog bite, and Bateman's Pectoral Drops. These remedies were available from the publishers of the papers in which they were advertised, and clearly indicate the integration of Bristol into the national market from the 1730s onwards. In slight contrast to the Hull evidence cited by Loudon, it is hard to find advertisements for *local* patent remedies in the Bristol press, but purveyors of such alternatives no doubt had other means of bringing these to popular notice. It is none the less of interest that, as with P.S. Brown's study of patent medicines on sale in eighteenth-century Bath, the overwhelming percentage of advertised remedies were both recommended and imported from exotic locales.[10]

Bristol in the late eighteenth century was a prosperous, semi-industrialised port with a large number of medical practitioners of the 'regular' sort to serve its population of about 80,000. In 1754, over 67 medical practitioners paid to be listed, and these included 5 physicians, 19 surgeons, 13 barber-surgeons, 1 surgeon-apothecary and 29 apothecaries. Twenty years later, Richard Smith computed from Sketchley's *Directory* a list of 8 physicians, over 20 surgeons, 32 apothecaries, 2 barber-surgeons, 6 chemists/druggists and 1 midwife.[11] It is perfectly possible that within this fairly large population of practitioners, medical practices of unusual kinds may have been carried on, but on the assumption that the severity of the attack on 'quackery' occurs early in the nineteenth century, it is hard to untangle regular from irregular practice. Another puzzle is the disappearance — at least from the newspaper sources, of low-order irregulars who specialised in cures for poor hearing. A 'Mr Duckett' of Fairford, Gloucester, who claimed he had been a licensed surgeon for forty-one years, advertised regularly in the *Gloucester Journal* in the late 1730s. In the same pages a John Penn of Melksham, Wiltshire, similarly offered cures for deafness. From mid-century, in both the Bristol and Gloucester papers, this type of practitioner vanishes. Is it possible that the extravagant quackery of Taylor *et al.* was in fact the takeover of specialisms of this kind in order to cash in on a wider commercial market from mid-century onwards, especially in the area of venereal diseases and diseases of the eyes?

If the real fringe in eighteenth-century provincial medicine is the spectacular theatre of itinerants — the extravagant display of Dominiceti's *Short and Calm Apology* of 1762, with its admissions to pretence, Papism and maintenance of 'gaiety and pleasures' in a Protestant city (as well as helping 3,296 patients!) — then the more fruitful area of research might be into the initiation, within 'regular' practice, of remedies that required 'puffing' simply on the ground that they were innovative. *An Apology to the Public for Commencing the Practice of Physic*, written in 1775 by Daniel Smith MD, provides an example. Smith appears to have been some kind of regular practitioner, active in Bristol, who devised unusual remedies for the cure of the gout. His first patient was the Reverend Mr Camplin of Bristol Cathedral, followed by 'Mr Paulin, of North Parade in Bath'. What makes Smith's pamphlet interesting is his flirtatious hinting at the secret of his remedies, which can only be purchased by meeting with Smith himself or by writing to Mr Francis Newbery, proprietor of Dr James's Powder, at 65 St Paul's Churchyard; and, second, his blaming the 'general itch of quackery' on the commercial sale of dispensatories, with their 'tens of thousands of receipts for curing diseases'.[12] 'Quackery', therefore, was a product of consumer self-help — at least in the eyes of this particular writer, anxious himself to avoid the charge.

This historically intriguing idea — that self-help was the real quackery — cannot easily be followed up, but chimes, albeit remotely, with Jewson's thesis, and the mysterious sleight-of-hand whereby patients slowly turned from commercially powerful consumers to nineteenth-century servile acceptors of medical orthodoxy. The area in which the eighteenth-century patient might exercise — even as a conspiratorial relationship — remarkable demands is indicated in the literature on smallpox. In his 1771 *Letter to a Surgeon on Inoculation*, John Blake defends his own practice of inoculation while berating quack inoculators for their series of false promises. But more importantly, he reveals that pregnant women would apply to these practitioners in the hope that abortion would ensue, rather than that they would be conducted through the 'disease with the greatest safety'. Thus, the charge against quackery was not simply that quack inoculations were injurious to pregnant women; it was the revelation that such desperate remedies were actually being sought by the patients themselves.[13]

The difficult task of tracking the fate of the collapse of consumer sovereignty can only be hinted at here, but the sheer growth in the number of medical practitioners, as well as the post-1790 attack on 'quacks', must be important factors. In neighbouring Bath, it could be said that the campaign to defend orthodoxy had started earlier, as local physicians built up a considerable literature on the unique qualities of Bath water, partly as a way of seeing off more unusual figures such as James Graham.[14] In Bristol, the growth of directory-cited regulars grew in the early nineteenth century, there being twenty physicians and eighty surgeons and apothecaries listed in 1808. And, as other writers have noted, the attack on irregularity comes, within a now dangerously overcrowded profession, in two waves. At the century's end, there are attacks on the wealth and the practice of apothecaries themselves. Then, in the period after 1815, a different series of pressures produced a different target, as the forces of increased costs of medical education and the overproduction of medical practitioners after the Apothecaries Act led to the dispensing druggist being named as the guilty party. The simple point to be stressed here is that the appeal to canons of medical honesty, as against quackery, was made to keep the 'profession' manageable, not necessarily out of deep concern for the dangerous activities of irregulars. The second wave of hostility is directed here, pathologising the activities of unwanted rivals, as the profession itself gets tightened up, via the 'College and Hall' qualification, the beginnings (clear in Bristol) of provincial medical education, the beginnings too of the professional idea of the general practitioner. Underlying both waves of panic is the historical engine that keeps the quackery issue alive, even to the present: the desire, on the part of the ordinary consumer, to get to the drugs with the minimum waste of time. The quest for the consolation of drugs is surely the popular demand upon which the running battle about who was, or was not, a quack has been historically founded.

But we must not assume that the attack on quackery came only from what we might call conservative medical writers. One of the most consistent and fiercest tirades in Bristol was the work of a constitutional democrat, anti-establishment radical, the physician and chemist Thomas Beddoes (1760-1808). Beddoes combined a political idea for a new order with a medical belief that chemistry could form part of a revolution in therapeutics; his hostility was sometimes directed at conservative doctors, but most frequently at 'apothecaries and their slops'.

In the debates of the 1820s and 1830s the imputation of quack activity was prevalent in areas that had once been the preserve of irregular empirics, particularly in diseases of the eye. This could be because the number of techniques available for diseases of the eye were few, and also that opthalmology, perhaps like midwifery, was an area that practitioners went into *faute de mieux*, and were particularly sensitive to the legacy of single-technique, 'quack' practices that had dominated this medical field. One noted Bristol eye surgeon, the Unitarian anti-slavery agitator John Bishop Estlin (1785-1855), was renowned for his hostility to irregular practice, and he came to include in his critique phrenology, homoeopathy and mesmerism. In Bristol he established a small specialist dispensary for eye diseases, having failed to secure an infirmary-based surgical post. The 'touchiness' of early (and recent) general practitioners described so well by Loudon, may have been particularly prevalent in areas such as the one Estlin was forced to specialise in.[15]

For behind the Wakleyesque cries of quackery, and its imputations, lies the harder social fact that in the rag and bone shop that was the humble historical birthplace of general practice, things could be tough and difficult. The real history of the quackery scare in the nineteenth century could be seen as the accusatory cry of medical men, whether in Southwark (an area that particularly concerned Thomas Wakley), or a small Somerset village, or the poorer parts of provincial cities, where remuneration was bad and prospects often worse. The unknown fates of many practitioners in the badlands of the 1820s, 1830s — even the 1840s — is the real historical landscape that sets the scene for the language of quackery and its various usages. By the 1840s, the profession of medicine — and this is absolutely clear in a city like Bristol — had a geographical distribution that was itself an index of class organisation. In the salubrious suburbs — Clifton, above all — dwelt the elite physicians and some of the surgeons. In the commercial areas of the city — especially the busy through road of Park Street — the area around the cathedral, and in the business section, dwelt the mass of surgeons and surgeon-apothecaries. Across the river, and to the east, in Bedminster, Old Market, St Paul's, the still unknown fates of many practitioners — whether dispensing druggist or unqualified surgeon-apothecary, doing whatever work was available — were working themselves out. Old Market, for example, was the home of William Herapath (1796-1868), respected chemist as well as politically radical and socially anti-elitist organiser of the Bristol Political Union. It is in that sense entirely unsurprising that when the 1840s brought the arrival of the evangelising Thomsonians — the Mormons of medicine — all the newcomers' activities and propaganda were aimed at proletarian Bristol, the suburbs of St Paul's and St Philip's above all. In the nineteenth-century presentation of medicine, battles were not simply about university backgrounds, infirmary elections, let alone theories of physic; rather, they concerned the most simple social fact of all: your address.[16]

If it is impossible to define exactly the place of fringe irregularities in a provincial city like late Georgian Bristol, then the opposite holds for the institutions of orthodoxy. The eighteenth-century infirmary was part of a network of smaller sites which went out of their way to emphasise social and ethical distance from any contamination by unorthodox physic. The main examples here were: from the 1830s, the Bristol General Hospital, which had been preceded by St Peter's Hospital (Bristol's unusual combined workhouse and lunatic asylum); the Bristol Dispensary; Clifton Dispensary; and a small number of other institutions for diseases of the eyes or for lying-in women.

These institutions varied in the number of patients they dealt with, and in their methods. What needs to be stressed is that all of them presented medicine within the hierarchical system of charitable recommendation that characterises so much eighteenth- and early-nineteenth-century medicine, and that 'medicine' or medical care thus dispensed spoke for the civic virtue and religious concern of the families and individuals who made up the main body of subscribers. As Jonathan Barry has noted, there was considerable Dissenting interest in the early history of the Bristol Dispensary and the Bristol Infirmary: my own view is that this eclecticism is much less apparent from 1810 or 1820 than it had been previously, and that the governors of the infirmary in these later years, or the people who set up the Clifton Dispensary in 1813, were, by a considerable majority, Anglican or Unitarian conservatives — in which category I include Whig elements — and had become distant from the Methodist, even Quaker, sources that had been there at the inception of eighteenth-century medical institutions. Many factors indicate that class segmentation was accompanied by religious segmentation: the years of political reaction; the number of conversions to Anglicanism within the city's elite; the domination of the city corporation by the Tories from 1812 onwards; the setting-up of a scientific institution in 1822-3 that expounded a conservative, natural theological series of doctrines, most famously the ethnology of the Tory Anglican physician James Cowles Prichard. Such considerations also show how the Wesleyan influence, both in medicine and social life, moved down into the general populace, while the city's wealthy and powerful citizens affiliated themselves to post-Napoleonic political and religious reaction. The classical texts of popular medicine may not have disappeared, since Wesley's *Primitive Physick* continued to be an influence on the 'fringe' in the middle of the nineteenth century. Within the medical hierarchy, however, Bristol had a physician elite that was almost entirely of Scottish, Oxbridge or continental pedigree, sometimes a mixture of each; a large surgeon and surgeon-apothecary corps; and a popular or self-help medical grouping that, at least up until 1851, remains something of a mystery. Some surgeons made quite good livings; others went to mixed futures. There can be little doubt that, particularly among the surgeons and surgeon-apothecaries, so-called 'quack medicines' were both dispensed and indeed kept as secret: John Webb's cordial, for example, to be had at the house of the surgeon John Dolman; or 'Essence of Coltsfoot', for a time the property of Thomas Goldwyn, surgeon. But especially with the organisation of medical education in the 1830s, the general respect for Parisian medicine, even the examples of commitment to 'heroic therapy' in some cases, we can surely agree that the medical elite, the members of the dining clubs, had some idea of orthodoxy.[17]

So, medicine was presented in nineteenth-century Bristol as a manifestation of civic philanthropy and social display, but in a context of increasing class differentiation and religious non-eclecticism. What was the place of quackery or, to put it more accurately, the place of quackery — real or ascribed — in the opinions of local medical authors?

First into the lists was the aforementioned physician and chemist Thomas Beddoes. Beddoes was a distinguished Edinburgh-trained physician with an interest in pneumatic medicine. He was a firm advocate of the medical philosophy of Erasmus Darwin and, in a modified form, of William Cullen's pupil John Brown (1735-88). In the late 1780s and early 1790s, Beddoes became a supporter of the constitutional phase of the French Revolution, and this adherence placed him in opposition to the government of the day and to the political delicacies of the senior members of the University of Oxford. What makes Beddoes's case of interest is that he was a radical: he was often deemed a quack himself — indeed, one could say that his medicine was seen by, say, the *Anti-Jacobin Review* as political quackery — and yet his commitment to the philosophy of Darwin and Brown, which he saw as revolutionary, was so intense that he seems to have regarded all those who spurned these views as risible and irresponsible.

This belief in the revolutionary impact of pneumatic medicine may even have stemmed from a deep exasperation with the disputes between Cullenians and Brunonians in Edinburgh medical circles. In a letter written during his years as a student, Beddoes foresaw the eventual collapse of both Cullenite and Brunonian medicine, and records that exasperation is likely to drive him into being 'a mere empiric'.[18] Beddoes could be said to have exposed the proximity of orthodoxy to quackery, by seeing that the collapse of theory, whether Cullenian or Brunonian, would leave an apothecary-based medicine as the only useful alternative. Except, of course, for pneumatics.

Beddoes was a man of considerable ambition, knowledgeable in

Plutonist geology, and impressively widely read in continental philosophy and continental medical writing. He felt able, for example, in a review published in Richard Griffith's *Monthly Review* in 1797, to dismiss Kurt Sprengel's *History of Medicine* (Halle: 1792-4) 'as a heavy, tasteless ill-arranged compilation, in which interesting and uninteresting things are detailed in nearly the same tone'. This arrogant assessment is certainly contested by modern historians of medicine, notably Charles Webster, who has deemed Sprengel's history 'as having lost none of its stature'.[19]

Beddoes's ambition, as his historians have agreed, overreached itself, and his overall scheme for a new kind of medicine was a disappointment. But as a denouncer of quackery, before the tirades of the *Lancet* era, he was indefatigable. In his introduction to a translation of John Brown's *Elements of Medicine* (1795), he denounces both elite physicians and quacks. Edinburgh Royal Infirmary is seen as mismanaged, and in the hands of 'political swindlers'; men who 'acquire the power of sporting with the wealth and blood of nations'. John Brown, famous for lecturing under the combined influence of whisky and opium, is — for whatever secret reason — protected by Beddoes, not merely as the revolutionary denied deserved recognition, but as a victim: 'a sharper', as Beddoes puts it, a 'speculator in public medicine' thought of marketing 'Dr Brown's exciting pill'. 'Poor Brown, needy as he was, spurned at the proposal.' Beddoes, unusually, sees quacks above *and* below. At the top of the profession are the 'unphilosophical doctors': here 'the caprice of fortune elevates her worthless favourites to the first eminence'; these intruders 'occupy the station due to physicians of enlarged views', blocking the way of doctors who have 'improved their ideas into principles'. Beddoes writes: 'the greatest repute in medicine affords scarce the slightest presumption of superiority', and then in the closing pages of his introduction, parodies the bullying, bacchanalian or solemn characteristics of doctors with good bedside manners but little else.

Some years later, in 1808, in *A Letter* to *Joseph Banks*, Beddoes's own concerns remain at the forefront: by this time the Pneumatic Institute had altered, becoming a more conventional preventive medical institution. But in writing to Banks, Beddoes sees rank quackery everywhere:[20]

if we are to judge by the usual signs of public confidence in medicine, has not a fellow who orders British gin from Bristol to Liverpool; colours and christens it *balm*, as much of this confidence as almost all the fellows of the three royal colleges put together?

So concerned is Beddoes with the extent of quackery, which at one point in the letter he explicitly compares with prostitution, that he even proposes the need to engage the Wesleyans in helping to stamp it out. But even here danger lurks, for what would happen if, 'following the example of John Wesley', people came to think that they could take their own bodies 'into their care'? It is instructive that Beddoes also attacks the world of what he calls 'corresponding medicine', marketed through advertisement, which allowed apothecaries to drench the world with their mixtures. He generally sees any kind of self-advertisement as bad, whether the sponsor be obsequious doctors anxious to give their patients what they ask for, or commercially minded apothecaries. Instead, society needed more medical students, taking five-year courses, with a broader curriculum and, if possible, continental experience. As for quack medicines, there was only one remedy: they should be made illegal. There should instead be more experimental hospitals, more preventive medical institutions, more centralised, statistically based information on public health. Beddoes was not a medical policeman, in the Viennese manner, but he certainly favoured a medicalisation of social life, to a marked degree.

Beddoes, as a critic of the fringe, appears to be concerned with, first and most obviously, the scale of apothecary medicine. Thus, if the itinerants and spectacular irregulars make up what historians wish to call the real 'fringe', it is noteworthy that he does not mention them. More importantly, as was seen with the brief notice of Daniel Smith, the essence of quackery is patient self-help, the conspiracy between buyer and seller that 'apothecary medicine' embodied. The medicalisation of society, along lines suggested by Johann Peter Frank, must require the destruction of this commercial relationship. Under the aegis of a notably aggressive view of the systematic emptiness of Cullen and to some extent Brown, Beddoes combines an apparent Jacobin orientation with an utter hostility to any form of popular medicine and indeed virtually any medical activity not engaged in by trained practitioners.[21]

Beddoes did make one interesting break with the subscriber recommendatory system discussed earlier: patients attending the preventive institution paid 2s. 6d. at the beginning of treatment, a sum which would be returned at the end of their period of attendance. And Beddoes, for all his dislike of common medicine, hoped that a gentler relationship could exist between doctor and patient:[22]

> The experience of former medical charities shows that the sick are constantly flying off before they have a chance of due benefit. I take

this to be a want of proper understanding. All has hitherto been conducted in a style of authority. It has been too much mere dumb show between doctor and patient.

These are the contradictions that surrounded Beddoes and his project: politically radical, yet hostile to popular medicine; violently anti-quackery, while verging on authoritarian continental models to replace the commercial druggists. This mixture, which is not unfamiliar in the annals of English Jacobinism, is also present in the thinking of Beddoes's acquaintance S.T. Coleridge: a democrat in his Bristol youth, Coleridge too came to denounce animal magnetism and phrenology as 'quackery, relying on mere . . . coincidence'.[23]

But this may be the essential point: that Beddoes was far closer, in his hostility to the murky underworld of 'apothecaries and their slops', to later figures — such as J.B. Estlin, working for long hours in his eye dispensary — than either man was to the harsh world where the poor avoided medicine altogether and trusted to wise women or the quackery of druggists. This is not to impugn either Beddoes or Estlin, since both — and particularly the latter whose constituency stretched far into South Wales — gave enormous service to their respective causes. But the levelling of the charge of quackery, whether against the apothecary in the first instance, or the sly druggist or his ophthalmological equivalent in the second, is in a sense an expression of frustration. For the real fringe could be said to consist of not the irregular practitioners themselves, but the mass of the public who avoided orthodox medicine altogether. The recognition of a 'fringe' is therefore a recognition of a class-based limit to the extent to which medicine could reach the general population at all, a fact that did not escape the notice of the Coffinites and Thomsonians before they themselves were absorbed into the regular world. Perhaps because of the relative failure of the reform movements in the 1830s, the politicisation of the fringe was one way to sharpen up the class conflict, and to include medical critiques as part of general frustration. This may have been the case even in a city such as Bristol, where Chartism was weak. The doctors had, to some extent, got the professional kudos that they wanted, had brought to an end the free market, had established their ethical codes and standards. But out in the darkness of the cities of which many of them knew so little, the mass of the population insisted on their ancient right to buy some solace in a bottle and to die among friends. The fringe, in that sense, is the shadow cast by the unextinguished right of the patient to ignore 'professional medicine'.[24]

52 Orthodoxy and Fringe

Victorian professional regulation in medicine needed to contradict the colourful laissez-faire world of the eighteenth-century market economy with its often strange alliances between patient and practitioner. Wakley's call in the *Lancet* for a career open to talents, and his attack on the corruption of the colleges and the quacks, was probably one good way of enforcing closure and spreading a sense of panic: the quacks — those ghastly skeletons from the cupboards of the 'age of agony' — had to be both evoked and dismissed, so that the liberal rhetoric of progressive individualism could conceal the hard business of restriction and demarcation, as part of the protection of now vulnerable 'general practitioners'.

As a result of this campaign which reached its height in the 1830s, the medical world of the 1840s does indeed see something new: complete *philosophies* of opposition to orthodox medicine; philosophies that had an explicitly political dimension, and which came to see orthodoxy as simply part of class interest. The Bristolian version of this nineteenth-century politicisation — much of it accompanied by a sarcastic, American-imported rhetoric, in the case of the Thomsonians — has been admirably discussed by P.S. Brown. Brown has conveyed a vivid picture of mid-century Bristol characterised by residual popular beliefs in magical practice, or astrology, and a rural constituency near the city among whom many folk ideas remained potent — not least an apparent belief in witches.[25]

Yet this glimpse into the survival of theoretically archaic beliefs only reinforces the historical sense as to how distant medicine, as an organised profession, had become from the 'fringe', medicine here meaning the new framework of training and regulation enforced from 1815. In the late Georgian period, any half-candid historian must surely admit to confusion, and even to an attraction to the 'conventional view', in that the phenomenon of 'regularity' is simply more impressive than a still mysterious quack world. Compared to the display of power managed by the surgeons of the Bristol Infirmary in the years 1750-1800, the history of (say) Chevalier Taylor is an aside.

However exotic some of the mixtures dispensed by apothecaries to their clients; however persistent the barber-surgeons may have been in places such as Bristol; however 'quackish' some of the practices of local practitioners might seem to the Victorian professional mind, the underlying theme of the sparse materials available is that patients should not be allowed to exist in a deregulated commercial market. Whether from a Beddoesian, continental viewpoint, or within the conspiratorial alliance managed by Oxbridge physicians to push out the rich apothecary, the true irregular turns out to be the 'consumer' who was now a 'patient'.

The real quack may, in the end, be the drug-taking self-helper.[26]

Notes

1. On the received history of quackery, see C.J.S. Thompson, *The Quacks of Old London* (London, Brentano's, 1928); Eric Maple, *Magic, Medicine and Quackery* (London, Robert Hale, 1968). For Taylor 'himself', see John Chevalier Taylor, *The History of the Travels and Adventures of the Chevalier John Taylor, Ophthalmiater* (3 vols in 1; London, J. Williams, 1761-2).
2. The protection of the reputation of the Bath waters is discussed in B. Schnorrenberg, 'Medical Men of Bath', *Studies in Eighteenth Century Culture*, 13 (1984), 189-203. See also Roger Rolls, 'Archibald Cleland c.1700-1771', *British Medical Journal*, 288 (1984), 1132-4.
3. The importance of Smith's 'Memoirs' is evident to all who have interested themselves in provincial medical practice in the eighteenth and nineteenth centuries; careful study of the materials from which remarks can be made on 'quacks' shows them to be scattered and sparse. Smith himself — a *very* curious figure, who has not been properly analysed as a medical collector — would not have been averse to adding materials of a strange kind on 'quacks' or indeed any other fringe world: the drawings of the toes of witches, or the shoes of Irish giants, to take only two examples, and perhaps more alarmingly, books bound in the skin of hanged men. For a more sober view, see A.L. Eyre-Brook, 'R. Smith, jnr. and his Times', *Bristol Medico Chirurgical Journal*, 84 (1969), 1-11.
4. George Winter, *A New and Compendious System of Husbandry* (London, T. Type, 1799); Winter also produced an interesting criticism of mesmerism, *Animal Magnetism, Origins, Progress and Present State* (Bristol, George Routh, 1801).
5. I owe this reference, and a number of others, to the kindness of Mary Fissell. Taylor visited the West Country on a variety of occasions, including 1743, 1748, 1758, 1761, 1763 as well as this visit of 1733, where, accompanied by 'his chariot and six, with numerous attendants', he called at Bristol, Bath, Gloucester and Hereford. It might be said that the technique of being too busy to be seen has a long subsequent history in the area of medical self-advertisement.
6. G. Munro Smith, *A History of the Bristol Royal Infirmary* (Bristol, J.W. Arrowsmith, 1917), 249-55.
7. R. Smith, 'Memoirs', I, 174. Both references from the newspapers are from *Felix Farley's Bristol Journal*, 28 September 1752, and 9 March 1754 respectively. On barber-surgeons, see G. Munro Smith, 'Early Bristol Medical Institutions', *Transactions of the Bristol and Gloucester Archaeological Society*, 44 (1922), 155-78. Roy Porter has pointed out to me that Partridge, in Henry Fielding's novel *Tom Jones*, ends up as a barber-surgeon.
8. For example: a Dr Speakman, 'to be found at Bush's Tiler and Plaisterer, Denmark Street', alleged he could cure the French disease 'for 2s 6d, without the knowledge of any friend'. It seems reasonable to see such a person as a non-itinerant, regular, locally based practitioner. See *Felix Farley's Bristol Journal*, 11 November 1754. Even Richard Smith had an understanding with venereally diseased patients, who could enter and depart from his premises via a hidden way. Compared to these local facilities, the visit of de Mainanduc in 1788 to lecture on animal magnetism (which so incensed George Winter) is a passing comet of fashion. A full discussion of the practice of apothecaries is available in J.G.L. Burnby, *A Study of the English Apothecary from 1600 to 1760, Medical History* Supplement no. 3 (London, Wellcome Institute for the History of Medicine, 1983). The author points out how Richard Smith saw apothecaries as greedy, dispensing enormous quantities of medicines that they induced patients to swallow, often by arrangement with a physician or surgeon.

54 Orthodoxy and Fringe

9. See R. Smith (note 7), I, 32, and the appearance of this story in G. Munro Smith (note 6), 247-8.

10. P.S. Brown, 'The Vendors of Medicines, Advertised in Eighteenth-century Bath Newspapers', *Medical History*, 19 (1975), 352-69; idem, 'Medicines Advertised in Eighteenth-century Bath Newspapers', *Medical History*, 20 (1976), 152-68.

11. R. Smith (note 7), I, 174.

12. Daniel Smith, *An Apology to the Public for Commencing the Practice of Physic*, 2nd edn (London, Carnan and Newberry, 1776), 24.

13. John Blake, *A Letter to a Surgeon on Inoculation* (London, W. Owen, 1771), 18-19.

14. For a full discussion of this issue, see M.R. Neve, 'Natural Philosophy, Medicine and the Culture of Science in Provincial England: The Cases of Bristol, 1790-1850 and Bath, 1750-1820', (unpublished PhD thesis, University of London, 1984), 79-98. James Graham was supported in his case for simple, as against Bath, water, by Philip Thicknesse. Thicknesse described Graham as a 'Great Empiric' who 'carried the art of healing to great heights'. Graham's attack on medical vested interest was an implicit criticism of the place of the hospital in the control of access to the waters.

15. The Smith 'Memoirs' (note 7) contain considerable deposits of Estlin material; see vol. VII, especially pp. 316-577.

16. The need to 'target' the poorer areas of Bristol for missionary purposes had already been displayed by Christian evangelicism in the 1810s and 1820s; on this see M.R. Neve, 'Science in a Commercial City: Bristol 1820-1860', in 1. Inkster and J.B. Morrell (eds), *Metropolis and Province* (London, Hutchinson, 1983), 179-204.

17. The lesson set to elite physicians in this matter (where Christian piety might exist alongside severe, 'physicalist' therapeutics) was that of J.C. Prichard (1786-1848), but the hitherto unrecognised presence of Parisian anatomical method featured elsewhere in medical discussion; see A. Desmond and M.R. Neve, 'The Civic Function of Science: Bristol in the 1830s', unpublished. On the strangely under-examined medical dining club, see G. Munro Smith (note 6), 223-46.

18. T. Beddoes, letter to C.B. Trye, 1785, held at Gloucestershire Record Office (D 303 C1/61). Mrs Dorothy Stansfield makes admirable use of this (regrettably brief) correspondence in her biography of Beddoes. *Thomas Beddoes, M.D., 1760-1808* (Dordrecht, Holland, Reidel, 1984), 23-8.

19. C. Webster, 'The Historiography of Medicine', in P. Corsi and P. Weindling (eds), *Information Sources in the History of Science and Medicine* (London, Butterworth, 1983), 32.

20. T. Beddoes, *A Letter to Sir Joseph Banks on the Causes and Removal of the Prevailing Discontents, Abuses and Imperfections in Medicine* (London, R. Phillips, 1808), 26.

21. Guenter Risse's account of the Royal Infirmary of Edinburgh, *Hospital Life in Enlightenment Scotland* (Cambridge, Cambridge University Press, 1986), gives information on Beddoes only as an activist in the student body known as the Royal Medical Society, without attending to his views on the teaching he received.

22. T. Beddoes, *Rules of the Medical Institution for the Relief of the Sick and Dropping Poor* (Bristol, J. Mills, 1804), 93.

23. On Coleridge's general position, see T.H. Levere, 'S.T. Coleridge and the Human Sciences: Anthropology, Phrenology and Mesmerism', in M.P. Hanen, M.J. Osler and R.G. Weyant (eds), *Science, Pseudoscience and Society* (Waterloo, Ontario, Wilfred Laurier University Press, 1980), 171-92.

24. Indeed, it could be historically the case that this world will never be accessible, in ordinary terms, least of all via public health historiography. On the particular bureaucratic remoteness of the Bristol example, see D. Large and F. Round, *Public Health in Mid-Victorian Bristol* (Bristol, Bristol branch of the Historical Association, 1974).

25. P.S. Brown, 'Providers of Medical Treatment in Mid-nineteenth-century Bristol', *Medical History*, 24 (1980), 297-314; idem, 'Herbalists and Medical Botanists in Mid-nineteenth-century Britain with Special Reference to Bristol', *Medical History*, 26

(1982), 405-20.

26. This extravagant claim is proposed simply because the revisionist history of quackery is in danger of losing a historical object, once it is acknowledged as a construction of the exclusionist era of early Victorian professionalisation. The 'patient's' own demands, and idiosyncratic conduct, may serve as a focus for the policing of self-medication, which was the target for orthodoxy, from Wesley onwards. Quacks played into the hands of the ultimate quack: the consumer-patient.

4 'I THINK YE BOTH QUACKS': THE CONTROVERSY BETWEEN DR THEODOR MYERSBACH AND DR JOHN COAKLEY LETTSOM

Roy Porter

Our grasp of the history of quackery[1] in England is rudimentary, and this is so for several reasons. On the whole, practitioners on the medical fringes did not leave behind them such large caches of records and papers as did leading orthodox physicians; or if they did, these were certainly not preserved with the same care, and worked up into multi-volume *Lives and Letters*. Furthermore, fringe doctors have received disproportionately less attention from medical historians, the lives of charlatans and mountebanks mainly being sketched in anecdotally, as cautionary tales or as light relief.[2] And not least, they have essentially been treated *individually*, seen as loners, eccentrics or, as with James Graham, cracked in the head. There is, of course, a certain truth in this; before the nineteenth century quacks did not tend to form schools or 'isms' and relied heavily on personal charisma. But it can be highly misleading to isolate a man from his times; and particularly if our aim is to pose the question: 'Where did quacks stand in relation to other forms of medical practice, and in the public forum?' As this issue is precisely the theme of the present volume, we must analyse the careers of the quacks in context of the complex and shifting relations between medical fringe and medical orthodoxy as a whole.

To do this properly for the whole tribe of fringe practitioners would involve scholarly labours on a scale hardly yet attempted.[3] Given that rich and full private papers, account books and the like seem to survive for hardly any quack doctors before the nineteenth century, piecing together the jigsaw of their career structures, business ventures, the swings of their finances, fame and fortunes will require the assembling and assimilating of vast numbers of fragments of information from widely dispersed sources: from patients' letters and diaries, from newspaper advertisements, from court cases, from contemporary squibs, prints, journalism and the like.[4] In the meantime, however, some small steps forward can be taken using sources which are relatively coherent and readily available. Even many highly illuminating printed materials have in fact been surprisingly little used as yet. For example, the most famous 'quack' oculist of the eighteenth century, John ('Chevalier') Taylor, actually published a three-volume autobiography. This is enormously revealing both for tracing his career profile and also (and equally importantly) for what it shows of Taylor's self-perception — his image, ambition and business acumen. Yet it has never been subjected to rigorous scrutiny.[5]

The following paper represents one such 'interim' measure. It draws on relatively easily accessible materials (mainly pamphlets and newspapers) to trace and interpret the significance of one of the more spectacular head-on collisions occurring in the eighteenth century between a quack and a scion of medical orthodoxy, the confrontation between Dr Theodor von Myersbach and Dr John Coakley Lettsom in the 1770s. For a time at least, Myersbach was a prominent practitioner (his clientele included David Garrick who assured his friend Ralph Lodge, 'I feel myself at this moment better for your recommendation of Dr Mierbach' [sic]).[6] According to public gossip, at one stage he was pulling in 'about one thousand guineas a month' in fees.[7] In view of his notoriety, it is odd that this acrimonious dispute has received so little attention. In fact, the only substantial discussion of it has treated it essentially from Lettsom's viewpoint (Lettsom is, not unreasonably, regarded as victor and hero).[8] But the dispute is also of wider interest for what it reveals of the dynamics and ideology of quack/orthodox interplay in the public arena.

I have argued elsewhere that it can be very misleading to view eighteenth-century quacks and medical regulars as black and white, polar opposites.[9] Their relations were more complex, and what they had in common was in various respects as important as what differentiated them and (polemically at least) made them antagonists. Not least, certain irregular practitioners enjoyed good relations with members of the faculty; and their services were often regarded by the public as complementing regular medicine. If this is so, then the slanging-match controversy between Myersbach and Lettsom is probably somewhat of an exception to this rule — indeed, is one of the few cases in the eighteenth century in which a quack drew not just the usual volley of exposés, satires and squibs, but incurred the public wrath of one of the faculty's big fish. How, then, was this slanging-match conducted between the protagonists? And how was it received by that late Georgian public which (it has been claimed) was rather knowledgeable about medicine?[10] I shall reconstruct the controversy in order to tease out these issues.

Dr Myersbach — his doctorate was purchased from Erfurt — first achieved prominence in London in the mid-1770s, where he set up as a practitioner specialising in the technique of uroscopy. What information we have about his earlier career comes only through his opponents. According to hostile pamphlet and newspaper reports, he had started life as a lowly post office clerk in Germany, then had emigrated to Amsterdam, and, not succeeding there, had moved on to London.[11] There he had contemplated making his way in the world as a rider at Angelo's equestrian circus, but was judged too short of stature. Lacking a source of income, and utterly ignorant medically, he finally received some coaching in the palaver of urine-casting. Pro-Myersbach sources never denied the truth of this story. Rather, they countered it indirectly by arguing: so what? The notion that a man's humble background should disqualify him from exercising medical skills was a typical elitist argument of the faculty.[12] This suggests that the potted life story above cannot have been far from the truth.

Urine-casting had been a regular and respectable diagnostic procedure from antiquity through the Middle Ages and beyond; indeed, the man gazing at the urine flask became a stock image of the doctor in paintings and prose alike. Scrutinising urine made good sense within humoral medicine, which stressed how the body's fluids above all were crucial to health, and which relied heavily upon evaluations for diagnostic specimens.

Yet during the sixteenth and seventeenth centuries urine-casting gradually fell under a cloud. The belief that urine provided the key signature of disease was increasingly attacked as irrational and magical, and exclusive reliance upon urine-gazing for diagnostic purposes became the hallmark of a sub-species of 'empirics', mainly men without regular medical training, or, worse still, even women. Thus the craft of uroscopy underwent a decline, though it seems that certain of these 'pisse prophets' continued to make a living in more remote parts of the country right through the eighteenth century (though little is yet known about their survival).[13]

Anecdotal evidence suggests that popular faith in urine-casting outlived the approval of the faculty. For example, the story is told of Dr John Radcliffe that a cobbler's wife brought him some of her husband's urine for Radcliffe to diagnose his ailments. The exasperated Radcliffe responded in kind by offering her a sample of his own urine, so that her husband could make him a pair of shoes. Certainly all the indications are that when Myersbach set up in London he found no shortage of customers who had faith in the ancient art.

He quickly built up a practice distinguished both for quality and quantity. As well as David Garrick, already mentioned, his fashionable clients included the Duke and Duchess of Richmond, Lord Archer, Lord

Hawke, and Lady Harrington.[14] Certainly his detractors implied that he built up a substantial following of hypochondriacal High Society ladies ('Lady Hysteric, Lady Credulous, Lady Innoffensive [sic], Lady Widow-Weed, the Hon. Miss Pregnant and many others').[15] And his testimonials came from members of the propertied and professional classes, and included bankers, goldsmiths, attorneys, clergymen, and army and naval officers. He kept a 'spacious house' and premises in Berwick Street, Soho — then still quite a smart area — and his fees seem to indicate an affluent clientele, for he charged half a guinea for a consultation and several shillings more for medicines. Of course, if, as Lettsom alleged, Myersbach actually saw 'two hundred votaries a day',[16] he must also have had a high percentage of lower-class customers for whom most likely his charges were correspondingly lower.

Why did the sick go to Myersbach? Presumably many of the sick poor did so simply because he was cheap and available. But what of his more respectable and educated clientele? Did they have a positive faith in uroscopy itself? That is possible. But it seems much more likely (as is in effect admitted in the pro-Myersbach pamphlets) that the better class of customer typically visited Myersbach as a last resort after their regular doctors had failed to achieve cure or relief, or, as one pamphlet put it, 'on the brink of the grave [when] all hope is gone'.[17] This was certainly the case with David Garrick, who had suffered excruciating pain with gout and with kidney disorders for many years. Pro-Myersbach pamphlets make much of the claim that where regulars had failed, the water-doctor had eased pain and sped recovery, just as they explain that the reason why various of his patients had died was precisely because they had failed to consult him till they were at death's door. The drugs Myersbach dispensed may also help account for his popularity. One of these was a brandy and opium cocktail, which must have been agreeable in the short term for its pain-deadening and intoxicating qualities.

How precisely did Myersbach perform? Clients would either attend in person, bringing with them a flask of urine, or, if they were too ill to move, a urine sample would be brought on their behalf by a servant or relative. Myersbach would scrutinise their water, and claim that on the basis of that inspection only, and without questioning or other forms of examination, he could divine the essential events of their life (e.g. in the case of women, whether they'd had many children), discern the site, nature and severity of their disorder, and judge what treatment was indicated.[18] It was one of Myersbach's party pieces that, in the case of clients not attending in person, he laid claims to powers of judging from their urine their sex, age and life story.

Detractors of course regarded him as a rank fraud, and denounced his diagnostic procedures as a mixture of balderdash and trickery.[19] Myersbach could deceive his patients with the illusion of preternatural prophetic powers (enemies alleged), because his servants and porters were expert in the art of getting into casual conversation with sufferers while they were waiting in the anterooms: patients would prattle on about the details of their condition, and that information would speedily be conveyed to Myersbach himself in time for the consultation. In the case of socially eminent clients, who would make advance appointments, the delay would allow plenty of opportunity to Myersbach's servants to gather information through discreet local enquiries.

To disclose the knavery of this urine-gazing, Myersbach's detractors sent along their friends as stool-pigeons, carrying with them flasks of cows' urine which they then pretended belonged to their wife, and allowed the doctor to dig his own grave by his absurd prognoses. One such exposé of Myersbach's boloney appeared in the *Gazetteer* newspaper for 26 August 1776:[20]

> Being thus introduced, I stepped forward and presented the sagacious Doctor with my vial, which contained no other than the urine of a young gelding. He looked at it with much seeming attention, and turning round, enquired whose water it was. Instead of giving him a direct answer to the question, I told him I came from my wife: this response, which by no means would have been deemed satisfactory to a cautious physician, well satisfied this water-doctor, who, very significantly shaking his head, and drawing up his shoulders, cried, with a kind of transport at his intuitive knowledge, Oh! I did tink it was a Lady's water — it be no good — she be very bad — Upon which the following conversation and particulars ensued.
> *Patient* What do you think is her complaint, Doctor?
> *Doctor* It be, Sir, — it be a disorder in her womb — her womb — her — her womb be somewhat affected — she have a pain across her loins — she be very bad — I do see she be very bad.
> *Patient* The water seems very clear, Doctor, doesn't it?
> *Doctor* Ah! Ah! It look so to you: but I do see — I do see a slime upon the kidneys she be very sick at the stomach — she have a pain in her head, and in her limbs. — Has she had many children?
> *Patient* Two, Doctor.
> *Doctor* Her pains in labour be very bad — be they not?
> *Patient* Why, Doctor, I think all women say labour-pains be very

bad: I cannot speak from experience.
Doctor No! No! No — your wife's temper be much affected by her disorder — it make her very peevish — very fretful — passionate — every little ting — (here he paused, and gazed once more on the gelding's urine, and turning round, cried) every little ting, I see, puts her in a passion — Does it not?
Patient Why, Doctor, she is as most women are, not always in the best humour.
Doctor Ah! Ah! There you do see — I did say so; she has had this complaint — yes, she has had this complaint these three years — I do perceive dat — and she always be coughing.

This last piece of presumption, in attempting to ascertain the precise time in which he supposed my wife to have been seized with these several chimerical disorders operated too powerfully on my passions to admit my remaining any longer the auditor of such ridiculous conjectures: and therefore requested him (in order to maintain the deception) to give me a prescription, which he did. I then gave him half a guinea; for which he returned me a most servile, unmeaning cringe, with a *God Almighty, he grant I may do your wife good, namely, the gelding.*

As well as urine-casting Myersbach had a further diagnostic technique. He professed to gauge the site and type of disorder by allowing his hands to hover quivering over the patient's body, moving them around until, experiencing the right rapport, he would cry, in his broken English: 'It is here, it is here.' Doubtless, many patients were impressed by what seemed like magical insight. But his opponents exposed it as just another of his tricks. By running his hands fast enough over a sufficient expanse of the body, and by keeping up a non-stop patter interlarded with 'It is here, it is here,' he would sooner or later discern the painful part, befuddling the dazed client into believing that he'd hit upon the spot through arcane skills.

Myersbach's opponents further claimed another mark of both his medical ignorance and his charlatanry — that his diagnoses were all words and no sense, involving a specious farrago of pseudo-technical jargon. Female patients would be told they had a 'disorder of the womb' — a diagnosis so vague as to have a fair chance of ringing true; and 'sick in the stomach', 'slime in the blood' or 'slime in the kidneys' were further instances of his diagnostic mumbo-jumbo.

Having made his diagnosis, Myersbach then wrote out a prescription which was made up by his own apothecary. When he embarked upon investigating the activities of the 'Urinarian', John Coakley Lettsom began to collect his prescriptions, to ascertain whether he was indeed — as Lettsom suspected — poisoning his patients. Lettsom discovered that Myersbach's 'green drops', 'sweet mixture', 'silver pills', 'red powder' and so forth kept fairly close to the official *pharmacopoeias*, but were dispensed randomly and recklessly. Many of the preparations were innocuous anodynes (such as water in which toasted bread had been steeped), but others were potent and potentially harmful, some containing heavy concentrations of opium and others solutions of sugar of lead (lead acetate), both of which produce a temporarily beneficial effect on a patient by quelling internal pains, but which would only compound intestinal disorders if taken repeatedly.[21]

Indeed, it was through the effects of such drugs that Myersbach first attracted hostile attention. After having been permitted to practise for two or three years in peace, without any action from the Royal College of Physicians, Myersbach fell under Lettsom's gaze when the latter found patients coming to him with iatrogenic disorders which a little detective work enabled him to trace to the medicines prescribed by Myersbach. Always a passionate polemicist in the cause of righteousness, Lettsom privately investigated Myersbach's activities, by taking testimony from his patients and by planting friends as clients of the water-doctor; and on the basis of what he discovered, he launched into print with a public denunciation in a 42-page pamphlet entitled *Observations Preparatory to the Use of Dr Myersbach's Medicines, in which the Efficacy of Certain German Prescriptions . . . is Ascertained by Facts and by Experience.*[22] This appeared in two editions in 1776, the first anonymous (though it was apparently public knowledge that Lettsom was the author), the second acknowledged. Moreover, through much of 1776 he also sent volleys of letters and insertions to the London newspapers, in particular the *Gazetteer*, the *Morning Chronicle* and the *Public Ledger*, exposing the quack.[23]

Lettsom's attack received support from other quarters. Two other pamphlets were published in the same year. One — *An Essay on the Inspection of the Urine; Shewing the Impossibility of Being Acquainted with the Diseases Incident to the Human Body, by the Inspection Only*, published under the heading 'By a Physician' — was fairly brief and content mainly to ridicule urine-casting as an almost worthless diagnostic test. The other — *The New Method of Curing Diseases by Inspecting the Urine Explained: as Practiced by the German Doctor. Intended for the Serious Perusal of Physicians, Surgeons, Apothecaries, and the Public in General* — was a more substantial work, exposing Myersbach for a fraud.

Unsurprisingly, Myersbach hit back, not (it seems) in his own person — it was said his English was too shaky — but presumably by hiring one or more hack controversialists. Counter-volleys of articles appeared in the newspapers, taking Myersbach's part, signed with such pseudonyms as 'London Spy' and 'Sally Sly', and two quite extensive pamphlets came out in his defence: one the 44-page *An Answer to a Pamphlet Written by Dr. Lettsom, Entitled 'Observations', Preparatory to the Use of Dr. Myersbach's Medicines*; the other, running to over 100 pages, *The Impostor Detected or the Physician the Greater Cheat: Being a Candid Enquiry Concerning the Practice of Dr. Myersbach: Commonly Known by the Title of the German Doctor. Containing a Faithful Account of Many Remarkable Cures Performed by Him which Have Been Deemed Incurable, and Therefore Declined by Physicians of Eminence. Being a Full Refutation of the Sophisticated Arguments, and Invidious Reflections of Dr. Lettsom and Others. And Shewing his Practice to be Defensible upon Natural and Philosophical Principles*.

Nor did the controversy, once it got into full swing, remain restricted to the antagonists and their immediate champions. Newspaper insertions proliferated through 1776 and into 1777 from readers who were, or who at least professed to be, impartial bystanders, signing themselves with such pseudonyms as 'Amicus' and 'Veritas'. Thus the affair ceased to be simply the defeat and demise of an arrant quack, as Lettsom had hoped, and turned into a general debate, in which larger issues were at stake, not least the whole question of medical authority, and the relative standings of the profession and the public in authorising medical procedures. Lettsom had bitten off more than he had bargained for, by opening up questions of the social sanctioning of medical knowledge which threatened to leave him almost as vulnerable as the 'Urinarian'.

One reason for this lay in Lettsom's own rather ambiguous position *vis-à-vis* medical orthodoxy. He made no bones about invoking the full authority of regular medicine to denounce Myersbach, plastering his credentials as a Fellow of the Royal Society and as a member of the College of Physicians on his title page. Yet was Lettsom's own stance really so clear? He was, after all, a Quaker, denied access to Oxford or Cambridge and therefore regular access to the Fellowship of the Royal College of Physicians. An outspoken opponent of professional exclusiveness and closed corporations in his own professional life, Lettsom was the leading light in the Medical Society of London, which he had helped found as an alternative, more liberal association of medical men than the College of Physicians.[24] In the controversy, Lettsom was thus himself left in danger of being caught in the crossfire; through using the authority of medicine to destroy the quack, he was easily and frequently accused of being an arch-defender of those very forms of oligarchy and monopoly which he himself deplored.

I shall not rehearse here in detail the wearisome war of words which unfolded in the press in 1776 and early 1777 — it ran to well over 100 newspaper insertions, most of them repetitive and vituperative. The substance of the case made by Lettsom and his friends has already been outlined: Myersbach was medically ignorant and incompetent, an adventurer, a fraud and, above all, a danger to life and health. Lettsom had some special trump cards up his sleeve, as when Myersbach's apothecary's assistant, Haussman, defected and testified to Lettsom that Myersbach knew nothing of medicine and was a total swindler. But basically, Lettsom spelt out at length, in his pamphlet and in the press, horror stories of patients whose health had been ruined by Myersbach's vile ministrations, e.g. this account in the *Gazetteer*:[25]

JANE REILY, of St. Mary at Hill, applied to Dr. Myersbach, with a vial of urine, on the 21st of May 1776, and was told by him that she had a disorder in the womb. At that time she laboured under a dysentery, which induced her to ask him, if her purging arose from the disorder in the womb? The Doctor avoided answering this question, by saying, that he could soon cure her; and gave her the silver pills. In a fortnight afterwards, the patient again applied, and told the Doctor that the purging was augmented, and her strength and constitution were greatly impaired; he assured her, however, she was getting better: and added, that he now perceived by her urine, that there were little kernels in the womb which he would soon remove. He then gave her the green drops, the red powder, and the sweet drops; but after attending three months, the kernels which Doctor Myersbach discovered in the womb were not removed, and her real disorder, which was a dysentery, continued, with additional violence, when I saw her on the 25th of September.

Time and again, Lettsom drew two main conclusions. The first was that such episodes proved the evils of medical 'empiricism'; indeed, as he put it, 'the history of empiricism affords no parallel of deception so general as that which actuated the votaries of this imposter for upwards of two years'. It was impossible to tell, he added, just how many patients had been 'murdered by empiricks'.[26] The only protection for the public was to put themselves solely in the hands of regular physicians, those who had been through an authorised education and training and who, by possessing due knowledge of anatomy and the animal economy, could make rational diagnoses.

This was especially important on account of his second *bête noire*, the total gullibility of the English people. 'It has been an observation', he informed readers of the *Gazetteer*, 'no less true than common, that the English are the greatest dupes of novelty and deception under the sun'; however gross the charlatanry, 'no people will swallow the bait with less reluctance than the English,' who were in medical matters a 'weak people', beset by 'national folly and credulity', and currently suffering from the contagion of 'Urinomania'.[27] Lettsom's supporters underlined this same point. The author of *The New Method of Curing Disease* spelt it out as follows:[28]

> To explain this matter more clearly and satisfactorily; to investigate the cause of such absolute folly and madness in the people, is not difficult. Let us recollect the South Sea scheme and bottle conjurer, Elizabeth Canning's story, the Cock-lane ghost, and the knavish trick of Le Fevre, the reputed Doctor, for curing the gout, and many other such like impositions; not to mention the two lotteries, for the disposal of houses and trinkets, which received parliamentary sanction; and for which the fortunate holders of prizes of five hundred pounds were offered by the *honest* projectors about sixty. Here are indisputable proofs, that not only the illiterate caught the alluring baits of designing artists; but the polite and well educated had implicit faith in doubtful schemes, or the most improbable fables.

But were these the right tactics to use in an appeal to the public? It must be doubted. Lettsom seemed to be following three contradictory strategies all at once. First, he was arguing the supreme authority of the regular medical profession; second, by laying his case before the public, he was also inviting them to judge and vindicate that authority; but then, third, he was telling the public what fools they were. The paradoxes in this position were, not surprisingly, exploited to the full both by Myersbach's defenders and (so far as one can tell) by neutral bystanders without an axe to grind.

It could be nothing but obfuscating (claimed Myersbach's vindicators) to attack the German doctor for his lack of regular medical training, degrees and membership of learned societies. For that created a fetish of forms, and made possession of skills in dead tongues such as Latin and Greek into a form of medical magic. Neatly reversing the standard anti-quack thrust (which denounced quacks for being all words and no skills), the author of *The Impostor Detected* declared the boot was on the other foot:[29] it was 'tools of the faculty' such as Lettsom who out of self-interest were equating medical skills with magical words. Myersbach's merit, the pamphleteer claimed,[30]

> depends upon the knowledge of nature, and of things, and not of words; . . . To think otherwise, is to suppose every physician must be a magician; seeing medicines are incapable of healing, unless accompanied with the knowledge of the import of certain sounds, or the signification of words of certain languages, to which they have no relation, but what is given them by the arbitrary appointment of man.

Yet such recourse to the authority of arcane and exclusive knowledge was, of course, to be expected from physicians who paraded their membership of closed societies such as the Royal Society and the College of Physicians,[31] groups whose interest lay in setting the 'false dignity of the faculty', the 'low arts of a craft' and the 'private police of a corporation' above those real objects of true medicine, 'the life and health of the human species'. Thus (it was alleged) Lettsom was exposing his own false colours, for 'the true dignity of the profession can never be supported by means that are irreconcileable with its true objects'.[32]

Of course, medical mystagogy needs to be exposed, argued *The Impostor Detected*; but who was the true mystery-monger here? It was Lettsom who hid behind the name of the faculty:[33]

> An affectation of mystery in their writings, conversations, and whole demeanor; a shew of deep erudition and profound knowledge relating to their profession, discoverable to none but the adepts in the science, an air of absolute confidence in their own skill and abilities; and a deportment stately, solemn, and superlatively expressive of self-importance are among the arts they practice.

The faculty might thereby hope (argued the controversialist) to 'captivate the ignorant', but the great British public would not be taken in by this mummery.[34]

Thus paper qualifications were at best a side-issue, at worst yet another form of professional mystification.[35] Medicine's acid test (argued Myersbach's supporters) was: Does it work? Which practitioners actually have the best track record? In other words, they claimed, empiricism, far from being the threat to medical standards which Lettsom made it out to be, was in reality the heart of the matter. Elite physicians (alleged *The Impostor Detected*) had wrapped and trapped themselves in systems and hypotheses, but these had proved a hindrance to healing:[36]

> The greatest obstacle to the improvement of the medical art, has been an inattention to its principal end and design, which is the convenience and happiness of life; to preserve health, to prolong life, and to cure diseases. But this most valuable object has been sacrificed to vanity and ostentation, and the acquisition of a fortune by craft, artifice, and mean adulation.

Facts must take priority over theories, and the true empiric was the practitioner who put his trust not in system-building, but in that crucial technique of the advancement of learning — the experiment. As the pamphleteer phrased it.[37]

> An attachment to novelty, however, is productive of some good, to systems and hypotheses none; the first from experiments communicates some real truths to the stock; the latter, are unproductive of any real knowledge.

Thus the question the public must ask (argued Myersbach's defenders) was this: On whose side were the facts? Lettsom published his own case studies of patients sent to the grave by the 'Urinarian's' treatments. Myersbach's minions responded by defending him in the same coin:[38]

> To suppose that Dr. Mayersbach is infallible would be to run into the contrary extreme and render one as deservedly ridiculous as Dr. Lettsom. His knowledge, as a physician (in the technical sense of the word) may be as slender as some of his enemies; but from many of the cases following, it is undeniably certain, that he has cured many which the faculty could not cure, and to deny it is to belye and affront the common sense of mankind. Here then is clear irrefragable proof that he has (in some cases at least) more skill, or nostrums, of greater medicinal virtues than they have any knowledge of.

And if the issue was thus a matter of facts, and the public was to judge, then Myersbach could present a clutch of testimonials from satisfied customers to match Lettsom's disaster stories.[39] *The Impostor Detected* paraded an impressive roster of happy clients and their cases:[40]

A list of persons who have received benefit from Dr. MAYERBACH'S [sic] advice and medicines, either in their own persons, families, or friends. The particular case referred to is denoted by the figure following the name.

JOHN Willan, Esq; Mary-le Bon, Case 1.
Thomas Limbery Sclater, Esq; Tangier park, Hants, 2.
Robert Johnson, Esq; Bath.
Mr. Pybus, Banker, in New Bond Street.
Mr. Parker, Glass Manufacturer, Fleet Street, 5.
Mr. Stephenson, Goldsmith, Ludgate Hill, 11.
Mr. Wolfe, his acquaintance.
Mr. Chinnery, Writing Master, Gough Square.

And not only did the pamphleteer chronicle these and eleven other cases, but some of these patients then also wrote (presumably of their own volition) to the newspapers testifying to Myersbach's skill and integrity, as witness this letter from John Willan which appeared in the *Gazetteer*:[41]

For the GAZETTEER
To Dr. COAKLEY LETTSOM.

WHEN I first entered upon a vindication of Dr. Mayersbach's character, which I saw wantonly and grossly attacked, by the pen of self-interested ill nature, I had not the most distant thought of a personal altercation with you; but the shameful abuse, and glaring untruths you daily advance against the object of your envy, call aloud for the pen of truth to stand forth in the vindication of injured innocence.

Where Dr. Mayerbach acquired his knowledge I will not pretend to determine; I have however the greatest right to say that he knows more than many of the most skilful of the faculty for he saved my life when they could not; and I might justly be thought the most ungrateful of wretches, if I should refuse to declare to the world that I owe my being entirely to his judgment as a physician; as a man I see him *traduced, vilified and belied*: excuse the expression, you call for it and you have it.

I every day read the most glaring falsehoods attested by your name: I therefore have a right to call you by the worst appellation which the promoter of untruths deserves.

Your asserting, that Dr. Mayersbach made use of the preparation of lead in his prescriptions, is publicly confuted by the affidavits of the Doctor and Mr. Koch, before the Lord Mayor, which were inserted in the Gazetteer of Monday last.

In the same paper you advance the most *impudent* and *barefaced falsehood* I ever met with.

You there assure the public, that 'Lady H. sent a message last Tuesday to the Urinarian, desiring him never more to enter into her Ladyship's house.' Now I assure the public and pledge myself for the truth of what I say, that it is a palpable and direct falsehood, which I have it in my power to prove in one moment, to any one who has credulity enough to put the least confidence in Dr. Lettsom's infamous assertions, and chuse to have those erroneous opinions removed by self-evident convictions.

A pamphlet which makes its appearance this day, will, I doubt not, afford the world sufficient proof of Dr Mayerbach's knowledge as a physician, and of the shameful intention of the prostituted pen of Dr. Lettsom.

Maryle-bone, Oct. 17. JOHN WILLEN.

Both Lettsom and Myersbach thus presented themselves to the public as champions of the public good. But whom was a reader of the public press to credit? With hindsight, we can feel pretty sure that Myersbach was a cheat, and no one doubts that Lettsom was a physician of the highest probity. But would a reader have discerned this? It is not clear that Lettsom actually got the better of the argument. For one thing (as was pointed out in the *Gazetteer*) the whole controversy was simply affording Myersbach a mass of free publicity: 'Doctor L. and the whole College may write against him, they'll only expand his fame, together with their own ignorance.'[42] For another, the rather unsavoury vituperations led to questions being raised about Lettsom's own motives and conduct. If he really had the public interest at heart, why didn't he activate the College of Physicians' machinery for examining unlicensed practitioners? That would have been the course of public justice, and, if Myersbach had been found guilty, his punishment would have afforded real protection to the public. Wasn't Lettsom's newspaper campaign, then, essentially a piece of self-advertisement and a mode of attack on a rival practitioner which lacked candour? This point was well put by 'Amicus' in the *Gazetteer*:[43]

To Dr. LETSOM.

In perusing the daily papers I have often observed the animadversions on Myersbach's practice and impositions on the public; and without being an advocate for this outlandish water-conjurer, to give him no harder epithet, I would just hint, that if he is in truth deserving public censure, (which he very probably may be) would it not be more effectual, and withal be more convincing to the world, that Dr. Letsom possesses a pure generosity, and liberality of sentiments, if he were to bring a fair open accusation for mal-practice before the Censors of the College of Physicians, who solely, in their judicial capacity (when an accusation is brought before them, and not before) are by law appointed the competent judges of the practice of physic in London and seven miles around, with full power to fine, imprison, and coerce all detected unwarrantable practice, than to let the Gazetteer be the weekly channel of vague accusations against this (as Dr. Letsom terms him) water-caster.

This would be a convincing proof that Dr. Letsom was not aiming to build up his own fame upon the ruins of a more favoured opponent, but that the public welfare and safety were his aim and greatest ambition.

Oct. 15.
I am with respect,
AMICUS.

Above all, the controversy brought to light the core contradiction in Lettsom's argument. If he chose to make a public appeal, the public had a right to decide for themselves; and here authority must make way for fact. As the 'London Spy' put it:[44]

Will Doctor L. and his colleagues have the effrontery to attempt to disprove matters of fact by argument, and to insist the old gentleman who was thus surprisingly restored to health and seeming rejuvenescency, had, in fact, received no benefit at all, but was imposed upon by a 'plausible tale, and an application they call suitable,' which is destitute of all sense and meaning?
Aug. 29.
The LONDON SPY

Or as another correspondent — possibly a bewildered, disinterested bystander — summed up the dilemma:[45]

To the PRINTER of the GAZETTEER
I have perused two late publications, the one by Dr. Lettsom, and the other is an answer to it.
Dr. Lettsom asserts, and quotes the opinion of Dr. Heberden and others, that it is exceedingly difficult to judge diseases, by urine . . .
He next states, though mostly in initials, several cases where

Dr. Mayersbach gave a very erroneous account of disorders, and therefore insists on it that Dr. Mayersbach is ignorant of what he pretends. As I intend impartially to survey these publications, I shall take it for granted what he has asserted, and the cases he has stated to be strictly true.

Dr. Lettsom's antagonist, to controvert the above, has published cases *authenticated* by the person's own names, that Dr. Mayersbach in their several disorders judged perfectly right by urine, though different from what the opinion of their former physicians had been. If I admit what Dr. Lettsom says to be true, must not I do the same here? What then is an impartial man to conclude? Facts are superior to opinion. Those well-authenticated cases clearly prove Dr. Mayersbach's skill in finding out disorders by urine, and Dr. Lettsom's, that in those cases he was mistaken; *errare humanum est*; saying himself a great part of this city crouded to have Dr. Mayersbach's advice, can it be otherwise but what he must be sometimes out? Do not then Dr. Lettsom's own assertions prove Dr. Mayersbach a regular-bred physician, a great anatomist, and a very skilful man?

All mankind take medicines against inclination; pay physicians fees and apothecaries bills with reluctance. Whatever stress Dr. Lettsom lays upon the effect of tales once propagated, was not Dr. Mayersbach obliged to deceive every patient separately?

He therefore must be of opinion that, contrary to their inclinations, Dr. Mayersbach had that art to deceive a great part of one of the greatest cities of the world. If my first conclusion be wrong, this must be right.

Haussman's evidence is inadmissible: revenge occasions duels, and often murder.

Oct. 30, 1776   J.S.

The paper war raged unabated for several months. In fact, it seems to have ended only when the editor of the *Gazetteer* declined to print any further contributions by Myersbach's leading defender (the 'London Spy') on account of his anonymity. This decision wears a certain arbitrary appearance — after all, many other insertions had been anonymous or pseudonymous, and for a long time Lettsom himself had used the pseudonym 'Cassius'. The author of *The Impostor Detected* hinted that pressure had been put on the editor by Lettsom's cronies.[46]

But the controversy didn't end before it had got out of the hands of the initial antagonists. For a kind of secondary debate sprang up, in which both parties fell under the lash of those who deplored how the whole debate was simply discrediting medicine in general. Thus the *Public Ledger* for 30 September 1776 ran a long poem by 'Galen', whose main theme was 'I think ye both quacks.' It consisted of a wrangle between Myersbach and Lettsom, the last section of which ran:[47]

> Dr. L. and Dr. M. talking confusedly
>   together,
> Pray, who are my betters? Why I am — yes,
>   I Sir,
> You *mistake* in good French, but in English
>   you lie, Sir,
> I appeal to this friend, I submit to another
> Why thou Talk'st like a fool, neither one
>   thing nor t'other.
> I will and I won't, and you can't and you
>   dare not,
> Either this Judge or that Judge, by heav'n
>   I care not:
> He'll pronounce thee an ass, my good
>   friend, never fear it,
> If he proves you a fool, I'll be happy to
>   hear it.
>   Friend says,
>   Gentlemen,
> At a club once established, for drinking and
>   dining,
> Two amazing great wits were determined on
>   shining
> They contended, who most like a
>   blackguard could quarrel,
> Who scolded the best was to bear off the
>   laurel.
> They curs'd and talk'd bawdry, and shouted
>   and thunder'd
> And so equal their parts, the spectators all
>   wonder'd.
> And the umpire himself, who was fix'd on to
>   hear'em.

> Vow'd no Billingsgate whores, Sirs, could
>   ever come near'em.
> With one it was art, with the other 'twas
>   nature,
> But that both were such blackguards, he never
>   saw greater.
> Now permit me to say, that it's hard to
>   determine
> In a case that concerns, Sirs, such physical
>   vermin:
> But I think ye both quacks, who prescribe
>   in the dark, Sirs,
> By trusting to p—s p—s, and opium, and bark,
>   Sirs.
>
> GALEN

'Galen' was then answered by 'Hippocrates' in the *Morning Chronicle* (9 October 1776), who, in a rather similar way, suggested that Lettsom and Myersbach appeared for all the world like Tweedledum and Tweedledee:[48]

> For a man and a frog,
>   Are two *chips* of one *log*,
> That equally merit the saying;
>   Dr. M. is a *block*,
>   Of some Jesuit's *flock*,
> But poor Dr. L. is a *shaving*.
>   Dr. M. Doctor L.
>   Sirs I wish ye both well
> I protest I have spleen against neither,
>   But whenever I'm sick
>   May I go to old Nick
> If I take a prescription from either.
>   I beg yet to mark
>   that both *opium* and *bark*,
> Ask for genius and skill to employ 'em.
>   That *p—s p—s* will cure
>   Neither rich man nor poor,
> Then Doctors why should you *destroy 'em*.
>
> HIPPOCRATES.

What is particularly remarkable is that even Lettsom's colleagues seem to have recognised that his attacks were damaging both the case against Myersbach and also the standing of regular medicine. The dignified Dr John Fothergill, who had earlier lent his support to Lettsom, even went so far as to publish an anonymous letter early in 1777 whose message was effectively 'a plague on both your houses'. In the context of the national war against the rebel American colonies, he called for an end to the infantile mud-slinging:[49]

> To the PRINTER of the GAZETTEER
> At a time when the fate of this great empire is depending, and a contest of such a magnitude as the world never saw is undecided, . . . It shocks me to think that a nation can be interesting itself about trifles, while their all is at stake, and that either public diversions or private quarrels, should fill up, as they do, the channels of public information.
> Let the two lawyers contend in Westminster-hall as long as they please. Let Mayersbach endeavour, like the scuttlefish, to hide himself in ink, and raise an army of credulous hypochondriacs in his defence; but do not let the public be pestered with such uninteresting combats. If Mayersbach has any thing to say against Dr. Lettsom let them fight in Warwick-lane.

How should this affair be viewed? In the short run it seems as if it proved a victory for Lettsom, for under the glare of publicity Myersbach upped stumps and returned to Germany. Nevertheless, according to Lettsom's biographer, 'the man returned, however, after a year, and so little had the exposure damaged him, and so short was the memory of the public, that he soon regained all his old popularity'. Lettsom himself confirms this. Writing thirty years later, he stated:[50]

> in less than twelve months he [Myersbach] returned and was again as much followed as previously to his emigration. The physician who had taken so active a part against the enterprise was dissatisfied with the conduct of the College; he was likewise insulted by a numerous herd of anonymous writers in the public prints; and having become an object of their envy, he avoided further interference.

Moreover, later in his career, Lettsom was to rediscover that vituperation in the public press was a highly dubious technique for hounding quacks. In 1804 Lettsom launched a series of anti-quack exposés in the *Medical and Physical Journal*. The third of these pilloried Myersbach, who was by then dead.[51] The fifth hurled a stream of abuse against the empiric Dr William Brodum, author of *A Guide to Old Age or a Cure for the Indiscretions of Youth*, and vendor of a Nervous Cordial. Lettsom dubbed Brodum an itinerant orange-seller, a renegade Jew, a footman, a mountebank, and alleged that he had tricked Marischal College, Aberdeen, into giving him his MD. Brodum sued the magazine, and the upshot of much backstairs legal negotiation was that Lettsom was forced to issue a public recantation — which effectively served as a puff for Brodum and his Nervous Cordial — and to pay costs.

But the wider significance of the war of words is worth reflecting upon, for what it tells us of the shifting standing of regular and quack medicine in the Georgian age. Unlike in the late Stuart period, by the 1770s the state and the law were supine in the face of quackery; the Royal College did nothing. Hence a ferret of quacks like Lettsom had to appeal to the public, using the press to drum the quack out of business. But could Lettsom simultaneously invoke the authority of the regular profession while also appealing to the public as judge and jury? There was no way out of that paradox: if a public appeal was to be made to pass judgement on Myersbach, Lettsom's own credentials would also come under public scrutiny.

If the public could be in a position to judge, it would judge by results, and so some form of empiricism must necessarily be ratified. The open world of late Georgian medicine was not yet a comfortable place for the regulars in their attempts to crack down on quacks and assert professional authority.

Notes

1. Throughout this paper I shall use the term 'quack' simply to refer to those practitioners who were commonly called quacks in their own time. My use implies no automatic judgement about their skill (or lack of it) or their morals (or lack of them). To avoid confusion, however, I shall state now that in my opinion Dr Myersbach was a fraud and was medically incompetent.

2. See for example E. Jameson, *The Natural History of Quackery* (London, Michael Joseph, 1971); B. Hill, 'Medical Imposters', *History of Medicine*, 2 (1960), 7-11; L. Harris and L. Knowles, 'The Golden Days of Dr Quack', *History of Medicine*, 6 (1975), 76-81; H. Burger, 'The Doctor, the Quack and the Appetite of the Public for Magic in Medicine', *Proceedings of the Royal Society of Medicine*, 27 (1933), 171-6.

3. A good start is made by R. Hambridge, 'Empiricomany, or an Infatuation in Favour of *Empiricism* or *Quackery*. The Socio-economics of Eighteenth Century Quackery', in S. Soupel and R. Hambridge, *Literature and Science and Medicine* (Los Angeles, Clark Memorial Library, 1982), 47-102. See also J. Crellin, 'Dr James's Fever Powder', *Transactions of the British Society for the History of Pharmacy*, I (1974), 136-43;

M.H. Nicolson, 'Ward's Pill and Drop and Men of Letters', *Journal of the History of Ideas*, 29 (1968), 173-96.
   4. Useful here are J.J. Looney, 'Advertising and Society in England, 1700-1820: A Statistical Analysis of Yorkshire Newspaper Advertisements' (unpublished PhD thesis, Princeton University, 1983), and the essays in Roy Porter (ed.), *Patients and Practitioners: Lay Perceptions of Medicine in Preindustrial Society* (Cambridge, Cambridge University Press, 1985). I explore some of these issues in 'Before the Fringe', in R. Cooter (ed.), *Alternatives: Essays in the Social History of Irregular Medicine* (London, Macmillan, 1987).
   5. 'Chevalier' Taylor, *The History of the Travels and Adventures of the Chevalier John Taylor*, 3 vols (London, J. Williams, 1761-2), I, 47. Taylor styled himself on the title page of his autobiography: 'Chevalier JOHN TAYLOR. OPHTHALMIATER: Pontifical — Imperial and Royal — The Kings of Poland, Denmark, Sweden, The Electors of the Holy Empire, The Princes of Saxegotha, Mecklenberg, Anspach, Brunswick, Parme, Modena, Zerbst, Loraine, Saxony, Hesse Cassel, Holstein, Salzborg, Baviere, Leige, Bareith, Georgia, &c. pr. in Opt. C. of Rom. M.D. — C.D. — Author of 45 Works in different Languages: the Produce for upwards of thirty Years, of the greatest Practice in the Cure of distempered Eyes, of any in the Age we live — Who has been in every Court, Kingdom, Province, State, City and Town of the least Consideration in all Europe, without exception'. For a brief discussion of Taylor, see D.M. Jackson, 'Bach, Handel and the Chevalier Taylor', *Medical History*, 12 (1968), 85-93.
   6. D. Little and G. Hahrl, *The Letters of David Garrick*, 3 vols (London, Oxford University Press, 1963),III, 1090. Myersbach's name was variously spelled at the time.
   7. Lettsom himself collected the pamphlets and newspaper clippings relating to his war against Myersbach in three volumes of 'Fugitive Pieces' (London, Wellcome Institute for the History of Medicine, MS 3246, vols 1-3). This comment appears in Lettsom's hand at the beginning of I.
   8. See J.J. Abraham, *John Coakley Lettsom 1744-1815* (London, Heinemann, 1933), 187ff. For further materials see T.J. Pettigrew, *Memoirs of the Life and Writings of the Late John Coakley Lettsom*, 2 vols (London, Nicholas, Son & Bentley, 1817).
   9. See note 2.
   10. N. Jewson, 'The Disappearance of the Sick Man from Medical Cosmology 1770-1870', *Sociology*, 10 (1976), 225-44; idem, 'Medical Knowledge and the Patronage System in Eighteenth Century England', *Sociology*, 8 (1974), 369-85; Roy Porter, 'Lay Medical Knowledge in the Eighteenth Century: The Evidence of the *Gentleman's Magazine*', *Medical History*, 29 (1985), 138-68; and idem, 'Laymen, Doctors and Medical Knowledge in the Eighteenth Century: The Evidence of the *Gentleman's Magazine*', in Porter (note 4), 283-314. Note that Lettsom wrote pieces for the *Gentleman's Magazine*.
   11. '*The New Method of Curing Diseases by Inspecting the Urine Explained: as practiced by the German Doctor. Intended for the Serious Perusal of Physicians, Surgeons, Apothecaries, and the Public in General.* "Mundus vult decepi, ergo decipiatur." "If ye understand not the urine, ye know nothing." London. printed for J. Bew, No. 28 Paternoster Row. Price one shilling.' In a MS note to his copy, Lettsom states that he did not know its author. See also Lettsom's own entries in the *Public Ledger* newspaper, to be found in 'Fugitive Pieces', II 73-5.
   12. See *The Impostor Detected; or The Physician the Greater Cheat: Being a Candid Enquiry Concerning the Practice of Dr. Myersbach: Commonly Known by the Title of the German Doctor. Containing a Faithfull Account of Many Remarkable Cures Performed by Him which Have Been Deemed Incurable and Therefore Declined by Physicians of Eminence. Being a Full Refutation of the Sophisticated Arguments, and Invidious Reflections of Dr. Lettsom and Others. And Shewing his Practice to be Defensible upon Natural and Philosophical Principles*. London. Printed for J. Wilkie, No. 71 St. Pauls Churchyard. 1776. Price one shilling and sixpence.
   13. See T. Brian, *The Pisse-prophet* (Northridge, Cal., Rilker labs., 1968; reprint of first edition, London, R. Thrale, 1637); L.J.T. Murphey, 'The Art of Uroscopy',

Medical Journal of Australia, 2 (1967), 879-86; J.H. Kiefer, 'Uroscopy, the Artists' Portrayal of the Physician', *Bulletin of the New York Academy of Medicine*, 40 (1964), 759-66; 'Piss-pot Science', *Journal of Medical History*, 10 (1955), 121-3. In 'Fugitive Pieces', I, introduction, Lettsom notes that in the Yorkshire of his youth, various lay practitioners still practised the art.

14. *The Impostor Detected*, xi.

15. See *The New Method of Curing Diseases by Inspecting the Urine Examined* (London, J. Bew, ?1776), 2. One hint here is that Myersbach was also an abortionist.

16. Lettsom (note 7), III, introductory note in MS.

17. *The Imposter Detected* (note 12), 13.

18. All this was a familiar enough form of performance. Cf., on an earlier piss-prophet, [Daniel Turner], *The Modern Quack* (London, J. Roberts, 1724), 127: 'he puts on his Conjuring *Cap*, lifts up the Urinal, shakes his Head, and begins very gravely his Speech, Dis person very *bad*; Yes, indeed Doctor replies the old Woman, so *he* is: Hence he gathers it is a man's Water, and goes on; *Dis be de Man's Water, good Woman is it not*? Yes, Sir, answers the Messenger. Then very demurely looking thereon again, he runs over his commnon Catalogue us'd at all times, as thus: *Here be much Pain in de Head*, then looking wishfully in the Woman's Face, to see if she contradicts him, if she say, not much, Sir, in the Head, *then here be great pain in de Breast*: Very much indeed, Sir, replies old Nurse: *Me see here be very great Disorder in de Breast, and also in de Stomach.*'

19. *An Essay on the Inspection of the Urine: Shewing the Impossibility of Being Acquainted with the Diseases incident to the Human Body, by the Inspection Only. "Urina est meretrix et mendax."* By a Physician. London. Printed for the Author, and Sold by J. Wilkie, St. Paul's Churchyard, and may be had of all Booksellers, and News Carriers in Town and Country. 1776.

20. This is reproduced in Lettsom (note 7), II, 11.

21. Lettsom carefully preserved scores of these prescriptions in *ibid.*, III.

22. [John Coakley Lettsom], *Observations Preparatory to the Use of Dr. Myersbach's Medicines: in which the Efficacy of Certain German Prescriptions (given in English) is Ascertained by Facts. . . with Cases Tending to Shew the Possibility of Acquiring a Knowledge of Diseases by Urine*. The second edition . . . enlarged. London, E. and C. Dilly, 1776.

23. Clippings of these make up the bulk of Lettsom (note 7), II.

24. See A. Marcovich, 'Concerning the Continuity between the Image of Society and the Image of the Human Body. An Examination of the Work of the English Physician, J.C. Lettsom (1746-1815)', in P. Wright and A. Treacher (eds), *The Problem of Medical Knowledge* (Edinburgh, Edinburgh University Press, 1982), 69-86.

25. *Gazetteer*, 2 October 1776.

26. Lettsom (note 7), III, MS note at beginning. For 'murdering empirics', see *Gazetteer*, 26 August 1776.

27. The *Gazetteer*, 26 August 1776. Cf. Lettsom (note 7), II, iv.

28. *The New Method of Curing Disease* (note 15), 22.

29. See Roy Porter, 'The Language of Quackery in England 1660-1800', in Peter Burke and Roy Porter (eds), *Language and Society* (Cambridge, Cambridge University Press, 1986).

30. *The Imposter Detected* (note 12), 3.

31. Defences of Myersbach make much of the 'gilt chariots' of the faculty. Cf. The 'London Spy', in *Gazetteer*, 19 September 1776.

32. *The Impostor Detected* (note 12), 3.

33. *Ibid.*, 2.

34. *Ibid.*

35. The author of *ibid.* brought in the parallel of the bone-setter (p. 10).

36. *Ibid.*, 7.

37. *Ibid.*, 9.

38. *Ibid.*, viii.
39. The author of *ibid.* further alleged that one of the main reasons why regular physicians enjoyed a good success rate was that their patients were rarely ill in the first place (p. 92); 'Regular physicians, have few of those difficulties to encounter with. Their patients are the flower of the flock, who seek for relief before the disease has rivetted itself in the constitution, and have had its force augmented by the aid of unskilfulness. One half of the disorders they encounter are imaginary, which are best palliated by imaginary remedies, provided they are pleasing to the palate, and acceptable to the stomach. This, if not an estate in fee simple, is at least a leasehold for life, by which, with true physical economy, an estate in fee simple may be acquired. These patients seldom injure the physicians's reputation, and it is thought there are not quite ninety-nine out of a hundred, who suffer much from remorse of conscience. Why should they? it can be no crime to take lawful game; if the patient be only *imaginery* ill, the doctor would be really mad to undeceive him; seeing that would be to cheat his patient of his happiness, and himself of the choisest and best fruits of his possession. Poor Dr. Mayersbach, little of this rich game falls to thy lot.'
40. *Ibid.*, xi. See the case of Mr Willan, 13-14: 'The testimony of a very intimate and worthy friend, Mr. Willan, of Marylebone, induced him to consult Dr. Mayersbach, in behalf of a relation, and the effect of that consultation was an entire belief of his knowledge of diseases, by the inspection of the urinal.

' "On his looking at the water, without hesitation, without any previous questions having been asked, or any kind of artifice made use of, that could give him the most distant hint of the disorder, or situation of the patient, he described not only the disease, but the cause which had produced it. That the water was a lady's, that she was elderly, had a large swelling in her body: of the dropsical kind, but not in a situation to be tapped; that her chief pain was in her side, with various other symptoms, as exact, as if he had attended her through every stage of her complaint; that the case was very desperate, and that he could not say whether he could be of any service to her or not, till he had tried the effect of some medicines for a few days. He made the experiment, found it was to no purpose, and declined taking any more fees."

'His opinion and conduct on the above occasion are particularly dwelt upon, for two reasons; in the first place, to prove his knowledge of the disorder by urine, and in the next place, to acquit him of any mercenary views; for if he had had the least intention of that kind, he had nothing more to have done than to have declared the disease curable, and continued taking his fees for six weeks longer.'
41. See Lettsom (note 7), II, 69.
42. 'The 'London Spy', *Gazetteer*, 29 August 1776.
43. *Gazetteer*, 15 October 1776.
44. The 'London Spy', *Gazetteer*, 29 August 1776.
45. Lettsom (note 7), II, 102.
46. *The Impostor Detected* (note 12), 76.
47. *Public Ledger*, 30 September 1776. Cf. Lettsom (note 7), II, 29ff.
48. *Morning Chronicle*, 9 October 1776.
49. *Gazetteer*, 3 January 1777 (Lettsom (note 7), II, 139). The identification is by Lettsom.   50. Lettsom (note 7), II, introductory notes in MS; Abraham (note 8), 387, 171. The Lettsom quotation is from the *Medical and Physical Journal*, 12 (1804), 215.
51. See H. Cook, *The Decline of the Old Medical Regime in Stuart England* (Ithaca, Cornell University Press, 1986).

5 PROPERTY RIGHTS AND THE RIGHT TO HEALTH: THE REGULATION OF SECRET REMEDIES IN FRANCE, 1789-1815

Matthew Ramsey

The complexities of the relationship between fringe and orthodox medicine in the late eighteenth and early nineteenth centuries are nowhere more apparent than in the history of proprietary remedies, or *remèdes secrets*, as they were known in France. Such remedies were neither officinal (standard preparations from the *pharmacopoeia* that the apothecaries kept in stock) nor magistral (compounded according to a physician's prescription for a particular case). As the French term indicates, their formula was a trade secret; and as the English term suggests, this secret was the property of the inventor or other owner who exploited it commercially. (In England a small number of proprietors took out patents for their concoctions under the Statute of Monopolies of 1624: hence the term 'patent medicines' applied indiscriminately in common usage to all such preparations.)[1] This form of enterprise might seem by definition to lie entirely outside the domain of official medicine, and indeed special remedies have always been a stock in trade of empirics great and small. The classic mountebank of the early modern era derived most of his profits from the sale of remedies, rather than from consultations; and with the passing of the old-style charlatans, new merchants of patent remedies, using newspaper advertisements, mail-order schemes, and a variety of retail outlets, stepped in to exploit the possibilities of the modern marketplace. They created a great parallel pharmaceutical industry.[2] Yet as recently as the last century — not to mention the one before — the unorthodox status of secret remedies was far from clear. Physicians prescribed them to patients; some developed and promoted their own proprietary formulations; and although by the end of the eighteenth century the body of 'enlightened' medical opinion was clearly against secrecy in therapeutics, medical men could be found who staunchly defended the practice of allowing an inventor the exclusive right to exploit his pharmaceutical discovery while veiling its composition from clinicians as well as commercial rivals.[3]

To the 'enlightened physicians', as they liked to style themselves, reforming the remedy trade appeared as urgent a task as establishing and enforcing a professional monopoly in the medical field. Ideally, many would have prohibited secret remedies, hoping simultaneously to strike a blow at 'quackery' and delineate a clearer boundary between official and parallel medicine; only apothecaries would sell medicines, and they would sell only officinal and magistral compounds. Since an absolute prohibition was not a practical possibility, the reformers accepted, as a *pis aller*, state regulation — a system of licensing that would separate the good remedies, which would be encouraged, from the bad, which would be suppressed. Even regulation of the remedy trade, however, was neither uncontroversial nor particularly successful. The history of the debates over secret remedies, and of the attempts by the medical profession and the state to control them, has much to tell us about the difficulties of sorting out fringe from orthodox and the limits of professionalisation in medicine.

This essay forms the sequel to an earlier article, which traced the efforts to regulate secret remedies in *ancien régime* France, culminating in the work of the Société Royale de Médecine.[4] The society received its letters patent in 1778. In theory all existing privileges would be annulled, and henceforth only remedies approved by the society could be sold in France. Although enforcement predictably proved difficult, the Société Royale did impose a new standard, formally licensing only a handful of remedies among the hundreds submitted to it for examination. This was not the only such attempt in eighteenth-century Europe, but in its scale, the zeal of its protagonists, and its influence abroad, it was arguably the most important. By the time of the Revolution of 1789, however, a significant number of enlightened physicians had become convinced that the Society had failed — not so much because it had not carried out its mandate, but because its programme was essentially flawed. Under its statutes, the Society could not publish the formula of a remedy it approved; only the members of the commission that examined the remedy would know its composition, which they were obliged not to divulge out of respect for the property rights of the inventor or owner. To the Society's critics, such a compromise was now unacceptable. Secrecy was inconsistent with the practice of rational medicine. Moreover, the delivery of royal warrants, however limited in number, could only lend prestige to empiricism in all its forms. Many of the society's own members and correspondents came to share this view; in the end, then, the Enlightenment project emphatically called for abolition rather than regulation.

The present essay traces the subsequent history of this project, from the initial hopes for implementation at the outset of the Revolution through its final failure under the Empire.[5] Though the revolutionaries took an active interest in medical reform and indeed proclaimed a right to health,[6] the regulatory institutions inherited from the *ancien régime* fell foul of two more fundamental principles: the right of property (which in 1789 the Declaration of the Rights of Man pronounced 'inviolable and sacred') and freedom of trade and enterprise. Far from enacting new regulatory measures, the revolutionary assemblies embarked on a programme of deregulation, which abolished the old medical faculties and colleges, made medicine a free profession, and effectively ended systematic control of the remedy trade. New legislation on medicine and pharmacy, debated under the Directory regime of 1795-9, had to await Bonaparte and the Consulate. In 1810, finally, the imperial government struck out boldly for the promised land of which the Revolution of 1789 had afforded only a Pisgah glimpse: a society free of secret remedies, in which the state would purchase and publish all valuable new formulas while prohibiting the sale of all proprietary compounds. This endeavour miscarried; what is interesting is not its failure (which the history of prohibitory legislation in general would lead us to expect), but the way in which it was compromised from the start by the government's respect for the inventor's or owner's interest in his remedy. In Napoleonic France, the right of property remained 'inviolable and sacred'; it could and often did outweigh the claims of public health. Although the régimes that followed the First Empire were to create other regulatory institutions, this retreat from the Enlightenment commitment to end secrecy in therapeutics set the pattern for the rest of the century and beyond.[7]

The Intellectual Background: Secret Remedies, Pro and Contra

Some acquaintance with the eighteenth-century debates on secret remedies is essential for understanding the positions that health reformers took in 1789. Although such remedies had been licensed by a royal commission since 1728 and in principle were subject to systematic evaluation, it remained an accepted feature of French law that owners of approved remedies, whether laymen or professionals, could sell them without divulging their formula. The widespread use of such remedies, however, ran counter to several fundamental tenets of the learned medical tradition.

First, the secret remedy was almost invariably said to cure a specific disease in all patients. Official medicine distrusted specifics, though it recognised a few (such as quinquina for the treatment of intermittent fevers).[8] The official medicine of the Enlightenment derived, in its broad outlines, from the Hippocratic tradition. Physicians generally viewed diseases as a congeries of symptoms which might appear in different permutations in different patients, or in the same patient at different stages of the disease. Starting in the middle of the eighteenth century, medical writers produced 'nosographies' that systematically classified symptoms of disease as Linnaeus had classified the distinguishing characteristics of plants; one of the last great treatises in this vein was Philippe Pinel's *Nosographie philosophique*, published in 1797.[9] Each pathological state, according to this view, manifested itself in external signs. The clinician, as Michel Foucault has suggested, had to be a semiologist, an observer of signs that the various senses could detect. Each drug substance would modify the signs, and the patient's underlying condition, in different degrees (reducing fever, for example).[10]

It followed that successful medical practice required an extensive knowledge of the course of different diseases and of the pharmacological effects of various remedies, together with an intensive knowledge of the individual patient and his idiosyncrasies. Only a quack would claim that a specific remedy, sold by its inventor, could take the place of a balanced course of treatment prescribed by an experienced medical man. But secret remedies were generally sold by laymen to other laymen.

The third great defect of the secret remedy was that its ingredients and therefore its mode of action were unknown. In support of his specialty the promoter argued *post hoc ergo propter hoc*: patients improved after taking it. The reasons for its success remained an enigma. Enlightened therapeutics, however, demanded what might be called transparency and rationality. Transparency implied that all curative means should be visible and known, rather than concealed and mysterious. Rationality implied that all ingredients should be included for a reason, derived from known pharmacological principles; it was not sufficient that in practice a certain hodgepodge appeared to work.

To be sure, sceptics (including some physicians) challenged the assertion that physicians knew how remedies worked. On one level, they were right: medical men could not precisely explain a drug's action in terms of its observable or measurable chemical and physical properties. But as the physician-*cum*-philosopher Georges Cabanis replied in his anti-Pyrrhonist tract of 1788 (published in 1798), *Du Degré de certitude de la médecine*, physicians did not need to know the inner 'nature' of remedies in order to understand that certain substances produced consistent physiological changes in patients.[11] Recognised remedies had known 'virtues', rather like the *virtus dormativa* that Molière's learned medicaster attributes to opium in *Le Malade imaginaire*. (This ascription of a pharmacological 'quality' to a substance may seem less ridiculous if we bear in mind how difficult it is even now to explain the action of a drug. The physician Lester King, in a recent study of the medical philosophy of the eighteenth century, suggests to his readers, 'as an exercise', that they 'try to find out why opium does put you to sleep, according to modern views of pharmacology and neurophysiology. The search will not be easy, nor necessarily satisfactory.')[12]

Some drug substances, it is true, accumulated quite long lists of supposed properties — what Gaston Bachelard, in a classic study of scientific epistemology, castigated as a 'prolix empiricism' associated with 'backward sciences' such as medicine: 'A medicament, in the eighteenth century, is literally covered with adjectives . . . The "simples" are particularly complex.' At the same time, a given remedy might comprise numerous different ingredients, often with overlapping properties.[13] Could such a therapeutics be considered rational? The enlightened physicians would have responded that this prolix empiricism and polypharmacy had been uncritical, and that scientific pharmacology would now establish new standards. One English work on vulgar errors from the end of the eighteenth century, for example, drew a sharp contrast between the inelegant use of sometimes quite repellent hodgepodges in the traditional armamentarium and the reformed pharmacy of the late Enlightenment, which sought to isolate active ingredients and determine a rigorous nosology:[14]

> Is it not a most disgustful thing to cram a sick stomach with a load of the filthiest things in nature, while chemistry affords us medicines of similar but superior virtues in doses of a few grains only? A few grains of sal ammoniac in solution being to the same intentions a more efficacious and a cleanlier medicine than a quart of the infusion of stonehorse dung, though sufficient care had been taken that the dung was dropped in the cleanest napkin . . . Of late, many wheel-barrows full of herbs, roots, barks, weeds, &c. &c. have been thrown out.

More work along these lines might transform therapeutics from an erratic art into a reliable technology.

In the case of a secret remedy, though, how could one determine the effective ingredients? True, the Société Royale de Médecine would not give its approbation unless its commissioners received the recipe; but this limited disclosure aided neither the medical scientist nor the clinician hoping to adjust a course of treatment to suit the needs of his patients.

In the end, a fundamental difference in outlook separated the proponents and antagonists of proprietary remedies. For the one side, nature was infinitely rich and mysterious, yielding up its secrets to anyone who was willing to be guided by experience. To ignore such contributions was to deprive humanity of a precious resource. The enlightened physicians, for their part, derided this vulgar notion of experience. In the words of a treatise on popular errors in medicine, 'it consists in having for many years applied such and such a remedy to certain diseases that seemed similar, without ever having been able to examine the proximate or remote causes, or to reason about their divers characters'.[15] Philosophical medicine required both broader acquaintance with clinical cases and a deeper understanding of physiology to distinguish between real regularities and superficial resemblances. The enlightened physician predictably took his watchword from Hippocrates: practice must be based on experience guided by reason.

Moreover, the naive empiricism of the untutored supposed that genius or serendipity randomly favoured professional and layman alike, whereas in the enlightened physicians' view, both the brilliant insight and the serendipitous discovery usually rewarded the trained intelligence. Only a few new permutations of recognised drug substances could be expected to make pharmacological sense; the amateur put his faith in the most improbable concoctions or hailed as a novelty a preparation that he might have found in his grandmother's recipe book, had he taken the trouble to consult it. Genuine discoveries, of course, were always possible; contact with the New World had brought to Europe previously unknown botanicals whose value was now well established. But even when promising remedies emerged, rational development of the actual medication implied careful analysis of the drug's properties and a good general grounding in pharmacy.

These ways of thinking about therapeutics helped shape the divergent attitudes of Frenchmen towards secret remedies. Many patients, perhaps most, used such remedies; they believed (if they thought about the question at all) that the details of the formula meant nothing beside the remedy's record of success or failure. For the professional elite, however, secrecy was unacceptable. In 1778, the respected *Gazette de santé* decided to reject all advertisements for secret remedies;[16] and in the end the Société Royale de Médecine concluded that a remedy's formula would have to be revealed not only to its commissioners, but also to the world at large. Enlightened medicine could not be occult, and the secret remedy was quite literally a *res occulta*, or hidden thing. Medicine had to be, so far as possible, a visible realm, in the interests both of science and of public health.

The Revolution and the Question of Secret Remedies

With the Revolution, the controversy over secret remedies came to a head, for the not always consistent promises of 1789 had something to offer each side. On the one hand, physicians had reason to hope that the National Constituent Assembly, charged with drawing up a new political constitution for the kingdom, would provide France with a new medical constitution as well. Realising 'man's right to health' entailed not only making medical assistance more widely available, but also suppressing abuses in the medical field that threatened public health. On the other hand, remedy-owners could take comfort from the Revolution's strict adherence to the principle of private property, proclaimed in the Declaration of Rights of 1789 (and later reaffirmed in the declaration that preceded the Jacobin constitution of 1793). No one could be deprived of his property without his consent, except out of public necessity and after payment of appropriate compensation. Was not a proprietary remedy a form of property? Moreover, as the Revolution turned more radical, restrictions on the development and distribution of secret remedies seemed inconsistent with the basic principles of intellectual and economic freedom. Even before the Revolution, amateurs had attacked academies like the Société Royale de Médecine as bastions of corporate privilege that perpetuated the status quo and stifled originality and true genius. Remedy-sellers whose panaceas had been spurned by the Society identified with egalitarians like the radical Jean-Paul Marat, amateur scientist and sometime student of medicine, whose criticisms of Newton's optics had failed to win the approval of the Academy of Sciences, and who now denounced all academicians as charlatans.[17]

In the debates of 1789, then, the apologists for secret remedies — chiefly proprietors with a vested interest — insisted that the composition must be kept secret if property rights were to be respected, and that remedies were best prepared by their 'inventors', rather than by pharmacists who took the formulas from published recipes. The physician Louis-Etienne Gachet, for example, who offered a professedly 'impartial' consideration of the question in his *Problème médico-politique: pour ou contre les arcanes, ou remèdes secrets* (c. 1789-90), was also the promoter of an elixir against gout that had been rejected by the Société Royale de Médecine[18] and the author of a handbook, *Le Manuel des goutteux*, describing how patients could treat themselves with his specific. Gachet argued that since a remedy's mode of action was uncertain, an exhaustive description of its formulation — assuming that it were possible to arrive at one — would mean less than a record of cures. 'What does it matter what knowledge one may have of it, provided that it is efficacious?' In the case of arcana, moreover, the inventor himself would bring greater zeal than anyone else to preparing his remedy. 'Does one ever expect from a mercenary nurse the same care, the same precautions, the same pains, the same sacrifices for the child that is entrusted to her than [from] the actual mother?'

This was only half of Gachet's argument. The other half was a plea for liberty in science and equity for the unrecognised genius — essentially the terms that Marat used in his critique of the royal academies: no one's creative faculties should be restrained by the law or by any official company. Gachet insisted further on the inventor's right to his intellectual property, a right that the National Assembly had recognised for authors of literary works. The only acceptable solution was to allow inventors complete freedom to exploit their remedies. This innovation would not open the floodgates to charlatanism; on the contrary, Gachet suggested, echoing the classic liberal argument for laissez-faire, free competition would allow good remedies to win public confidence and expose bad remedies to the opprobrium they deserved. Indeed, it was the system of endorsements and approbations that had encouraged charlatanism in the first place.[19]

This last point reappeared on the opposing side, in the arguments of the most hardened critics of secret remedies. One such was Alexandre-André-Philippe-Frédéric Bacher, doctor-regent of the Paris Medical Faculty and editor of the *Journal de médecine*. Bacher's father, Georges-Frédéric, had won celebrity as the inventor of tonic pills for the treatment of dropsy, but he had obligingly sold his formula to the Crown.[20] The younger Bacher complained that the examination system served only as free publicity for secret remedies, whether or not they were approved; that the examinations were not always reliable and were subject to fraud; and finally (parting company here with the apologists for secret remedies) that a physician could not properly prescribe a compound when he did not know its ingredients, even if it carried the seal of approval of a medical academy. Warrants for secret formulas should be suppressed, and the composition of all useful preparations published, after payment of appropriate compensation to the inventor — for 'a good remedy is a property for its inventor: he has the right to derive all the advantages from it that may be reconciled with the public interest and safety'.[21]

Between deregulation and automatic publication lay a middle ground, occupied by defenders of something like the status quo. François Thiéry, for example, in his *Voeux d'un patriote sur la médecine en France* (1789), proposed that 'all persons whatsoever be prohibited from selling and distributing any remedies if they have not been approved by a commission established for that purpose'.[22]

The discussion of secret remedies in the *Nouveau Plan de constitution pour la médecine en France*, which Félix Vicq d'Azyr presented in 1790 to the National Constituent Assembly on behalf of the Société Royale de Médecine, must be viewed against this background. The evaluation of remedies, the *Nouveau Plan* insisted, should remain the responsibility of the Société Royale, or a body very like it; in answer to those who suggested that the society had encouraged charlatanism by licensing proprietary remedies, the proposal cited the very small number of preparations that had actually received an official approbation. On the most crucial point, however, the society's plan reversed the existing practice: if approved, all new remedies would be published, and in the future no one would be allowed to sell a remedy whose formula remained a secret. Secrecy in medicine created 'veils of mystery. This mystery excites the enthusiasm and sustains the credulity of the people. It leads to uncertainty in distinguishing the circumstances and inexactitude in applying a [remedy] that one uses without being acquainted with it.'[23] This view had emerged as a consensus of the enlightened physicians in the society's debates on medical reform, starting in the summer of 1789.

In September of 1790, at the instigation of the physician Joseph-Ignace Guillotin, deputy from Paris, the National Constituent Assembly created a special committee on health, or Comité de Salubrité, comprising the seventeen physician members of the assembly and an equal number of laymen. Guillotin as chairman and Jean-Gabriel Gallot as secretary linked the committee to the Société Royale.[24] In May of the following year, the committee debated the question of secret remedies and unanimously adopted a resolution calling for a strict prohibition of their sale.[25] The committee's final report on medical reform, which Guillotin drafted in August, called for a law that would ban the sale of such remedies even by pharmacists, under penalty of a 500-livre fine.[26]

The Constituent Assembly, however, was dissolved on 30 September, leaving Guillotin's report in limbo, and none of the subsequent assemblies produced a new plan. Indeed, what followed could best be described as deregulation. The Société Royale de Médecine, like all the academies and faculties, came under fire as a privileged corporation, though it continued to evaluate secret remedies.[27] (One inventor's proposal from the year of the Jacobin dictatorship conveys the anti-professional sentiments of the radical revolutionary: if the government simply turned to citizens with effective remedies, he suggested, the result would be 'a popular medicine infinitely preferable to, and more certain than, all the often erroneous practices of our physicians'.)[28] In the summer of 1793, the Convention formally abolished all the academies, including the society.[29] The legislators, it is true, left standing a law of April 1791, which stated that the old legislation on pharmacy would be upheld;[30] and the College of Pharmacy, the one *ancien régime* medical institution to weather the Revolution, sometimes received formulas referred by the government for evaluation. But the examination of remedies had always been conducted under the supervision of physicians.[31] Without the Société Royale and the faculties, regulation could proceed only on a piecemeal basis.[32]

Much depended now on the initiative of local pharmaceutical societies (as in Rouen)[33] or of government authorities who had received requests for warrants and authorisations. Thus in the capital, the Bureau Central du Canton de Paris reported in 1798 on citizen Colas's elixir of long life, which it deemed unoriginal but none the less suitable for sale to the public.[34] Some local officials used their administrative powers to impose *ad hoc* measures. In the Department of the Seine, for example, which included Paris, the College of Pharmacy proposed a text for regulating secret remedies to the prefect of police, Nicolas-Thérèse-Benoît Frochot, who promulgated it as a prefectoral decree (6 Germinal Year X, or 27 March 1802).[35]

At the national level, the debate on secret remedies gathered momentum in 1797 and continued through the two remaining years of the Directory regime, without producing new legislation, or even a consensus on how the problem should be resolved. In a report to the Council of Five Hundred on behalf of the Committee on Public Education, Jean-Marie Calès (a physician from Toulouse who as a Jacobin member of the revolutionary Convention had voted for the death of Louis XVI) argued that if the law were to forbid the sale of secret remedies, vendors would escape surveillance altogether. It would be better to require them to present their remedies to a 'society of enlightened men'; if a formula were approved, the proprietor would then receive the right to sell his preparation.[36] The physician-legislator Jean-François Barailon (former Girondin member of the Convention) also proposed to the Council of Five Hundred an arrangement similar to the one that existed at the end of the *ancien régime*. The owner of an approved secret remedy would be allowed to sell it and would be assured that his secret would be kept until his death; sellers of unauthorised remedies would receive stiff penalties. No previous warrants, except those of the Société Royale de Médecine, would be recognised.[37] Other proposals, however, such as the one that Antoine-François Hardy (a physician from Rouen and another former Girondin *conventionnel*) presented to the Council of Five Hundred in the November of 1798, called for an outright ban on secret remedies.[38]

In the end, a compromise prevailed. Under the Consulate, an opinion of the Council of State (9 Germinal Year XI, or 30 March 1803) prohibited pharmacists from selling secret remedies and obliged them to conform to the dispensaries.[39] This principle was retained in the new legislation on pharmacy adopted later that month, on 21 Germinal (11 April); but all secret remedies were not outlawed as such.

The Régime of Germinal

The Germinal law, which followed a few weeks after a law regulating medical practice (adopted on 19 Ventôse or 10 March), primarily concerned the education and licensure of pharmacists and the repression of illegal practice of pharmacy. It mentioned secret remedies twice. Article XXXII banned pharmacists from selling them. Another, somewhat confusing article (XXXVI) was directed mainly against itinerant empirics: 'The retail sale by dose, any distribution of drugs and medicinal preparations from stages or displays in public squares, fairs, and markets, [and] any advertisement or printed poster that indicates secret remedies, by whatever name, are strictly prohibited.' The law did not expressly ban the sale of secret remedies altogether (it was arguably still legal for non-pharmacists to sell them in shops or homes if one overlooked, as contemporaries generally did, article XXV, which prohibited unqualified persons from 'preparing, selling, or distributing any medicament'); but neither did the act make any special provision for evaluating and certifying them.[40] A subsequent police ordinance reinforced the prohibition on advertising secret remedies or hawking them from stages; a supplementary law prescribed penalties (a fine of 25-600 francs, plus three to ten days in prison for recidivists).[41] In addition, an imperial decree (25 Prairial Year XIII, or 14 June 1805) clarified and in effect attenuated the legislation by confirming the rights of vendors whose approbations antedated the new measure. It also extended the same privilege to persons whose remedies had since been approved by the government following the recommendation of a medical school or society. Both the proprietor and his agents might sell the approved remedies in Paris and the provinces if they were authorised by local officials; they would not be obliged to divulge their secret.[42]

Napoleon's decree simply confirmed the existing *ad hoc* system of regulation, conducted now under the aegis of the Ministry of the

Interior. The government took a decision on whether to permit the distribution of a remedy after consulting an official medical body — usually the Paris School of Medicine (one of three medical schools established in 1794-5 to meet the need for new personnel after the suppression of the old faculties); in promising cases, trials were conducted in military hospitals and elsewhere.[43] A petitioner who at the end of the *ancien régime* might have written in supplication to Vicq d'Azyr, permanent secretary of the Société Royale de Médicine, now wrote to the Minister of the Interior.[44] At the local level, a major role was played by the *jurys médicaux*, departmental commissions created under the Ventôse law on medicine, whose principal tasks were to examine and license health officers (the new lower grade of medical practitioner) and inspect pharmacies. In the Yonne, for example, a tailor at Saint-Sauveur who had a remedy for scrofula, an 'infallible secret' inherited from his father, was forbidden by the mayor to distribute it until the medical jury had approved. it.[45] The health council of the Seine, created by the prefect Louis-Nicolas-Pierre-Joseph Dubois in 1802, also contributed to policing secret remedies in the capital and was frequently consulted by the prefect. In February of 1810, for example, it reported that Halin's jelly — an 'essence of sugar and fowl' — was not harmful, but that it did not, as its proprietor claimed, possess the properties of prolonging life and restoring the stomach.[46] Thus despite the absence of a central organisation comparable to the old Société Royale de Médecine, France under the First Empire made a serious effort to regulate the remedy trade.

Anthelme-Balthasar Richerand, the talented young physician who in 1807 — at the age of twenty-seven — was named a professor of medicine in Paris, left a description of the work of the Paris School (or, after 1808, Faculty) of Medicine. Each year, he wrote, the faculty was charged by the Minister of the Interior with examining several hundred discoveries and secrets submitted by 'retired military men, village mayors, honest and charitable persons living in the countryside, ecclesiastics, pious women, and sometimes even medicasters'. Most of the formulas, he suggested, came straight out of readily available printed sources; the petitioners had not even taken the trouble to modify the composition.[47]

The archives bear out Richerand's description. A certain Castellan, for example, extolled the virtues of his 'aquillea millefeuilles' (i.e. *achillea millefolium*: the milfoil, or yarrow) for treating sores and ulcers, whose secret he said he had learned from a 'good botanist'; but the faculty, in May of 1810, dismissed it as commonly known.[48] The previous year, a correspondent from the canton of Fribourg in Switzerland had proposed to the Minister of the Interior a specific against inflammation of wounds and ulcers; the Ministry of War, he said, had already had it analysed — and found that it had the same properties as an ointment commonly used in military hospitals.[49]

Like the Société Royale de Médecine before it, the Paris Faculty of Medicine insisted that petitioners disclose the formula of their remedy (to its examiners, under a pledge of confidentiality): and like the society, it encountered resistance. A Paris parasol dealer, Coutelet, 'blessed for forty years with a family secret [transmitted] from father to son', asked the minister's authorisation to sell a remedy for ulcers and sores. When the faculty required a formula, Coutelet refused. No further details on the remedy reached the minister. He did, however, receive a tearful supplication from a woman suffering from *lait répandu* (a condition supposedly caused by unsecreted milk that spread from the breasts to other parts of the body); the disease had begun to affect her face, the author wrote, and she implored the minister — apparently to no avail — to allow Coutelet to undertake the treatment.[50]

The unfortunate remedy-owner whose formula was rejected as unoriginal or worthless suffered a double blow. Not only was he deprived of the prestige of an official endorsement; by continuing to sell and administer an unapproved remedy, he also opened himself to charges of illegal practice of pharmacy and medicine, which vendors of approved remedies generally escaped under the provisions of the decree of 25 Prairial Year XIII. This fate befell a Belgian from the region of Liége named Carouge de Rocquemonty, proprietor of a 'true elixir of long life', which he said had been handed down from father to son; since the revolutionary Convention had annexed his homeland to France, he found himself obliged to conform to French law in selling his remedy. The Paris professors determined that his compound resembled a commonly used elixir and concluded that as a layman he should be forbidden to distribute it. Carouge de Rocquemonty asked the Minister of the Interior to let him benefit from the decree of Prairial on the grounds that his remedy was not new and therefore did not require approval, and that his experience combined with that of his ancestors would be a sufficient guarantee that the remedy would be properly prescribed, even though he was not a physician. Without a confirmed property right, however, he had no redress and could in theory have been prosecuted for violating the law of Germinal.[51]

It has been seen that the legislation of Germinal and the interpretive decrees that followed it revived, in disjointed fashion, the regulatory functions of the Société Royale de Médecine, while confirming the property of the remedy-owners in their preparations. Like the law of Ventôse on

92 *Property Rights and the Right to Health*

medical practice, which recognised the rights of *ancien régime* practitioners and of many persons who had begun practising after the abolition of the old corporations, the regime of Germinal represented a compromise between established interests and the demands of public health.

The Decree of 1810 and the Commission on Secret Remedies

Despite the best efforts of the authorities, the secret remedy trade continued to flourish in all its forms during the Empire; not only the old approved remedies (like Laffecteur's vegetable 'rob' for syphilis)[52] but also many hundreds of unauthorised preparations sold well, often in violation of the existing regulations. Physicians and administrators alike found the law insufficiently rigorous. Too many remedy-vendors and inventors could claim valid privileges. Some had registered their remedies under the patent law of 1791; although such patents merely recognised priority, many persons (even officials) took them as conferring permission to exploit the invention.[53] Despairing of winning convictions in court, the authorities turned to administrative measures to restrain offenders.[54]

The government's response to the problem came in the form of an imperial decree, promulgated 18 August 1810 with the declared purpose of disseminating knowledge of good remedies while discouraging the sale of bad ones. The state would buy and make public the recipes of useful compositions: 'it is a duty for the owners of such secrets to co-operate in having them published'. All previous permissions would be nullified. Proprietors would submit their recipes to the Minister of the Interior, together with an account of their use and a record of clinical experience to date. The minister would name a special five-member commission on secret remedies, including three professors from the faculties of medicine. The commission would determine whether the remedy was harmless; if harmless, whether it was useful; and if useful, what price should be paid to acquire it, depending on the merit of the discovery, the possible advantages to be derived from it, and the gains that the inventor had realised or might expect to realise. In the event of a dispute, the minister would name an appeals board. Once a remedy had been approved, the minister would negotiate an agreement with the inventor; after confirmation by the Council of State, the formula would be published immediately. No inventor would receive an approbation if he insisted on keeping his remedy secret.[55] The law's larger intent, as the preamble made clear, was not only to protect the public health, by preventing the use of drugs that had no value or contained unknown substances, but also to 'spread enlightenment' and 'discourage charlatanism'. A month later, a police circular instructed the prefects to enforce the law strictly and to use the occasion of the new legislation as an opportunity to attack quackery more generally.[56]

In October, the commission was organised, and a set of instructions prepared for owners of secret remedies who now had to comply with the new law.[57] The abrogation of permissions was to take effect on New Year's Day 1811. A subsequent decree (26 December 1810) extended the grace period to April (the date was later postponed to July) and further provided that any proprietor who before the adoption of the decree had had his remedy examined by a 'commission' (presumably the Faculty of Medicine, consulted by the Minister of the Interior), would be exempted from a new examination if the commission had pronounced the remedy harmless. Finally, on 5 April 1811, the Council of State felt it necessary to reaffirm the right of access to the appeals board, against the recommendation of the Minister of the Interior, 'so that the property rights of inventors or proprietors of secret remedies will be guaranteed, as His Majesty wished, and that a single commission will not be their absolute judge without [any] recourse'.[58] Thus the decree of 18 August, which had been promulgated in the interest of spreading 'enlightenment', promoting public health, and fighting 'charlatanism', had to yield some of its force to a competing concern for property.

The commission duly began its work, headed by the distinguished anatomist François Chaussier, professor at the Paris faculty and an authority on medical jurisprudence. As will be seen, the threat to property never materialised; the programme of 1810 collapsed, and the government returned in practice to the system of the Year XIII (the reinterpreted law of Germinal). But the experiment — the last systematic attempt in France to review all proprietary remedies across the board — is not without interest. Perhaps even more than the re-examination of privileges conducted after 1778 by the Société Royale de Médecine, it produced a clash over the conflicting rights of remedy owners and the public. In the course of this dispute, the proprietors and medical bureaucrats raised fundamental questions about who was entitled to practise medicine and pharmacy and what sorts of therapies they might apply.

Richerand's brief account suggests,[59] and archival documents confirm,[60] that the commission began its work under a cloud of hostility. To understand the proprietors' attitude, one need only recall that the 1810 decree imposed a sweeping review of all privileges for the first time since 1778-81, and that the proprietors of 1810 faced a more awesome bureaucratic machine than their counterparts had thirty years earlier. Even in the 1780s, many officials in the provinces did not quite understand the workings of the Société Royale de Médecine; some refused to recognise the authority of its letters patent or were ignorant of their contents. Imperial legislation carried more weight, and under Napoleon, the network of prefects and subprefects posed a more serious threat than had the intendants, subdelegates, and municipal officials of the *ancien régime*. As for the commission itself, it appears to have been no stricter than the Société Royale, though even that degree of rigour would have seemed harsh to the beneficiaries of the system of the year XIII. But perhaps the most important consideration was that in principal no remedies would be allowed to remain 'secret', a drastic reform that the Société Royale had advocated in the early years of the Revolution, but which no previous government had actually attempted to implement. No one, whether pharmacist or layman, would be allowed to sell secret remedies; official approbation of a remedy would mean publication, loss of monopoly, and prolonged haggling over compensation.

Not surprisingly, many proprietors proved uncooperative. One petitioner, a certain Péroutet, wrote a plaintive but stubborn letter to Minister of the Interior Montalivet, explaining: 'I will do whatever Monseigneur may order but I will not give recipes, because I need them in order to live.'[61] Another patiently explained that his secret was of the sort that could not be revealed to just anyone, and that he would have to maintain his silence:[62]

> Not only do I persist in this, but I renew the vow that I made (to the person who made me the repository of this recipe) that no one will ever know my secret until my death; and then I must still find someone worthy of my confidence. It is my property, and I am sure of being the sole proprietor. I have done my duty in making myself known [to the commission].

The law went against one of the most hallowed traditions of popular medicine. Although for the medical entrepreneur a remedy was simply a commercial property, for many popular healers the secret was a confidence and sacred trust; indeed, in the hands of the wrong person the remedy might not work.

The petitioners' anxieties about disclosing their marvellous recipes proved well founded. When the commission did receive the formula, it often responded harshly, and it was quick to suggest that any layman who continued to sell a remedy, whatever its merits, was probably practising pharmacy and medicine illegally. A certain Warmon, in the Belgian department of the Escaut, sent a manuscript listing a series of proposed remedies; the commission rejected them as having been culled from commonplace works, or else as ridiculous and even dangerous.[63] When Salmon-Maugé, a remedy-proprietor and former merchant of Paris, sent a longish manuscript on the treatment of venereal disease, the commission ruled, first, that his proposed remedy resembled other treatments and that Salmon-Maugé therefore deserved no recompense, but also that his remedy, while it might be useful in some cases, should be prescribed by a physician.[64] Such responses left many proprietors feeling deeply embittered. One letter to the Minister of the Interior epitomised their reaction: 'given the manner in which I have been treated by the members of the commission on secret remedies, I do not wish to have anything to do with them; and I refuse all of them'.[65]

Despite their obvious lack of relish for the task, the commissioners continued to make their way through the piles of recipes, many of them familiar therapies from the grab-bag of empirical medicine. This encounter between traditional and official medicine was not much of a dialogue, for the physicians rarely offered a lengthy explanation for their decisions: but they did at least listen. A certain Sourget offered a remedy for intermittent fevers: take freshly laid eggs, steep them for twenty-four hours in a local white wine, with three or four leaves of chicory. The commission pronounced this remedy null and insignificant.[66] A certain Vincent wrote to propose a topical remedy for hernias (also good for wens and sores, among other things), the secret of which he had learned from his father. The recipe included lard, the leaves and flowers of Aaron's rod, and more; as proof of its efficacy, he cited the remarkable cure of a young man from Epinal who suffered from priapism for two weeks after attempting to consummate marriage with his new bride, 'who was too narrow for him'. After all the physicians confessed themselves baffled, Vincent *père*, summoned by a modest and wise surgeon, applied the balm and succeeded in moving the recalcitrant prepuce back to its normal position. Vincent added a personal plea: as a former clerk whose post had been eliminated, he needed the money. The sceptical commission solemnly announced that the remedy consisted merely of rancid grease prepared with a few leaves and flowers of Aaron's rod, and that the cure of an ordinary case of phimosis could have been obtained without any lubricant at all.[67] Another remedy-owner, a bootmaker of Paris, sent the recipe for a plaster (consisting chiefly of resin and rue) for treating prolapse of the uterus, together with a covering letter that conveyed more clearly than anything else its author's shaky command of

French grammar and orthography. The remedy was to be applied to the lower abdomen; the commission observed that a simple description sufficed to show that it would not work.[68] A similarly unpromising topical remedy, for hernia, was prepared by a tax agent (*employé des droits réunis*) in the *arrondissement* of Brussels. He said that the Revolution had deprived him of the 'honest comfort' he had once enjoyed, but that he still administered his remedy gratis. The recipe called for using a new earthen pot, glazed on the inside; a bottle of red wine, as old as possible; a pomegranate with sweet fruit, cut in four; a quart of white soap of Marseilles; a quart of superfine olive oil; and a quart of fresh unsalted butter. The commission drily noted that successful treatment of a hernia required a surgical procedure.[69] Predictably, the commission received at least one recipe for an omelette for victims of the bite of a rabid animal (three eggs, nut oil, and powder of dogrose root, part to be applied to the wound, and part consumed by the patient in the morning on an empty stomach). This infallible remedy, the author suggested, had been used for more than a hundred years at Charenton. A simple description, the commission replied, was sufficient for them to recognise that the recipe did not deserve attention.[70] Some remedies, finally, seemed intended for treatment of unrecognisable or imaginary conditions. A certain Vaubaillon (a former preacher of the gospel, according to his letter) wrote to complain that the commission, which had rejected his remedies for retention of urine, 'sciatic gout', dropsy and other disorders on the ground that they were already public knowledge, had failed to consider his additional claims to cure epilepsy, scrofula, haemorrhoids, fluxions of the blood, loss of blood, and other disorders besides:[71]

> I am furthermore bold enough to assert that there exists a disease whose name I do not know, which physicians only rarely cure, of which I cured several persons after their worthless remedies [had failed] and in this disease there are winds . . . one belches frequently, the body cries out and sometimes roars. One has bubbles [*boulles=bulles*?] in the body, vomiting everything that one consumes. Others cannot eat.

The commission let this one pass.

The commission thus kept its distance from a wide range of traditional medications. Moreover, the decree of 1810 and the subsequent regulation of secret remedies helped resolve a major point of conflict between the traditional and 'enlightened' view of remedy-vending.

Physicians and administrators consistently rejected *ad hominem* pleas based on personal need or a history of public service as justifications for illegal practice of medicine and pharmacy. The commission did not entirely ignore the issue of petitioners' claims to charity or public assistance; it did, however, insist on separating this question from its judgement of a remedy's merits and its proprietor's qualifications.

Nevertheless, the commission's own charge required it to consider the compensation due to a remedy-proprietor for the financial loss incurred through the state's exercise of eminent domain; it quickly became embroiled in economic and legal questions that had nothing to do with medicine and tended to shift attention from the question of public health to the question of property rights. This process can best be illustrated by a case involving one of the most celebrated remedies of the *ancien régime*, Belloste's pills — one of the very few preparations to receive the official approbation of the Société Royale de Médecine. In 1781, following evaluation and approval of their remedy, the heirs of Michel-Antoine Belloste (son of the inventor) obtained a new privilege valid for thirty years; the edict of 1810 thus took effect just as this privilege was about to expire, and the current owner had no choice but to submit it to the commission.[72] The petitioner was Armande-Geneviève-Elisabeth Lechat, widow of Jean-Baptiste Belloste, a Paris physician who in the 1780s had pestered Vica d'Azyr with requests for the Société Royale to affirm his rights as against those of his siblings. According to a notarised attestation prepared in 1806, she was the sole proprietor. The commission, simply echoing the findings of the Société Royale, recognised that the 'correctives' introduced in the formulation of this remedy made it preferable to other mercurial preparations; but in view of the warrant of 1781 and an earlier one issued in 1758, both of which had been fully exploited, it recommended against paying any further recompense. If the widow were needy, she might perhaps be paid a small indemnity — provided she revealed the formula. (Under the charge given to the commission, the question of need might conceivably arise, but only after it had disposed of the question of the remedy's safety and efficacy.)[73]

The widow appealed the decision, questioning the commission's statements about the profits she had derived from the remedy. She suggested that among the various beneficiaries of the warrant of 1781, her mother-in-law (the widow of Michel-Antoine Belloste) had gained the most; but 'no one is unaware of the way in which she sold her remedy, often at half price and sometimes gratis, even giving her money to patients so that they could use her remedy appropriately'. Her husband, the eldest of the Belloste children, had shared the secret with the youngest brother but had also been obliged to make regular payments as stipulated in an agreement among the co-heirs:

> [As a result of] discharging these same obligations, after having sustained losses during the Revolution, as much because of the sluggishness of trade as because of the depreciation of paper money, I was forced to use up my dowry to raise my son, who studied medicine; what finally ruined me was having to take care of my invalid husband for a long time. *The only means of existence now remaining to us is our property, the sale of our pills; I ask to retain it.* [Original italics.] To deprive us of it would be to leave us without bread for the benefit of a few individuals who do not need it.

The widow added that she had duly administered her remedy for dartres, effusions of milk and scrofula only, in keeping with the terms of her authorisation. She had taken the patients' means into account, especially when they had brought a recommendation from a physician, which happened often; and despite her lack of credentials, she paid each year a pharmacist's *patente* (the tax on trade and industry), 'which authorises me to sell [my remedy] without being bothered during the course of the year'.[74]

The appeals board, like its predecessors, routinely observed that the remedy was distinct from the mercurial pills listed in the Codex or in Baumé's *Eléments de pharmacie*, and it noted without disagreement that the commission had deemed it suitable for 'divers alterations of the lymph'; but it differed with the commission on the question of compensation. The government should purchase the remedy; in view of the earlier privileges the indemnity would be limited, but the widow should still receive 24,000 francs 'because of the obligations she has contracted to her co-heirs in the Belloste succession'. Moreover, she should receive the right to sell her pills for life, concurrently with the pharmacists — a concession at variance with the law of Germinal, strictly construed. The widow expressed her willingness to accept this arrangement.[75]

The Minister of the Interior was prepared to adopt the conclusions of the appeals board, but the Council of State hesitated to follow suit and turned to the Paris Faculty of Medicine for a third opinion. In the meantime, the minister was to authorise the widow to continue selling the remedy on a temporary basis. Frustrated by the government's inability to agree on an indemnity, she now offered to give the government her secret without any compensation, provided that it were published only after her death, and that she were allowed to sell her remedy throughout her lifetime.[76]

The Paris Faculty of Medicine prepared a report in the summer of 1813. On the question of the remedy's safety and efficacy — the only real medical issues in the case — the faculty simply parroted the opinions of its predecessors. The bulk of the report was devoted to the issue that lay outside its special competence — the nature and amount of compensation. The size of any indemnity, the authors suggested, would depend not only on the remedy's value, but also on two key economic considerations: on the one hand, the profits that the proprietor had already derived from exploiting the secret (which diminished the government's obligation); and, on the other hand, the additional earnings that might accrue in the future if the formula were not published (which increased the obligation). On the first point, the reporters maintained that Elisabeth Lechat had benefited handsomely from the royal privilege of 1781. It was true, as she argued, that the contract signed that year by the four children of Michel-Antoine Belloste had divided the rewards: after their mother's death, the physician Jean-Baptiste (Lechat's husband) was to exploit the remedy together with Antoine, and they would have to pay an annual *rente* of 2,000 livres to each of their siblings. They had the option, however, of acquiring the interest of the two passive partners for 24,000 livres apiece. Nothing now proved that Jean-Baptiste's widow had not bought out all the other heirs — indeed she must have, if (as her notarised document attested) she could deal with the government in her own name. (The authors added, somewhat sheepishly, that the government could not enter into all the details of these private arrangements, and that they had cited a few only 'because it is a question of establishing the amount of an indemnity for the cession of a thing that has no real value, and because in order to reconcile as much as possible the different interests, it is necessary to gather as much evidence as possible'.) The government, the report concluded, owed no more favours to a remedy-owner who had already gained so much; an indemnity of 24,000 livres seemed too high. If, however, one considered the second point — the loss of income resulting from publication of the formula — it did not seem possible to reduce the widow's compensation below 12,000 francs, or an annual *rente* of 1,200, without 'hurting her interests'.[77]

The collapse of Napoleon's regime in 1814 prevented a definitive resolution of the problem under the Empire, but the case is an interesting one, for it suggests the extent to which the question of conflicting property rights could submerge what in principle was the overriding issue — promoting and defending public health. In the various exchanges between Elisabeth Lechat and the medical commissions, the merits of Belloste's pills figured only incidentally. Lechat feared that her livelihood was about to be expropriated, and that the various boards would not give sufficient consideration to her personal circumstances. The bureaucrats, for their part, bickered over the compensation to which her 'property' in the remedy entitled her. Nor did the authorities seize the opportunity to strike a blow against unqualified practice of pharmacy; in the end, they seemed willing to stretch the law and allow her to continue selling the remedy, as the decree of Prairial allowed.

The commission on secret remedies was disbanded in 1813, leaving responsibility for assessing new remedies in the hands of the Paris Faculty of Medicine. The programme of 1810 had fallen far short of the goal of publishing good remedies and suppressing bad ones. Secret remedies were not abolished, though the campaign to regulate and control them continued, drawing on the resources of the faculties, the departmental *jurys médicaux*, the health councils in Paris and major provincial cities, and, after 1820, the newly created Académie Royale de Médecine. The government had in effect reverted to the limited toleration of the Year XIII.

Why did the project collapse? The view of therapeutics on which it was based no doubt contradicted the prevailing assumptions of French patients and many of their doctors. In 1812, Richerand could still cite with approval the observation of the eighteenth-century physician Johann Georg von Zimmermann: 'For the majority of physicians, as for the people, . . . practical medicine is nothing other than the good fortune of possessing a recipe for each ailment.'[78] The main obstacle in the path of the abolitionists, however, was not a medical concept, but a legal one: the inventor's property rights in his formula. On this one point the petitioners, beaten back on every other issue, held their own. In the regulation of medical practice, the physicians had been able to cite both the interests of public health and a sort of property right in medical practice, acquired through their expenditures for training and certification and guaranteed by their diploma; but in the regulation of the remedy trade, as in other branches of commerce and industry, these claims conflicted, and the government's reverence for property favoured the entrepreneur. Total elimination of secret remedies would have meant the wholesale expropriation of the vast majority of proprietors whose preparations did not win professional approval. In the end, the French continued to draw a chaste veil over trade secrets in medicine.

Notes

1. See A.C. Wootton, *Chronicles of Pharmacy*, 2 vols (London, Macmillan, 1910), ch. 21, 'Noted Nostrums'. Wootton comments: 'The term "patent medicines", as now popularly used, means generally secret medicines, and the meaning is therefore in exact contradiction to the expression. Truthfully to declare the composition of these proprietary compounds would ruin their sale' (II, 162).
2. Indeed, discussions of 'medical quackery' in the twentieth century typically focus on the nostrum peddlers. The fullest general histories of patent medicines deal with the United States: James Harvey Young, *The Toadstool Millionaires: A Social History of Patent Medicines in America before Federal Regulation* (Princeton, Princeton University Press, 1961); idem, *The Medical Messiahs: A Social History of Health Quackery in Twentieth-Century America* (Princeton, Princeton University Press, 1967).
3. For an example of toleration of secret remedies (including some condemned by the medical faculties), see Olivier Faure, *Genèse de l'hôpital moderne: les hospices civils de Lyon de 1802 à 1845* (Lyons, Presses Universitaires de Lyon, 1982), 100, 232.
4. Matthew Ramsey, 'Traditional Medicine and Medical Enlightenment: The Regulation of Secret Remedies in the Ancien Régime', *Historical Reflections/Réflexions historiques*, 9 (1982), 215-32.
5. A still useful survey of the problem can be found in Louis Faligot, *La Question des remèdes secrets sous la Révolution et l'Empire* (Paris, E.H. Guitard, 1924). For the history of regulatory legislation: Marcel Bouvet, 'La Législation des remèdes secrets de 1778 à 1803', *Bulletin de la Société d'Histoire de la Pharmacie*, 4 (1923), 204-16. For a brief overview of regulation in the nineteenth century: Alex Berman, 'Drug Control in Nineteenth-century France: Antecedents and Directions', in John B. Blake (ed.), *Safeguarding the Public: Historical Aspects of Medicinal Drug Control* (Baltimore, Johns Hopkins University Press, 1970), 3-14.
6. See Dora B. Wiener, 'Le Droit de l'homme à la santé: une belle idée devant l'Assemblée Constituante, 1790-91', *Clio medica*, 5 (1970), 209-23.
7. Significant reform did not come until 1926. See André Narod Narodetzki, *Le Remède secret: législation et jurisprudence, de la loi du 21 germinal an XI au décret du 13 juillet 1926* (Paris, Librairie Générale de Droit et de Jurisprudence, 1928).
8. For a statement of the critique (from the early nineteenth century), see Anthelme-Balthasar Richerand, *Des Erreurs populaires relatives à la médecine*, 2nd edn (Paris, Caille & Ravier, 1812), 126; or Jean-Jacques Salet, *Essai sur les moyens de perfectionner l'exercice de la médecine dans les campagnes* (Valence, M. Aurel, 1810), p. 41. Salet suggests that the people think that 'each disease has its remedy, and that the art [of medicine] is restricted to knowing what it is'.
9. See Lester S. King, *The Medical World of the Eighteenth Century* (Chicago, University of Chicago Press, 1958), ch. 7.
10. Michel Foucault, *The Birth of the Clinic: An Archaeology of Medical Perception*, trans. A.M. Sheridan Smith (London, Tavistock Publications 1974), chs 1 and 6. Charles Rosenberg provides a convenient overview of the relationship between medical theory and therapeutics in 'The Therapeutic Revolution: Medicine, Meaning and Social Change in Nineteenth-Century America', in Rosenberg and Morris J. Vogel (eds), *The Therapeutic Revolution: Essays in the Social History of American Medicine* (Philadelphia, University of Pennsylvania Press, 1979), 1-25.
11. Pierre-Jean-Georges Cabanis, *Du Degré de certitude de la médecine*, in *Oeuvres complètes*, 5 vols (Paris, Bossange Frères, 1823-5), I, 474-6.
12. Lester S. King, *The Philosophy of Medicine: The Early Eighteenth Century* (Cambridge, Mass., Harvard University Press, 1978), 189.
13. Gaston Bachelard, *La Formation de l'esprit scientifique: contribution à une psychanalyse de la connaissance objective*, 6th edn (Paris, Librairie Philosophique J. Vrin, 1969), 112.

14. John Jones, *Medical, Philosophical, and Vulgar Errors of Various Kinds, Considered and Refuted* (London, T. Cadell, Jr. & W. Davies, 1797), 6-7.
15. J.-D.-T. de Bienville, *Traité des erreurs populaires sur la santé* (The Hague, P.F. Gosse, 1775), 132-3.
16. Faligot (note 5), 22.
17. Jean-Paul Marat, *Les Charlatans modernes, ou lettres sur le charlatanisme académique* (Paris, Imprimerie de Marat, 1791). See Roger Hahn *The Anatomy of a Scientific Institution: The Paris Academy of Sciences, 1666-1803* (Berkeley and Los Angeles, University of California Press, 1971), chs 5-8.
18. *Journal de médecine, chirurgie, pharmacie &c.* (1788), 573-4.
19. Louis-Etienne Gachet, *Problème médico-politique pour et contre les arcanes ou remèdes secrets . . . discussion impartiale* (Paris, the author, nd), 19, 23, 36-7, 38, and *passim*. See also *idem, Manuel des goutteux et des rhumatistes, ou l'art de se traiter soi-même de la goutte, du rhumatisme . . .* (Paris, M. Gachet, 1785). Cf. the pamphlet by Jean-Stanislas Mittié, doctor-regent of the Paris Faculty *A l'Assemblée Nationale, sur le traitement de la syphilis par les végétaux* (no place or publisher, 1789), which protested the failure of the Société Royale to recognise his vegetable treatment of venereal disease and denounced the society as a 'company of physician aristocrats' (p. 5).
20. Albert Couvreur, *La Pharmacie et la thérapeutique au XVIIIe siècle vues à travers le* Journal Encyclopédique *de Pierre Rousseau, à Bouillon*, 2nd edn 2 vols (Paris, Vigot Frères, 1953), I, 68.
21. 'Des Secrets en médecine', *Journal de médecine* (January 1789), 5-43; quotation, p. 5. Cf. *Aux Représentans du peuple français: plan général pour l'enseignement, la pratique, et la police de la médecine* (nd), copy in Archives Nationales, Paris (henceforth A.N.), *AD VIII 33, tit. 4, art. 6*. For a sharp critique of the programme of the Société Royale: Noël Retz, *Exposé succinct à l'Assemblée Nationale, sur les facultés et les sociétés de médecine* (Paris, Chez Devaux, 1791 (reprinted from vol. 7 of *Annales de l'art de guérir*)), 13-15.
22. François Thiéry, *Voeux d'un patriote sur la médecine en France où l'on expose les moyens de fournir d'habiles médecins au royaume, de perfectionner la médecine et de faire l'histoire naturelle de la France* (Paris, Garnery, 1789), 78.
23. Société Royale de Médecine, *Nouveau Plan de constitution pour la médecine en France* (no place or publisher, 1790), 125-32; quotation, 127.
24. A general history of the committee, which functioned until the end of the Constituent Assembly (September 1791), may be found in H. Ingrand, *Le Comité de Salubrité de l'Assemblée Nationale Constituante* (Paris, Paris Medical Thesis, 1934, no. 432). Toby Gelfand has called attention to the exchanges between the committee and the Société Royale de Médecine, preserved in Box 4 of the archives of the Académie Royale de Chirurgie, at the Académie Nationale de Médecine, Paris.
25. A.N. AF I*23, *procès-verbaux* of the committee, fol. 83^R, 28 May 1791.
26. 'Projet de décret sur l'enseignement et l'exercice de l'art de guérir, présenté au nom du Comité de Salubrité, par M. Guillotin, député de Paris', *Journal de médecine* (October 1791), 51 (tit. 5, art. 28 of project). See Faligot (note 5), 42.
27. For the society's work on secret remedies during the Revolution, see MS 15, Académie Nationale de Médecine, table of inventors (last entry, p. 316) and archives of the society, Box 199, Dossiers 30-38, 1792/93. Cf. the last records of the Paris Faculty of Medecine, 'Commentaires', MS vol. 25.
28. A.N. F^{17} 1146, Dossier 4, Cardon, Petition to National Convention; see *Archives parlementaires*, 1st series, vol. 79, pp. 337-8, 26 Brumaire Year II = 16 November 1793. Cf. Jeudy de Lhoumaud, *Adresse et conseils patriotiques, à l'Assemblée Nationale, sur l'importance de la réforme de la médecine et du charlatanisme en France . . .* no publisher, (Paris, 1791); the owner of a remedy for venereal disease, the author suggested that the only true charlatanism was the ignorance of the physicians, and that only men of genius should be admitted to the medical field.

29. Hahn (note 17), ch. 8.
30. *Décret de l'Assemblée Nationale, du 14 avril 1791* . . . (Paris, Imprimerie Nationale, 1791).
See Georges Dillemann, 'Le Monopole pharmaceutique et le décret du 2 mars 1791 [on professional freedom]', *Revue d'histoire de la pharmacie*, 27 (1980), 235-7.
31. Bénédicte Dehillerin. 'Le Collège de Pharmacie de Paris: du régime des corporations au régime de germinal, ou de l'étonnante vitalité du modèle parisien', *thèse de 3e cycle* (University of Paris I, 1981), chs 1 and 2 (p. 40 on analysis of remedies).
32. The only remaining central authority that could exercise some sort of oversight was the committee on public education of the revolutionary assemblies, which had jurisdiction over medical affairs. Some isolated materials (including petitions from remedy owners) for the years III-VI (1794-8) can be found in A.N. F^{17} 2273-76.
33. Faligot (note 5), 57.
34. A.N. F^{17} 2273, 9 Messidor VI=27 June 1798.
35. Faligot (note 5), 55.
36. Calès, report of 12 Prairial year V=31 May 1797, in Alfred de Beauchamp (comp.), *Médecine et pharmacie: projets de lois*, 5 vols (Paris, Imprimerie Nationale, 1888-95), I, 279-80.
37. Baraillon, *Motion d'ordre . . . au Conseil des Cinq-Cents, sur les établissements relatifs à l'art de guérir*, 14 Nivôse year V=3 January 1797, 3rd resolution (on police of medicine), title 5, in Beauchamp (note 36), I, 249-50; cf. Baraillon, *Rapport . . . au nom de la Commission d'Instruction Publique . . . sur la partie de la police qui tient à la médecine*, 8 Germinal Year VI=28 March 1798 (Paris, Imprimerie Nationale, Year VI), pp. 18-19.
38. *Rapport fait par Hardy au nom des Commissions d'Instruction Publique & d'Institutions Républicaines réunies, sur l'organisation des écoles de médecine*, 1 Frimaire Year VII=21 November 1798 (Paris, Imprimerie Nationale, Year VII) p. 16.
39. Faligot (note 5), 58.
40. Text of law in *Bulletin des lois*, 3rd series, 8 (Paris, Imprimerie de la République, Year XI), no. 270.
41. Ordinance of 17 Frimaire Year XII=9 December 1803 (Faligot (note 5), 66): law of Pluviôse Year XIII=18 February 1805, cited in Adolphe Trébuchet, *Jurisprudence de la médecine, de la chirurgie, et de la pharmacie en France* . . . (Paris, J.-B. Baillière, 1834), 366.
42. Text in *Bulletin des lois*, 4th series, 3 (Paris, Imprimerie Impériale, Year XIV), no. 813. A further ordinance on remedies that had already been approved was promulgated on 10 Thermidor Year XIII=29 July 1805 (see Faligot (note 5), 68). Some local officials had interpreted the original legislation to mean that approval by any physician or district notable would suffice.
43. See, for example, the material on the evaluation of Mettemberg's 'antipsoric' remedy in the archives of the Paris Faculty of Pharmacy, Register 52 (1810).
44. The archives of the cases considered by the Ministry of the Interior are mainly in A.N. F^8 149-67, arranged alphabetically by name of petitioner. Some material can also be found in A.N. F^{15} 141.
45. Archives Départementales (henceforth A.D.) de l'Yonne, 5 M 7/1, nos 78-81, January 1808.
46. Conseil de Salubrité de la Seine, report to Conseil d'Etat, 11 February 1810; papers in Archives de la Préfecture de Police, Paris.
47. Richerand (note 8), 310-11.
48. A.N. F^8 151, minutes of meeting, Paris Faculty of Medicine, 17 May 1810.
49. A.N. F^8 152, 9 April 1809. According to the petitioner, the Minister of War nevertheless suggested that the remedy was simple to use and might perhaps be recommended to country priests.
50. A.N. F^8 152, minute of deliberation by Ecole de Médecine de Paris, 25 Brumaire Year XII=17 November 1803; testimonial from Sophie de Muray, 1 Germinal Year

XII=22 March 1804.
  51. A.N. F⁸ 151, nd (beginning of First Empire).
  52. See Boyveau-Laffecteur, *Recueil de recherches et d'observations sur les différentes méthodes de traiter les maladies vénériennes* . . . (Paris, The Author, new edn 1810).
  53. 'Loi relative aux découvertes utiles, et aux moyens d'en assurer la propriété aux auteurs, donnée à Paris le 7 janvier 1791', in *Lois et actes du gouvernement* (Paris, Imprimerie Nationale, 1806), vol. 2, pp. 323-9. See Adolphe Trébuchet, 'Des Brevets d'invention délivrés pour remèdes secrets', *Annales d'hygiène publique et de médecine légale*, 29 (1843), 203-11.
  54. See, for example, A.N. F⁷ 3763, police bulletin, 13 June 1809, on Pinel woman, wife of Le Boulanger, who sold a 'sovereign water' and falsely described herself as a midwife: the responsible *conseiller d'état* proposed an administrative penalty of a month's detention, since the defendants found ways of escaping the legal penalty when brought to court.
  55. Text in *Bulletin des lois*, 4th series, 13 (Paris, Imprimerie Impériale 1811), no. 5874.
  56. *Conseiller d'état* for 2nd arrondissement, Police Générale, 13 September 1810; copy in A.D. Yonne 5 M 7/1, no. 91. See Matthew Ramsey, 'Sous le Régime de la législation de 1803: trois enquètes sur les charlatans au XIXᵉ siècle'. *Revue d'histoire moderne et contemporaine*, 27 (1980), 486-94.
  57. 'Projet d'organisation et plan de travail pour la commission des remèdes secrets' and 'Instruction pour les propriétaires des remèdes secrets' (15 October 1810), in Trébuchet (note 41), 636-41.
  58. *Ibid.*, 641-2.
  59. Richerand (note 8), 312, describes the challenges to the commission's legal jurisdiction and the impartiality of its judges.
  60. Most of the relevant documents are in A.N. F⁸ and F¹⁵ (see note 44). Some additional material can be found in the papers of the commission on secret remedies of the Académie Royale de Médecine, created in 1820; see Box 65 (and subsequent Boxes for the period after 1824), Académie Nationale de Médecine, Paris.
  61. A.N. F¹⁵ 141, Péroutet (or Péroutel), nd.
  62. *Ibid.*, Pierre-Daniel Formel, 10 May 1813.
  63. A.N. F⁸ 167, Warmon to Minister of the Interior, 21 November 1810, with commission's response.
  64. A.N. F⁸ 162, Minister of the Interior to Salmon-Maugé, 5 November 1811.
  65. A.N. F¹⁵ 141, 16 March 1813 (illegible signature).
  66. A.N. F⁸165, extract from the commission's deliberations, 11 January 1811.
  67. A.N. F⁸ 167, Vincent to Minister of the Interior, 26 May 1811; extract from commission's deliberations, 26 July.
  68. A.N. F⁸ 165, Seltez to Minister of the Interior, 17 September 1810; commission's reply (extract from Register, 25 May 1811).
  69. A.N. F⁸167, Villars recipe; commission's reply, 2 September 1811.
  70. A.N. F⁸ 162, Saillet remedy, extract from commission's deliberations, 4 January 1811.
  71. A.N. F¹⁵ 141, Minister of the Interior to Vaubaillon, 26 September 1812; Vaubaillon's response, 20 December 1812.
  72. For the *ancien régime* privileges: archives of the old Paris College of Pharmacy, Paris Faculty of Pharmacy, Register 12, nos 44 (1758) and 46 (1781), and archives of the Société Royale de Médecine (Académie de Médecine, Paris), Box 96, dossier 102. The complete dossier is in the archives of the commission on secret remedies of the Académie Royale de Médecine, Box 68; the documents cited below are from this file. For a summary of the case: *Archives générales de médecine*, 22, (1830), 418-19. On the history of the remedy, see Maurice Bouvet, 'Les Pilules de Belloste', *Bulletin des sciences pharmacologiques* 35 (1928), 246-59 and 296-312.
  73. Notarised attestation prepared by J.-C.-T Guenoux, 1 April 1806; commission

decision, 25 January 1811.
 74. Belloste widow to appeals board, 9 July 1812; to Minister of the Interior, same date.
 75. Reply of appeals board, 24 September 1812; signed statement by Belloste widow, 21 January 1813.
 76. Minister of the Interior to Faculty of medicine, 27 April 1813, and to Belloste widow (same date); the council's decision was dated 19 March. Widow to Faculty of Medicine, 26 March 1813.
 77. Faculty report of August 1813.
 78. Richerand (note 8), 307.

6 'THE VILE RACE OF QUACKS WITH WHICH THIS COUNTRY IS INFESTED'

Irvine Loudon

The Quack Perceived

It was, as one would guess, an angry doctor who provided the title for this chapter. Although it may be obvious who said it, however, it is much more difficult to guess when it was said. It might have been at any time between the late seventeenth and twentieth centuries (in fact it was 1846)[1] because the conflict between the regular, on the one hand, and the irregular practitioners, on the other, was long-standing and rich in invective, accusation and counter-accusation. This conflict, or at least one aspect of it, is my subject — the perception of quackery from the point of view of the regular practitioners. To narrow it down even further, I shall concentrate especially on the way in which that perception shaped the development of the medical profession during the late eighteenth century and first half of the nineteenth — the so-called period of medical reform.[2]

If one looks behind the invective to discover who is being labelled as an irregular there is an obvious and well-recognised difficulty. Before the Apothecaries Act of 1815 and medical registration in 1858, the term 'qualified medical practitioner' had no precise limits. At opposite ends of the spectrum the physician with his MD and the itinerant quack of the market-place were clearly delineated. At the centre, however, was a blurred grey area in which the identification of an individual as a 'regular' or 'irregular' practitioner was often impossible, for it depended on the observer. In general, the further one goes back from the nineteenth century, the larger this blurred area becomes. Pelling and Webster, for example, in their account of medical practitioners in the sixteenth century, recognised the impossibility of a clear-cut regular/irregular distinction and used the term 'medical practitioner' to describe 'any individual whose occupation is basically concerned with the care of the sick'.[3] Physicians, surgeons, apothecaries and others all held their own views on who was and who was not a quack.

In 1712, the physician Francis Guybon broadly defined the quack as anyone who practised physic but lacked a classical education and knowledge of the classical texts, implicitly condemning the surgeon and apothecary who strayed into the field of physic.[4] In 1727, Coltheart, a surgeon, defined as a quack anyone who trespassed on the surgeon's monopoly in the treatment of venereal disease.[5] The fully apprenticed apothecary despised the grocer-apothecary who had served no apprenticeship and could not read a physician's prescription, while the latter looked down on the healers and midwives of the backstreets. They, in turn, might well have been deeply offended by such snobbery since, from their level, the quack was the shabby itinerant, a stranger, here today and gone tomorrow before he could be found out. In short, one can visualise all these people ranged on a flight of steps, the physician at the top, then the surgeon and so on down to the itinerant at the very bottom. At every level the individual shouted 'Quack!' at all below him.

Even this simile, however, makes no allowance for two other groups of practitioners. First, there was the regular practitioner (so defined in terms of training and formal qualifications) who adopted the manners and appearances of the quack. Chevalier Taylor MD is the most famous of these medical transvestites. Second, there were the gentry and members of the professional classes who were apt, for reasons of philanthropy or merely as a hobby, to 'take up' the practice of medicine, and usually did so with complete impunity. The Anglican clergy provided a number of examples[6] and James Clegg (1679-1755), Presbyterian minister in Chapel-en-Frith in Derbyshire, practised physic extensively in order to feed his growing family. He acquired the official label of 'physician' solely because, at the age of fifty, his success provoked the jealous anger of his Anglican colleagues.[7] Threatened with prosecution in the ecclesiastical courts, he bought an MD from Aberdeen to regularise his second occupation. But it was not only the clergy. George Winter, a 'practical farmer' (his own description) who lived near Bristol, published a *Compendious System of Husbandry* in 1797. With delightful insouciance he devoted the whole of the long preface to his practice as an amateur physician, which resulted from the chance inheritance of his physician uncle's manuscripts and medical texts. He spent his evenings reading them, was fascinated, and treated the local poor free of charge, three days a week, regularly.[8] Probably his neighbours, medical and lay, saw nothing more reprehensible in this than mild eccentricity.

Social class, in other words, made a difference. The gentleman farmer and gentlemen of the cloth who dabbled in physic were usually spared the lash of the regular-bred practitioners. As for the other irregulars, the degree of antagonism and the venom of the invective seems to have been related most of all to those periods in which one or more groups of medical practitioners believed their livelihood was seriously threatened by irregular practice. For any section or group of regular practitioners it became customary when times were hard to lay the blame at the feet of the irregulars. Get rid of the quack and all would be well. The quack was the enemy and also the scapegoat.

Thus, in the late seventeenth and early eighteenth centuries, when apothecaries were invading the practice of physic on a large scale, we find the physicians complaining incessantly about 'the increase in quackery' in the form of the apothecaries.[9] By the mid-eighteenth century medical practitioners, especially the rank-and-file practitioners, the apothecaries and surgeon-apothecaries, became notably more prosperous.[10] The antagonism of the physicians towards the apothecaries began to diminish and the period 1740-90 is on the whole remarkable for the absence of tracts and pamphlets vilifying the quack. Medical prosperity associated with the consumer revolution (medicine being one of the commodities in greater demand) allowed practitioners to ignore the quack. This was the period which Richard Smith of Bristol described as the 'Golden Age of Physic' and it was income, not learning, he had in mind.[11] But it was shortlived. In the final years of the eighteenth century and early years of the nineteenth there was an unparalleled outburst against the evils of quackery; only this time it was not the physicians but the surgeon-apothecaries and their successors, the general practitioners, who led the attack. The whole race of quacks was stigmatised, but the outburst was not due to any rise in the numbers or activities of irregulars as a whole: it was engendered by the growth of one group only — the dispensing druggists. The rise of the dispensing druggist occupies the centre of the stage in this essay. It was an event which brought into the open the whole question of irregular practice.

The Rise of the Dispensing Druggist

This increase occurred in the final years of the eighteenth century and continued into the first half of the nineteenth. Previously, druggists were nearly always wholesalers, supplying the apothecaries. When the change occurred, however, the druggist started to supply the public with medicine sold over the counter at a much lower price than that charged by medical practitioners. The latter, accusing the druggists of treating diseases about which they knew nothing, classed them as new members of the 'vile race of quacks'.[12]

We now think of the chemist and druggist as an eminently respectable, trained, professional person. When he first appeared in the 1780s and 1790s he was anything but that. He was seen as an untrained, ignorant opportunist, a mere grocer pretending to be an apothecary, guilty of invading the rightful territory of the regular practitioner. He was the most dangerous, the most threatening quack there ever was. Richard Smith gives a vivid account of the rise of the druggists in Bristol. It was a Mr Jackson who was the first to have a 'magnificent shop with coloured bottles in the window'. He did a thriving trade and his apprentices soon set up on their own account. Druggists appeared all over the city and undercut the regular apothecaries who were forced to reduce their price for a 6oz. bottle of medicine from 2*s*. 6*d*. to a few pence.[13] A wide variety of sources confirm this rapid rise of the druggist all over England. Some examples can be found in Table 6.1.

Table 6.1: Numbers of Dispensing Druggists and Regular Medical Practitioners, Late Eighteenth and Early Nineteenth Centuries (Southwest England)

Town	Date	Physicians	Surgeons and apothecaries	Druggists
Bristol	1775	8	56	3
	1793-4	18	52	12
	1819	21	89	29
	1835	22	104	56
	1845	25	108	61
Salisbury	1783	3	6	1
	1793-4	2	8	1
	1822	3	10	3
	1842	4	10	8
Devizes	1783	0	3	1
	1822	0	4	2
	1839	1	7	5
	1842	4	5	6
Dorchester	1793	1	5	0
	1823-4	0	3	3
	1855	1	9	5
Blandford	1793	1	5	0
	1823-4	1	2	2
	1855	1	9	6
Chippenham	1793-4	0	4	0
	1822	1	3	2
	1842	1	7	6

Sources: various trade directories and Bristol Infirmary biographical memoirs.

The effect on medical practitioners was sometimes devastating. Take Billy Broderip, the Bristol apothecary, for example. In the 1790s, when he had been long established as a popular and fashionable practitioner, he booked the extraordinary sums of £5,000 to £6,000 a year, and, after bad debts, obtained £3,500 to £4,500. He had his carriage and coachman, a town house and a country house (which the locals called Gallypot Hall), pictures, expensive furniture and all the signs of conspicuous wealth. In a few years the druggists had broken him. He took to the bottle, all his possessions disappeared, and he went bankrupt.[14] The druggists even colluded with the physicians, some of whom attended the druggists' shops, gave free advice, and split the profits on the medicine with the druggist. Others, no friends of the apothecaries, told their patients 'there was no need for their paying eighteenpence to an apothecary when the draught might be had for sixpence at the druggist'.[15] A father wrote to the *Monthly Magazine* in 1818 to say he had 'a family of four children and until I grew wiser I annually paid 20 to 30 pounds per annum for their little ailings, for which I now get medicine for about as many shillings at a neighbouring druggist'.[16] Such were the inroads made by the druggists (it was calculated that the average London apothecary had lost £200 a year as a consequence) that the ephemeral and ineffectual General Pharmaceutical Association of Great Britain was established in 1794.[17] It would be easy to mistake this by its title for an association of druggists. In fact, it was an association of apothecaries and surgeon-apothecaries, founded specifically to attack the druggists. Its only claim to fame is that it marked the beginning of the period of medical reform.

Not surprisingly, it was pointed out by several writers that the druggist of the 1790s was only imitating the apothecary of the 1690s:[18]

> The apothecary, who was formerly only a druggist, had become a physician . . . the druggists took possession of his vacant stool and thus excited the same jealousy in the new physician as the encroachment of the apothecary had done in the mind of the old physician . . . the apothecaries were certainly wrong for becoming grand, and shutting up their own shops, because they hastened the sad catastrophe: but we believe that nothing would have prevented it.

It may seem an apt analogy, but there was an important difference. The rise of the apothecary at the time of the case of the Royal College of Physicians of London v. Rose (House of Lords, 1704) by which the apothecaries won the right to visit, advise, and prescribe for patients (but only to charge for medicines), was the rise of a medical man

'The Vile Race of Quacks . . . '   111

expanding the scope of his activities. The apothecary was condemned not for practising medicine, but for stepping outside his shop, and then only by some London physicians. The druggist, however, was seen by all regular practitioners as an irresponsible, untrained quack: it was a situation that brought out into the open the whole question of irregular practice, not only by the druggist himself, but also by the fly-by-night itinerants, the local healers, the blacksmiths who did a bit of midwifery on the side, and even the clergymen-physicians. By 1800, quackery was brought into prominence not only as a threat to the economy of regular practice, but also as a blot on the fair name of English medicine.

Dr Harrison of Horncastle

This was the subject which dominated the first meeting of the Lincolnshire Medical Benevolent Society in 1804; the first president, Dr Edward Harrison of Horncastle, was persuaded to undertake on behalf of the society, the examination of the state of the practice of physic in England. He began in his own area.[19] The results are summarised in Table 6.2. Less well known, but even more important, were the replies received by Harrison to a questionnaire sent out to practitioners all over Britain, the first, if not the only, attempt at a quantitative estimate of the extent of irregular practice.[20] Some of the replies are summarised in the appendix at the end of this chapter (pp. 123-5). Medical practitioners, already disturbed by irregular practice, were shocked at its extent as revealed by Harrison's investigations. In round figures, it seemed there were nine irregulars (including, that is, midwives and druggists) to every regular: in other words, a whole army intent on taking the bread from the mouths of the regular fraternity and indifferent to the harm they inflicted on the public.

It was a scandal. Medical practitioners decided that legislation was needed to license all the regular practitioners and outlaw the quack, but so far, it may be said, the evidence produced had all come from the most biased source imaginable, the medical practitioners. Was there really such an army of irregulars? Were they really so outrageous in their practices? These are not easy questions to answer. It was not the habit of irregulars to leave much account of themselves, much less their feelings about their profession. We see them for the most part through the eyes of their enemies. Fortunately, however, they were great ones for pamphlets and self-advertisement, and a collection of such material tends to confirm the ubiquity of the irregular in just the historical period with which we are concerned.

Table 6.2: Numbers of Regular and Irregular Practitioners in the Horncastle and Market Razon districts of Lincolnshire, 1804-6

Physicians	5
Surgeons and Apothecaries	18
Druggists	34
Irregulars of both sexes over and above the druggists	37
Midwives	63

Source: E. Harrison, *The Ineffective State of the Practice of Physic*, (1806).

The Irregulars of Hull c.1780-1830

This source consists of a substantial collection of advertisements and pamphlets published in or near Hull between 1780 and 1830.[21] They provide a picture of the medical subculture of provincial England during this period. Admirers of Donnizetti may often have felt that Dr Dulcamara was a pardonable operatic exaggeration. Not a bit of it. In flamboyance and outrageous claims he had his contemporary rivals in Yorkshire.[22]

Roughly half of this collection is advertisements for medicines, and the other half pamphlets by irregulars proclaiming their skills. Medicines were sold under names designed to catch the eye and the imagination. Dr Solomon (of Gilead House, near Liverpool) produced the Cordial Balm of Gilead with its nice Old Testament touch.[23] It was recommended for those 'suffering from shattered constitutions, nervous and bilious complaints and phthisis pulmonalis'. The balm, at half a guinea a bottle, was obtainable at the 'Mercantile Gazette Office adjoining the Post-Office, Liverpool, also Mr Martin Keene, Bookseller, No 6 College Green, Dublin'. One notes in passing that the sale of medicine by booksellers and printers, which was usual throughout the eighteenth century, survived the early rise of the chemist and druggist, at least in the north of England, until the 1820s. There were constant references in this area both to booksellers and druggists as the places for purchasing patent medicines.[24] Sometimes the names of the famous were borrowed to boost a product; for instance, Dr Bateman's Pectoral Drops,[25] Dr Boerhaave's Red Pill, Dr Radcliffe's Elixir and Dr Anderson's or the Scotch Pill. More often, however, the name belonged to the real or supposed inventor of the remedy — Squire's Original Grand Elixir, Mr

'The Vile Race of Quacks . . . ' 113

Lignum's Royal Anti-scorbutic Drops, the True Daffy's Elixir and Dr Norris's Fever Drops. R. and L. Jordan were 'the inventors and sole proprietors of the Balm of Soriacum' and Dr Borthwick at his Botanical Establishment in Hull specialised in 'vegetable remedies'.

Whether a pamphlet advertised a specific remedy or the skill of an individual (or both in many instances) extravagant claims were often made of patronage by the famous. Cockle's Compound Anti-Bilious Pills were 'under the patronage of the Nobility and Clergy; Gentlemen in the Law, Medical Men, Officers in the Army Navy etc.'. This was modest. Splashed across the top of the advertisement for Dr Scott's Bilious and Liver Pills in the boldest type was the claim that they were used with good results by 'the Dukes of Devonshire, Northumberland and Wellington, the Marquesses of Salisbury, Angelsea [sic] and Hastings, the Earls of Pembroke, Essex and Oxford and the Bishops of London, Exeter and Gloucester' — three to each rank, and, seeing there was no Trade Descriptions Act, why not?

Letters from grateful patients recounting their amazing recoveries when all the regulars had failed were commonplace,[26] and these were usually designed to underline the long lists of diseases which the irregular claimed to cure — lists in which there was often a bizarre conjunction of the grave and the trivial, where the cure for cancer and smelly breath, for phthisis or typhus and corns on the feet, rubbed shoulders in the same sentence. Few exceeded Mr English, 'practitioner in physic', in this respect.[27] Even when a remedy was advertised as a specific rather than the usual panacea, it covered the whole of its special field. Dr Norris's Fever Drops were a certain cure not only for 'the Inflammatory and Putrid, the Malignant Epidemical or Endemical fever', but also for the 'slow commonly called Nervous, Miliary and Hectic fever, Typhus, Putrid Sore Throats and Ague'. Finally, in case you had missed the point, the drops were good for 'Fever'.

I tried to find some common factors in these lists of diseases and to discover what disorders were especially the prerogative of irregular practitioners and patent medicine sellers. The results were rather disappointing, mainly because the lists were so detailed and comprehensive — presumably on the basis that if you claimed to cure twenty diseases it might as well be forty. But there were a few pointers, both positive and negative. Children's diseases were almost never included, and childbirth was never mentioned except once when an irregular boasted of his knack for instant diagnosis of any and every disorder 'except childbed'. One notes, incidentally, that Dr Norris's Fever Drops cured all known fevers except puerperal or childbed fever. Obstetrics and paediatrics were not a part of the irregular's territory.[28] But there were some disorders which recurred with significant frequency. Deafness 'provided the tympanum or ear-drum is intact' was one, providing one of the few hints that chronic *otitis media* was probably, as one would expect, a common disorder. Ruptures or 'broken bellies' (either cured without a truss or by a special new piece of apparatus) were also prominent in the lists. Venereal disease, above all, was a quack's specialty, usually described euphemistically as 'a certain disease, however inveterate or long-standing, even if twenty years, cured in a week'. Dr Natras of 58 Carr Lane, Hull, not only specialised in the cure of venereal disorders but undertook the management of 'seminal weakness, unhappily so frequent and prevalent, arising either from early abuse, intemperance, excess of pleasure, mental sympathy or other injurious causes'.[29] One of the chief attractions of the irregular was the promise, implicit or explicit, of painless cures with non-injurious methods. Dr Johnson of 54 Old South End, Humber Street, Hull, presumably a rival of Dr Natras in the field of sexology, scorned the euphemisms and advertised openly the treatment of venereal disease with the guarantee of complete secrecy. Revealingly, he emphasised that his 'system is not injurious to the constitution as he avoids the use of *mercury* which has caused the death of thousands'.[30] Cancer cures were common in the vocabulary of the irregular, sometimes promised 'without operation'. The 'High German Dr Symon', as he called himself, included cancer among the diseases he cured and if you had a particle of doubt it could be eliminated by 'a cancer of the armpit of five pieces of 12 and one half ozs. weight which may be seen at the Doctor's House'. Proof positive. Scurvy, still treated by regulars and irregulars with medicines, more than fifty years after Lind's treatise, was the final specialty of the irregular — although the descriptions reveal the usual muddle between the possibly true cases with loose teeth and bleeding gums and other probably non-scorbutic conditions such as scabby skin eruptions (especially on the scalp) and a number of vague symptoms labelled as scorbutic.

If the irregular could be identified by the character of his pamphlets in these respects, he could also be spotted by his most famous characteristic of all — his itinerant lifestyle, even if this, like everything else, was sometimes embroidered. Dr Lambert ('from his dispensaries at 36 High Street, Borough, London, and 49 Queen Square, Bristol') claimed to visit regularly:

> The West Indies, the Isles of Scilly, London, Bristol, Birmingham, Leicester, Nottingham, Derby, Norwich, Lincoln, Boston,

Gloucester, Wolverhampton, Lichfield, Stourbridge and almost every other town in the Kingdom.

Perhaps he did, but the list lacks the ring of truth. Dr Gardner of 75 and 76 Long Acre, London, who had 'Under Divine Providence and by Royal Authority' achieved 'hundreds of extraordinary cures on patients of all ages from one month to 80 years' in London, Edinburgh, Glasgow and Dublin (where his skill had been proclaimed) was not the only irregular who provoked the obvious question: What are you doing in Hull, then?

These were extravagant claims; but the travels of the locally itinerant were obviously genuine. In 1815 Dr Taylor of Beverley announced that he had 'now made arrangements to attend at the Blue Boar Inn, Beverley, every Saturday from Ten till Four, every Wednesday at the Star Inn, Bridlington from Ten till Eight, and every Thursday at Driffield at the Bell from Ten till Four'. Patients only had to send their urine and he would tell at once if they were curable or not.[31] This glimpse of 'surgeries' or 'clinics' held regularly at inns (good, probably, for the innkeeper's trade as well) is not so very far removed from some rural branch surgeries held in the front rooms of cottages (where waiting-room and consulting-room were one and the same) as recently as the early years of the National Health Service. But the most local of all irregulars were the door-to-door variety. Many of the pamphlets in the Bodleian collection were designed to be pushed through the door with firm instructions to 'keep this paper clean' because the 'doctor' would call back to collect it. Dr Elcocks, for example, began his pamphlet by listing the usual diseases he cured, including the 'certain disorder, however inveterate', and then informed his reader: 'The Doctor who calls for this Bill will tell any person, male or female, their complaint or disorder without any examination or the least resemblance of their countenance, only by the smell of their handkerchiefs, or casting their urine.' Urine-casters, like bone-setters, were two a penny, but the handkerchief seems to be an original touch.

Who were the patients/clients of these ingenious men, and what were they charged? Where patent medicines were concerned, prices were remarkably uniform. The Cordial Balm of Gilead at half a guinea was expensive; most other preparations, whether balms, elixirs, cordials or fever drops, came in two or three sizes, the smallest at 1s. to 1s. 6d., the medium at 2s. 9d. and the family size at up to 7s. This seems expensive given that a labourer's wage was in the region of 5s. to 7s. a week. But an ointment specifically called 'The Poor Man's Friend ('Ulcerated

Legs if of twenty years standing and eruptions of every description . . . in the course of one week will be entirely cured') came in the same price range — the small for 1s. 1½d., the large for 2s. 9d. There seems little doubt that, for all their boasts of royal connections, these irregulars worked mostly among the cottages and tenements of the labouring classes, even when they had some devoted followers higher up the social scale.

A question that is not easily answered is whether a practitioner who would ordinarily be classified as 'regular' resorted to pamphleteering to increase his trade and was thus included in this collection. Many, after all, proclaimed themselves 'doctor' or 'surgeon'. Those who called themselves 'doctor' sometimes added 'MD' but seldom specified the university, although it was not their nature to hide their light under a bushel. 'Mr Innes, Surgeon', claimed a long career in the navy but was vague about whether he served as an ordinary seaman or as a paid-up naval surgeon. He also claimed attendance at Edinburgh where 'he was regularly graduated' and subsequently he attended 'the principal hospitals in England'. But he flourished neither 'MD Edinburgh' nor 'LRCS' after his name, and plain Mr Innes could be found at 'No 27 Blanket Row, Hull'.[32] At best, one suspects, these irregulars rubbed shoulders with medical students in a tavern or even, perhaps, attended a few lectures. But there is nothing to suggest this colourful collection of Hull irregulars included a self-advertising regular — not even one who served a full apprenticeship, let alone acquired a medical degree or licence from an established university or medical corporation.[33] Although the regular practitioners may on occasions have adopted some of the methods of the irregular, by the early nineteenth century the distinction between the two was usually clear. The irregulars stood out by the vigour of their pamphleteering, the extravagance of their claims to therapeutic skill and noble patronage and to some extent by the selection of diseases which they claimed as their territory.

The Irregulars and Medical Reform

The outstanding characteristics of the pre-Victorian irregulars, as the Hull collection of pamphlets shows, were their variety, individuality and salesmanship. Later in the nineteenth century, irregular practice tended to change from the flamboyant entrepreneur to groups of serious-minded practitioners who followed one of a number of heterodox systems of pathology or therapy. Often they claimed for their systems as much scientific respectability as orthodox medicine, but the medical profession tended to label them all as no more than a new series of fashionable but disreputable '-isms' and '-opathies', although some (notably homeopathy and mesmerism) dated from the late eighteenth or early nineteenth century.

As irregular practice became increasingly systematised in the 1840s it seems that the old-fashioned itinerant was dying out. In 1841 a medical practitioner noted that 'the regular imposing quack, with his farrago of receipts, who seldom visits the same neighbourhood but at very long intervals in order to avoid recognition . . . this class of practitioner is fast coming to a close'. Instead, he was being replaced by literate and educated empirics who read books. Together with the druggist they provided an even more formidable combination against the regulars.[34] In the early years of the century, however, the regular practitioners classified the irregulars into four clear groups — the druggists, the midwives, the itinerants and the local or 'stationary' irregulars. This last group included such exotic examples as water-casters, bone-setters, wart-charmers, 'curers by imagination' (a crude form of hypnosis) and the Greenland Doctors (see appendix at the end of this chapter, pp. 123-5). They were usually part-time healers whose main occupation or station in life included 'a collector of geese, failed grocers, workers in the leather line, a cobbler and a cutter, farriers, mechanics', and 'women who called themselves "doctresses" ' as well as the 'regularly educated surgeon-apothecary who acts in the manner of the empiric — to this person the ignorant flock in multitudes'. There was also the clergyman-physician: 'What think you Sir, of a clergyman receiving his pound note for a prescription whilst his wife goes daily to administer her nostrums to her neighbours?'[35]

It is easy to understand why the early general practitioners felt themselves surrounded by swarms of irregulars from a wide range of social classes, all intent on taking away their patients. And it is undeniable that, had none of the irregulars existed, the general practitioner would have been more prosperous. But one questions whether the difference would have been as great as the general practitioners imagined. The itinerant and local irregulars, like the later professors of heterodox systems of medicine, may have served different needs and different sections of the community. The cheapest irregulars found their custom largely among the very poor, unable to pay the regular practitioner. Above this level, it is clear that irregular practice had a special appeal to religious dissenters, political radicals, and certain sections of the aristocracy and royalty; strange bedfellows, but traces of such connections can still be observed today.

Regular practitioners, on the other hand, made their living chiefly among the middling sorts, from artisans and small shopkeepers to professional people. Childish ailments and the numerous common chronic conditions such as indigestion, rheumatism, constipation, menstrual disorders, bronchitis and leg ulcers were the basis of a regular practice of frequent attenders and a steady income. If the itinerant quack treated this group at all it was usually only fleetingly. The druggist, however, was different. His power was derived from being resident (and therefore unable to make unrealistic claims about his cures) and the tendency to use orthodox as well as patent medicines at much lower prices than the regular practitioner. It is clear that the druggists treated large numbers of the poor, as well as the middle classes. In 1844 H.W. Rumsey, a Gloucester surgeon, stated that 'one fourth of the population of Hull attend druggists and other irregulars', and in Southampton 'quite as many of the poor are prescribed for by druggists as by regular practitioners'. In Wakefield 'probably from 4000 to 5000 poor resort annually to the druggists', while in Lincoln 'all the retail druggists have considerable practice among the poor, both in chronic cases and in the early stages of acute complaints; minor operations are also performed by them'.[36] One notices again and again that when irregular practice was mentioned, druggists were put first. But it was the whole group of irregulars that were regarded as the enemy. What could be done to outlaw them?

The Attempted Suppression of Irregular Practice

The plan for medical reform devised by Edward Harrison grew directly from his researches into irregular practice. In essence, the plan was simple. The tripartite profession would be perpetuated. Each section would be subject to a process of standardised education, examination and licensing. Two advantages would result. The standard of medical education and practice would rise, and the distinction between the regular and the irregular would be clear and unmistakable. The public would be sensible and choose the qualified practitioner. The irregular would thus be put out of business. Harrison's plan, of course, was defeated by the London College of Physicians. Harrison was an Edinburgh-trained provincial physician, who showed no reverence for the College (of which he was not a member) even to the point of tactlessness. The College regarded Harrison as a rank outsider and set out to crush him. By December 1809 it had succeeded.[37] Harrison abandoned his plans and further measures for reform lay dormant until 1812 and the events which led up to the Apothecaries Act of 1815.

'The Vile Race of Quacks . . . ' 119

The Apothecaries Act was only a shadow of the original Bill conceived by the Association of Apothecaries and Surgeon-Apothecaries. As its president commented, 'that it is very unsatisfactory can be seen by comparing the Apothecaries Act as it is with the Bill first projected by the Association. Shorn, indeed, is the latter of its fair proportions'.[38] The original Bill was founded on the same basic premiss as Dr Harrison's plan for reform. Through a statutory process of medical education, examination and licensing, the general practitioner would be distinguished from the irregular. But the Bill went a good deal further. It was suggested that the power of awarding licences should be vested in sixteen district medical committees. After the appointed day no one would be allowed to practise as an apothecary, surgeon-apothecary or practitioner of midwifery without a licence; nor would anyone be allowed to practise as a midwife or 'compounder or dispenser of medicines'.[39] Midwives and druggists, in other words, were to be licensed as well and brought under the control of medical practitioners.

Membership of the association, initially about 200 and consisting of 'the first in rank, ability and character among the London Practitioners'[40] grew to over 3,000 in less than three years on the promise that, at last, irregular practice in all its forms would be controlled. By the time the Bill was modified and became the Apothecaries Act, however, the chemists and druggists had successfully petitioned Parliament and the clause to control them was removed, the clause for licensing midwives was dropped, and the administration was taken from the Association and given to the Society of Apothecaries. What was left was an ill-defined clause which made it illegal to practise as an apothecary after 1 August 1815 (unless established in practice beforehand) without the Licence of the Society.

Thoroughly disappointed at the outcome of the Act, general practitioners pinned their hopes on the penal clause and on the introduction at some later date of amendments to the Act. In both respects they were again disappointed. There were no significant modifications of the Act, except in the structure of the curriculum, and the penal clause was virtually useless as a means of preventing irregular practice. There were two reasons why it was a failure. First, it defined illegal practice in terms of practising as an apothecary. Irregulars who performed surgical cures were exempt from its penalties. Thomas Wakley, editor of the *Lancet*, went even further and, with faultless logic, maintained that in the legal sense 'acting as an apothecary' consisted solely of dispensing a physician's prescription, and nothing else.[41] This, of course, had never been one of the irregular's activities. The judiciary thought otherwise and, interpreting the spirit of the law, upheld a prosecution of a surgeon for treating a patient for a medical complaint.[42] The second reason was more important. The Society of Apothecaries could only take action as a result of informers, and when it did take action it had to bear the cost of the prosecution, often £300 to £400.[43] The Society, therefore, did all it could to avoid resorting to the law. By 1822 many informations had been laid but the Society proceeded only on four of them, of which only two were true irregulars. Instead, practitioners with the Licence of the Society were in the habit of laying information against their more successful medical colleagues who practised as general practitioners on the basis of an Edinburgh MD or LRCS, both evidence of a higher standard of education than the Apothecaries' Licence. The prosecution of these well-qualified Scottish-trained practitioners turned the operation of the penal clause into a farce.[44] One observer believed 'the future medical historian can scarcely believe that this is the state of physic in 1833'.[45]

Robert Upton, the Clerk of the Society of Apothecaries, responsible for the administration of the penal clause, admitted that although action had been taken on some informations, 'by far the greatest number of individuals [informed against] were of necessity left to pursue their practice undisturbed'.[46] This enraged a general practitioner who protested:[47]

> We complain of illegal practice at our own doors — practice which is robbing us of our legitimate reward of a long professional study — practice which you have publicly promised to check, but which you suffer to continue undisturbed, and it is nothing to us to know that you are engaged in stopping such practice elsewhere.

The irregular therefore continued to practise with as much impunity after the Act as before. The druggists thrived and, what was worse, it became increasingly difficult to distinguish between the medical practitioners and the druggists.

At first sight this seems an odd thing to say. One of the themes of the period of medical reform, stated openly not just by ambitious general practitioners but also by many physicians, was the new high standard of medical education and knowledge possessed by the general practitioner. In fact, it was often asserted that to all intents and purposes the general practitioner had become a physician with the added advantage of knowing surgery and pharmacy as well. The physician might boast of his 'liberal education' symbolised by his university degree, but that carried little weight when it was known how easily degrees could be bought, and when a knowledge of the classics was no longer the hallmark of the superior members of the medical profession. But the general practitioner was still separated from the physician by one small but unbridgeable gap, the dispensing of drugs with its stigma of trade. This was the area in which the druggist and the general practitioner walked side by side, and the public saw little to choose between them.

Although, therefore, the general practitioner aspired to the title of 'physician-in-ordinary' or 'physician in general practice',[48] as long as he dealt with drugs he was 'a mere poacher on the manor of the physician, the surgeon and the druggist'.[49] General practitioners despised the druggists as 'a set of small traders, ignorant of the property of medicines',[50] but in fact 'a great number of apothecaries [were] driven by necessity to become the actual chemists and druggists of the narrow streets and bye-lanes' pocketing 'the humblest coin', while the successful druggists of the 'Broadways . . . lined their tills with a more noble metal'.[51] Some of the London druggists — still household names today — were very successful in the early nineteenth century, and by 1820 the chemist's shop had become a 'social necessity'.[52] In every new area 'shops retailing drugs sprang up before the grocer, the butcher, the cheesemonger and put "Doctor" over their door'.[53] Some of these were druggists, others 'licentiates of Apothecaries Hall or Surgeon's College forced into retail trade in order to survive'.[54] If the 'medical man persists in identifying himself to the tradesman, he cannot expect the public to draw a distinction',[55] especially when some of the druggists took it on themselves to visit patients in their homes, practise surgery and even midwifery.[56]

In other words, as the general practitioner clambered up the ladder to get on a level with the physician, he noticed over his shoulder that the druggist below was steadily catching him up. The blurring, in the public's eyes, between the regularly educated general practitioner with his LSA (Licence of the Society of Apothecaries) and MRCS (Membership of The Royal College of Surgeons) and the druggist who put 'Doctor' over his door was one of the reasons why George Man Burrows, the President of the Association of Apothecaries and Surgeon-Apothecaries approved of the original plan to license the druggist. It had the advantage of 'defining that which was before undefined',[57] but it was a double-edged proposal. Licensing would have conferred a semi-professional status on the druggist. Therefore, the only remedy for the general practitioner (and it was one which was frequently advised) was to abandon the drug trade, send his prescriptions to the druggist like a physician, and charge only for visits and advice. Then there would be a clear difference between the regulars and all the irregulars. The general practitioner would not be held down by the 'shop', by the sale of bottles of medicines and boxes of pills, nor would the less respectable members of the profession be tempted to increase their income by selling articles of toilet and patent medicines. There was really no other way to put an unmistakable distance between the qualified medical practitioner and the unqualified druggist. It was, however, a solution which few general practitioners were willing to contemplate. In the nineteenth as much as in the eighteenth century, dispensing medicine was essential to his livelihood. It accounted, in most cases, for three-quarters of his income; sometimes even more.

Consequently, there was through the 1820s and 1830s a growing realisation that a monopoly of medical care could never be achieved; patent medicines and irregular practice could not be outlawed.[58] Guthrie saw in 1834 that if such proposals were put to Parliament members would stand up and claim they had 'been cured by Mr St John Long' or say, 'I was cured by Morison's pills when the regular doctors could not do it.' Patent medicines and irregular practice were fashions 'like brandy and French gloves and other things'.[59] The public would have them, say what you will. The only remedy was to educate the public in the hope of weaning them gradually from the irregulars.

Medical reform, which had started with the aim of defeating the irregular, now turned inwards from its prime objective and became, instead, an intraprofessional quarrel. The self-assertive general practitioner attempted to achieve the status of the physician and 'pure' surgeon and the Colleges of Physicians and Surgeons made sure that he failed. In an extraordinarily vicious and bitter conflict, the general practitioners were firmly kept in a subordinate position. In many ways it was all like a family quarrel. To outsiders (the lay public) it was mostly unknown or, if known, confusing and irrelevant. Parliament and successive Home Secretaries sympathised with Sir James Graham who, after strenuous attempts to achieve agreement in 1848 between physicians, surgeons and general practitioners, said that[60]

> Though he had sometime successfully shifted a hive of bees from a rickety stand to a safer spot, without much concern for a casual sting or two, he had made up his mind never again to try the experiment of lifting three hives at once or of concentrating them all under one glass.

By the twentieth century the compromises and inadequacies of the

Apothecaries Act and the bitterness of the period of medical reform were forgotten. As they receded into the distance they both received an aura of sanctity, because, it was said, they marked the division between old medieval ways and modern scientific medicine. The Act of 1815 was often referred to as one of the great reforming Acts of the nineteenth century. Since Holloway's notable papers in 1966, few now hold such rosy views.[61] Historians now tend to see the process of medical reform wholly in terms of the struggle of the general practitioner to achieve professional status, and the emergence of the consultant. The part played by irregular practice and the importance of the druggist, if recognised at all, tends to be in the background. It has been the purpose of this essay to describe the nature of irregular practice and the way it was perceived by regular practitioners, to stress its central importance in the initiation of the movement of medical reform, and to note the ineffectiveness of various attempts to eliminate the 'vile race of quacks' from English society.

Appendix

A selection of replies to a questionnaire sent out by Dr Edward Harrison of Lincolnshire in 1806 asking for data on the numbers of regular and irregular practitioners in various parts of Britain. The respondents were all regular medical practitioners.

The following were reported.

Suffolk (1)
'The chemists and druggists are of late become numerous . . . five in the principal town and in every town one or more.' Also a man who cured by 'imagination' and a person 'of much *reputation* in the cure of ulcerated legs'.

Suffolk (2)
Twelve quacks to every regular practitioner, but 'private quacks' much more numerous, such as clergymen and their wives who treated their flock for £1 each.

Cambridgeshire
'A failed grocer turned bone-setter and man-midwife'; urine-casters — 'generally very rich'; small-pox doctors, 'but Jenner has nearly ruined them'; 'The grocers in the villages sell drugs, which are always bad.'

Northumberland

Five empirics to every regular but nearly all of them part-timers.

Yorkshire

We have 'The "Greenland Doctors" . . . a set of failed mechanics who learn to bleed, and are then qualified for the place on board a Greenland ship. On their return . . . they go into the country until the next Greenland season.'

Durham

Physicians = 2; those practising surgery, midwifery and pharmacy = 5; druggists = 3; irregular and ignorant practitioners = 7; midwives = 2.

Nottingham

Four physicians all graduates of Scotland; 15 surgeon-apothecaries all practising midwifery; 13 druggists; 29 irregulars of both sexes over and above the druggists; 6 quacks; 11 midwives — all uninstructed; '78 persons exercise medicine for gain . . . of whom not one in four has previously been educated for the profession'.

Nottinghamshire District (Within 15 Miles of Nottingham, Excluding the City of Nottingham)

Thirty-five Surgeon-apothecaries and men-midwives; 14 druggists; 112 irregulars over and above the druggists; 123 midwives, all uninstructed; 286 persons exercising medicine for gain.

Sherborne

Twenty regular medical practitioners in radius of ten miles; 6 druggists; 1 or 2 irregulars — bone-setters and sellers of toads in bags as charms; 1 regularly educated surgeon-apothecary 'who acts in the manner of an empiric' — 'to this person the ignorant flock in multitudes'.

Stirling

'Regular quacks . . . who live entirely by quacking can hardly be expected to thrive in so poor a country as Scotland, and we have none of them here.'

Dorsetshire (Town not Specified)

'Surgeons without diplomas, instruments or knowledge'; 'apothecaries who have never been beyond the precincts of their parish'; 'accoucheurs ignorant of the shape and formation of the female pelvis'; 'grocers and stationers turned chemist and druggist'; 'quacks and empirics, both stationary and itinerant'.

Letters from Berkshire, Devonshire, Essex and Montrose in Scotland were exceptions in stating that irregular practitioners were outnumbered by the regular, and the correspondent from Essex was unique in believing they were decreasing in number.

Notes

1. J. Forbes, 'On the Patronage of Quacks and Impostors by the Upper Classes of Society', *British and Foreign Medical Review*, 21 (1846), 533-40.
2. The conventional chronological limits of the period of medical reform are from 1794, when the General Pharmaceutical Association of Great Britain was established, until the Medical Act of 1858.
3. M. Pelling and C. Webster, 'Medical Practitioners' in C. Webster (ed.), *Health, Medicine and Mortality in the Sixteenth Century* (London, Cambridge University Press, 1979), 166.
4. F. Guybon, *An Essay Concerning the Growth of Empiricism, or the Enlargement of Quacks* (London, 1712).
5. P. Coltheart, *The Quacks Unmasked* (London, for the author, 1727): 'We have the ablest Physicians and Surgeons in Europe and at the same time the greatest number of pretenders and ignorant quacks . . . a Coal-Porter, Tinker, Taylor, Midwife, Nurse etc, spring up like mushrooms in a night to be physicians and surgeons.'
6. Richard Napier, thanks to the work of Professor Michael MacDonald and Ronald Sawyer of the University of Wisconsin, is perhaps the best known and documented example from the early modern period. Richard Wilkes (1690-1760), Deacon of Stowe-by-Chartley, Staffordshire, was another clergyman who took up medicine without any formal training or qualifications and became a fashionable physician: N.W. Tildesley, 'Richard Wilkes of Willenhall, Staffs, an 18th century doctor', *Transactions of the Lichfield and South Staffordshire Archaeological and Historical Society*, 7 (1965-6), 1-10.
7. V.S. Doe, *The Diary of James Clegg of Chapel-en-Frith, 1708-55*, 3 vols (Derbyshire, Derbyshire Record Society, 1978, 1979, 1981).
8. G. Winter, *A New and Compendious System of Husbandry*, 2nd edn (London, 1797). He rationalised his eccentric preface by suggesting that knowledge of medical science would reinforce the science of husbandry, reflecting a broad eighteenth-century view of the unity of all scientific activities and thought.
9. C. Merrett, *A Short View of the Frauds and Abuses Committed by the Apothecaries*, 2nd edn (London, J. Allestely, 1670); Anon., *The Present State of Physick and Surgery in London* (London, 1701): 'The great increase of *Apothecaries* is evidently the cause of the present *Grievances* to the *Profession of Physick*, to *themselves* and to the *People*. They are become one *thousand*, including the *Partners*, more than ten to one *Physician*.' R. Pitt, *The Calamities of all the English in Sickness and the Sufferings of the Apothecaries from their Unbounded Increase* (London, J. Morphew, 1707).
10. This hypothesis is dealt with at length in I. Loudon, 'The Nature of Provincial Medical Practice in Eighteenth-century England', *Medical History*, 29 (1985), 1-32.
11. The memoirs of Richard Smith, junior (1772-1843), surgeon to the Bristol Infirmary, 'Bristol Infirmary Biographical Memoirs', 8 vols (Bristol, Bristol Record Office), II, 155.
12. Dr J. Power of Bosworth in 1806 described the druggists as 'persons who have served an apprenticeship to Grocers and Tea-Dealers . . . and are generally incompetent to judge betwixt good and bad drugs [and] many serious accidents have arisen from their selling one medicine for another, or giving them in improper dose': letter xvi, *Medical*

and *Chirurgical Review*, 13 (1806), clxxi-clxxii. See also J.M. Good, *The History of Medicine so far as it Relates to the Profession of Pharmacy* (London, C. Dilly, 1795); J. Bell, *Historical Sketch of the Progress of Pharmacy* (London, J. Churchill 1843); letter in *Medical and Chirurgical Review*, 13 (1806), clxxi-clxxii; J. Davies, *An Exposition of the Laws which Relate to the Medical Profession* (London, J. Churchill 1844), especially 40-1. Editorial 'On Medical Education. A Critical Analysis', *London Medical and Physical Journal*, 43 (1820), 500.

13. Smith (note 11), I, 94; and VI, 350.
14. Ibid., II, 152-64.
15. Ibid., II, 161.
16. 'C.H.', 'Increase of Medical Fees', *Monthly Magazine*, 44 (1817), 498-9.
17. J.M. Good (note 12).
18. *Letters to the President of the Associated Apothecaries and Surgeon Apothecaries of England and Wales on the Present State of the Practice of Physic and Surgery*, 1st series (London, Burgess & Hill, 1820), reviewed in *The London Medical and Physical Journal*, 43 (1820), 496-501. During his term as President of the Association, George Man Burrows received a very extensive correspondence from medical practitioners. It is therefore unfortunate that, so far, no copy of this important publication has been traced.
19. E. Harrison, *Remarks on the Ineffective State of the Practice of Physic in Great Britain* (London, R. Bickerstaff, 1806).
20. They were published as a preface to vol. 13 of the *Medical and Chirurgical Review* (1806). Copies of this are rare but one can be found at the library of the Royal College of Surgeons in London.
21. Oxford, Bodleian Library, 'Medical Advertisements', Gough Pamphlets 2919.
22. 'L'Elisir D'Amore' was composed in 1831 and first performed in 1832.
23. 'Is there no Balm in Gilead? Is there no physician there? Why, then, is not the health of the daughter of my people recovered?' (Jeremiah: VIII, 22). Dr Solomon was said to have made a fortune from the sale of his balm, whose formula was never known, but was said to be based on 'spirits of wine'. He was reputed to spend £5,000 a year on advertisements, maintaining that £100 of advertising brought £2,000 of profit, and when he died his fortune was put at between £300,000 and £400,000. It is hinted that he succeeded in getting the recommendations of two regular physicians and applied, successfully, to the University of Aberdeen for an MD: but he was widely recognised as a quack doctor. *Monthly Gazette of Health*, 8 (1823), 533; 9 (1824), 891; 10 (1825), 173; 11 (1826) 764.
24. See J. Alden, 'Pills and Publishing', *Library*, 5th series, 7 (1952), 21-30. The association between booksellers and the sale of patent or quack medicines dates back at least to the seventeenth century and was prominent throughout the eighteenth. But in 1806: 'Druggists are making their fortunes by pills which they compound and advertise, but they are not the only persons to do so, for there are booksellers and schoolmasters who have their pills and embrocations' (Anon., letter xi in *Medical and Chirurgical Review*, 13 (1806), xxxvi).
25. The Bateman referred to is probably John Bateman of the seventeenth century who recommended and purveyed scurvy grass, and not Thomas Bateman (1778-1821), physician to the Public Dispensary and the London Fever Hospital.
26. The names and addresses were seldom informative, but these letters often provided the only clue to the approximate date of the pamphlet.
27. His list included the cure of 'wounds of any part of the body, ulcers, cancers, King's evil, old running sores, the bloody flux, convulsions, fits, gravel and stone, all manners of deafness (provided the tympanum or drum of the ear is intact), agues, dropsy, disagreeable smells of the breath, yellow jaundice, hypochondriac, hysteric, vapours and nervous complaints, consumptions, asthmas, inward decays, fistulas, hard and soft corns on any part of the feet or toes, scald head, wens, cutaneous eruptions, the toothache, leprosy, scurvy, coughs and colds etc. . . . Advice will be given gratis.'

'The Vile Race of Quacks . . . ' 127

28. Although there are accounts of farriers, etc., who acted as midwives, often with disastrous results. These were local people following another occupation rather than itinerants. See for example E. Harrison (note 19), 12 and 18. See also D. Evans, 'A Series of Bad Cases of Midwifery and Surgery', *Transactions of the Associated Apothecaries and Surgeon-Apothecaries*, 1 (1823), 201-7.

29. Probably 'John Natras, 56 Corn Lane Hull, 1838, Surgeon, no qualifications' in J.A.R. Bickford and M.E. Bickford, *The Medical Profession in Hull, 1400-1900* (Kingston Upon Hull, City Council, 1983).

30. Probably 'Peter Johnston (1798-1844) surgeon of 3 Trippett Court 1834: 54 Humber Street 1838-42' in *ibid*.

31. Probably in *ibid*. 'Mr Walker, Surgeon and Bone-Setter attends at . . . ' and there followed a list of inns and stated times in Scarborough, Beveley, Burton-upon-Humber, Hull, Driffield and Bridlington. He travelled these considerable distances 'for the accommodation of the Public'.

32. Entered in *ibid*. as 'Thomas Innes, Surgeon, 27 Blanket Row, 1822'. No qualifications given.

33. A possible exception was a Dr Dunn who claimed to be a graduate of an ancient and honourable university and an MRCS, who advertised by pamphlet that he 'May be consulted every day at No. 2 Princes Street, near Trinity House Lane, Hull'. This statement was followed by the usual list of diseases characteristic of the quack. Bickford and Bickford (*ibid*.) list him as William Dunn, surgeon and apothecary who had apparently served a regular apprenticeship to a surgeon and who practised in the 1780s and 1790s, but they mention no university degree or MRCS. All the names which appeared in these pamphlets were checked against Bickford and Bickford's comprehensive account of regular practitioners in Hull. None was included apart from those mentioned in these notes, and Dr Solomon (note 23).

34. 'Omega', 'Remarks on Quackery', *Provincial Medical and Surgical Journal*, 1 (1840-1), 418-19.

35. These examples are all taken from the preface of the *Medical and Chirurgical Journal*, 13 (1806).

36. Evidence of H.W. Rumsey, *Select Committee on Medical Poor Relief*, PP 1844 IX, third report (531), Q.9121.

37. 'Those who held privileges, and those who held none; those who believed themselves deprived of rights and those who feared a change on the grounds that all change was dangerous, united into a phalanx, compact, formidable and impenetrable. Against this host, drawn together by various motives and feelings, but all looking to particular interests . . . it would have been unwise to contend; and Dr Harrison, judiciously perhaps, suspended his projected plan of reform' (leading article, *Medical and Physical Journal*, 26 (1811), 2-5).

38. *Transactions of the Associated Apothecaries*, 1 (1823), lviii.

39. *Ibid*. xxiii-xxix; and Guildhall Library, London, Records of the Society of Apothecaries of London, 'Papers Relating to the Proceedings of the Apothecaries Act', MS 8299.

40. G.M. Burrows, *A Statement of Circumstances Connected with the Apothecaries Act and its Administration* (London, Callow, 1817).

41. Leading article, *Lancet* (1826-7), ii 514-17.

42. See 'Important to Surgeons', *Medico-Chirurgical Review*, new series, 14 (1831), 570-1; and 'Miscellanies', *London Medical and Surgical Journal*, 7 (1831), 173-5.

43. *A Statement of the Society of Apothecaries* (London, Society of Apothecaries, 1844); evidence of G.M. Burrows, *Report of the Select Committee on Medical Education*, PP 1834 XIII (620), part III, Q.213-298.

44. *Select Committee on Medical Education* (note 43), part III, Q.100.

45. 'Repeal of the Apothecaries Act. Abuses in the Profession', *London Medical and Surgical Journal*, new series, 3 (1833), 341-2.

46. Guildhall Library, London, Records of the Society of Apothecaries of London,

'Minutes of the Act of Parliament Committee in Reference to the Proposed Changes in the Laws Affecting the Medical Profession' (1847), MS 8212.

47. *Ibid.*

48. 'Medical Statistics and Reform', *Medico-Chirurgical Review*, 20 (1834), 567-71.

49. 'Illi Ego Qui Quondam', *Lancet* (1836-7), ii 647-8.

50. *Medical Examiner*, 1 (1830), 105-7.

51. J. Davies, *An Exposition of the Laws which Relate to the Medical Profession* (London, J. Churchill, 1844).

52. Letter from D.O. Edwards, *Lancet* (1841), ii 779.

53. Leading article, *Lancet* (1833-4), i 722.

54. *London Medical Gazette*, new series, 2 (1842-3), 52-3.

55. *Medical Times*, 19 (1848-9), 594.

56. Some of the assertions have the flavour of apocryphal stories, but a few are convincing, e.g. correspondence from 'General Practitioner, North Wales', *Lancet* (1836-7), i 412.

57. G.M. Burrows (note 40).

58. Perversely, when in the 1830s the repeal of the Apothecaries Act was mooted, the Association of General Medical and Surgical Practitioners who had so bitterly criticised the Act opposed the repeal on the grounds that the slight protection it provided against irregular practice was better than nothing. See 'Report of the Association', *London Medical Gazette*, 12 (1833), 367-8.

59. *Report of the Select Committee on Medical Education* (note 43), Part II, Q.4902. Mr St John Long was a well-known irregular with a large and fashionable practice amongst the upper classes of London society.

60. Torrance McCullogh Torrens, *The Life and Times of the Rt. Hon. Sir James Graham, Bart* (London, Horst & Blackett, 1863).

61. S.W.F. Holloway, 'The Apothecaries Act 1815: Part 1, The Origins of the Act', *Medical History*, 10 (1966), 107-29; *idem*, 'The Apothecaries Act 1815: Part 2, The Consequences of the Act', *Medical History*, 10 (1966), 221-36.

7 THE ORTHODOX FRINGE: THE ORIGINS OF THE PHARMACEUTICAL SOCIETY OF GREAT BRITAIN

S.W.F. Holloway

One of the highlights of the Pharmaceutical Society's centenary celebrations in 1941 was the production by Donald Wolfit of H.N. Linstead's play *Jacob Bell and Some Others*. The play has been described as a vivid portrayal of the public meeting at the Crown and Anchor tavern in the Strand on 15 April 1841 at which the historic resolution to form the Pharmaceutical Society of Great Britain was adopted. Sir Hugh Linstead's title was apt: the Pharmaceutical Society was the creation of Jacob Bell, with a little help from his friends.

It is tempting to see the Pharmaceutical Society as a form of permanent organisation crystallising out of the series of public protest meetings of chemists and druggists which preceded it. Leslie Matthews in his *History of Pharmacy in Britain* implies such a development,[1] and Dr J.K. Crellin in an article on 'the growth of professionalism in nineteenth-century British pharmacy' is explicit. He writes that 'the time had become ripe for an organization devoted entirely to the interests of pharmacy', and he notes 'the success of the Pharmaceutical Society in unifying the chemists and druggists into a recognized professional body'.[2] In this interpretation the public meetings are seen as the first expression of that growing sense of professional solidarity which finds its logical culmination in the creation of the Pharmaceutical Society. This is precisely the impression that Jacob Bell himself wished to convey in his *Historical Sketch of the Progress of Pharmacy in Great Britain* written in 1842.[3] It was not just modesty that led him to underplay his part in the creation of the society. He wanted to show that the society represented the true aspirations of chemists and druggists; that it emerged naturally and inevitably to meet their needs; that he was merely the midwife, not the father. Such an interpretation, however, conceals more than it reveals.

From the beginning of the nineteenth century shortlived associations of chemists and druggists were formed whenever attempts were made to impose restrictions or taxes upon them. In 1802 a small group of metropolitan apothecaries, chemists and druggists secured a modification in the new Medicine Act. In 1829 the threat arising from the exaction of new penalties under the Medicine Stamp Acts led to the formation of 'The General Association of Chemists and Druggists of Great

Britain'. It survived little longer than it took for the grievance to be met by the Commissioners of Stamps. During the years 1813-15 'The Chemists and Druggists of the Metropolis' successfully fought off attempts to bring them under the control of the Society of Apothecaries. In 1819 a public meeting of chemists and druggists at the Globe Tavern, Fleet Street, gave their support to a Bill to regulate the sale of poisons.[4] In 1839 an unsuccessful attempt was made to form a benevolent society, 'The Druggists' Provident Association', with the aim 'of affording relief and assistance to its members in cases of sickness and distress, and of giving information to persons seeking to obtain situations in the trade'.[5] Finally, the introduction of Benjamin Hawes's Medical Reform Bill in 1841, which revived the proposal to put the control of chemists and druggists in the hands of the apothecaries, precipitated the events that led to the formation of the Pharmaceutical Society.

These ephemeral, *ad hoc* associations represent the emergence of the chemist and druggist on the political scene. But they should not be interpreted as expressions of an incipient occupational consciousness, nor as stepping-stones towards the establishment of a permanent professional organisation. Obvious features of these gatherings militate against such a view. They were protest meetings, reactions against interference, designed to restore the status quo. There were no calls for change, no list of radical demands, no programmes of reform, no desire for permanent organisation. All that there was, was a plea to be left alone, not to be interfered with, not to be unfairly taxed, not to be placed under grievous restrictions. Whenever their immediate interests were threatened, the London druggists would come together to stave off the attack: but there was no enthusiasm for projects of reform and regulation. When two of the most highly regarded London wholesale druggists, John Savory and W.B. Hudson, tried in 1830 to interest 'a considerable number of the Chemists and Druggists in London' in such a programme, they received 'so little encouragement . . . that the project fell to the ground'. Their proposal had been to petition the government to introduce a bill to regulate the practice of pharmacy.

> The memorial which was prepared contained a brief and appropriate exposition of the importance of Pharmacy to the health and life of His Majesty's subjects; the necessity of education and integrity in those whose duty it is to carry into effect the instructions of medical men; the prevalence of ignorant and incompetent persons calling themselves Chemists and Druggists, and the frequency of injury to the public from this source; the difficulty of detecting adulterations and the necessity of proper qualification in Pharmaceutists, in order to enable

them to perform their duty in this respect; the advantages resulting from Pharmaceutical education in foreign countries; the danger arising from the uncontrolled sale of poisons by ignorant persons; and, finally the absolute necessity of some sanitary regulations for the elevation of this department in the profession, and the protection of the public.

This petition represents a summary of the grievances and solutions which reformers were to repeat for the remainder of the century. In 1830, however, the memorial 'proved abortive, not from any doubt of its propriety or justice, but because the parties concerned . . . were not disposed . . . to coalesce and embark in an undertaking which would have involved a departure from the strictly *defensive* policy hitherto adopted by the trade'.[6]

A striking feature of the public gatherings of chemists and druggists was the speed and efficiency of their organisation. The response of the pharmacists to threats was like a reflex action. Advertisements in the press, well-attended meetings, resolutions passed unanimously, lobbies organised, counsel briefed, and subscriptions collected: these are the hallmarks of political organisation. The nucleus of this organisation was the Wholesale Druggists' Club, a commercial association of drug importers, brokers and wholesalers in the City of London, established to discuss and regulate the trade in drugs and chemicals. Its members included the wealthy City merchants who purchased imported organic drugs at the East India Company's fortnightly sales as well as those who supplied drugs and chemicals to apothecaries, hospitals, dispensaries, and retail chemists. They were men with influence in the City of London, and at Westminster, and with extensive contacts with retailers. The Wholesale Druggists' Club did not openly engage in political agitation.[7] It was the Druggists' Association, a body consisting of both pharmacists and apothecaries, which organised the opposition to new government taxation in 1802 and 1829. Its existence was less continuous than that of the Committee of Chemists and Druggists formed during the negotiations surrounding the passage of the 1815 Apothecaries Act. The 1814-15 committee continued to meet until 1841 as an organised body and 'kept a watchful eye on any proceedings or events which appeared likely to influence the welfare of their body'. It was this group which set in motion the opposition to Hawes's Bill in 1841 and which later transferred its funds to the newly founded Pharmaceutical Society.

The successful outcome of the protests of chemists and druggists in the first half of the nineteenth century was not due to the weight of numbers or the representative nature of their meetings, but to the personal influence of the leading druggists with members of the government. The public meetings in London taverns and the appeals to the provinces through press advertisements were stage-managed: designed to influence public debate but largely irrelevant to the crucial private negotiations.

Jacob Bell's great achievement was to seize the opportunity created by the proceedings against the 1841 Medical Reform Bill to establish the Pharmaceutical Society. It was a remarkable personal achievement involving much hard work, a degree of forcefulness and a great deal of tact. It involved transforming an occasional, informal committee of London druggists into a permanent professional organisation. It entailed persuading the metropolitan elite to move from a defensive, laissez-faire, position to one which sought actively to regulate and control the occupation. It meant the adoption of an aggressive professionalising strategy in place of the former protective trading policy. Jacob Bell has himself described the birth of the Pharmaceutical Society. During the numerous meetings of the committee appointed to oppose the progress of Hawes's Bill, 'the propriety of establishing a society was frequently suggested; but it was found impossible in an open committee to come to an unanimous decision on the details of so important a measure'. Nevertheless, 'the Committee saw plainly that nothing short of a permanent Association could secure the trade against a recurrence of the inconveniences and annoyances which it had from time to time experienced during the last half-century'. Such an opportunity 'might not speedily occur again; . . . in the excitement occasioned by the threatened blow at their independence minor considerations were forgotten'. The failure of all former attempts to form a society was due to the 'degree of coolness and distrust' which had hitherto existed; but 'in the present crisis, jealousy seemed to be forgotten'.[8]

> It was evident that Pharmacy must be placed on a more scientific footing . . . [for] the fact was notorious that no institution existed in this country for the systematic education and examination of Chemists and Druggists . . . It was, therefore, the policy of the Druggists . . . to give a practical answer to all objections by establishing a system of government for themselves.
>
> But the task was one which required the most mature deliberation and unwearied perseverance. The members of the Committee were not unanimous either as to the details of the plan or the mode of accomplishing it, and there was every reason to anticipate still greater

The Orthodox Fringe 133

difficulty in amalgamating the various opinions of the body at large on so intricate and momentous a question.

On 20 March 1841 Jacob Bell invited those members of the committee who agreed with his proposals to a 'pharmaceutical tea-party' at his house in Oxford Street and there they worked out their future strategy. 'Several other meetings of this unofficial character took place, at each of which other members were added to the number, until twenty-four of the Committee were unanimous on the general principles of the Association.' The historic meeting at the Crown and Anchor on 15 April 1841 followed. The transformation of a trade-protection society into a professional association was not yet complete. On Monday 1 November 1841 a public meeting took place which was important both financially and symbolically for the newly formed society. The subscribers to the 1814-15 fund decided to present the balance in hand to the Pharmaceutical Society. The resolution declared

> That the original object of this fund being the protection and advancement of the interests of Chemists and Druggists, this meeting . . . desires to recognise in the establishment of the Pharmaceutical Society of Great Britain a permanent and legitimate means of accomplishing such object; namely, by a general union and organisation for the protection of present privileges and the education and improvement of the future members of the trade.

Jacob Bell's comments on this meeting are very instructive. The transfer of £862 18s 2d. connected the Pharmaceutical Society with the chemists and druggists who, twenty-five years earlier, had won a major victory in the struggle over the Apothecaries Act. Yet it was the differences rather than the similarities that were more important:[9]

> On the former occasion the proceedings of the trade were directed to a defensive resistance of threatened encroachments, and contemplated merely the preservation of accustomed rights and privileges by legal means and parliamentary influence. In the establishment of the Pharmaceutical Society . . . the extension of pharmaceutical knowledge and the further improvements in the qualifications of the trade individually and collectively, became the basis of the defence which was set up against future innovations or restraint.

A comparison of the successive statements of the aims and objectives of the society shows how gradually the references to the protection of the present privileges of the trade gave way to an emphasis on science, education and the elevation of the profession. The general committee of 5 April 1841 agreed on the aims of the society which they hoped to form:

> To benefit the public, and elevate the profession of Pharmacy, by furnishing the means of proper instruction; to protect the collective and individual interests and privileges of all its members, in the event of any hostile attack in Parliament or otherwise; to establish a club for the relief of decayed or distressed members.

The historic resolution at the public meeting ten days later merely declared:

> That for the purpose of protecting the permanent interests, and increasing the respectability of Chemists and Druggists, an Association be now formed under the title of the 'Pharmaceutical Society of Great Britain'.

By July 1841 the newly formed council saw 'the general advantages contemplated in the Society' as:[10]

> the union of all members of the body, for the purpose of self-government and self-protection; the establishment of a uniform system of education, which will promote the advancement of science and the elevation of the profession of Pharmacy; the restraint which will be placed upon the incompetent for the benefit of the public; and lastly the alleviation of the suffering of the unfortunate.

However, by February 1843, the Royal Charter of Incorporation proclaimed that the Pharmaceutical Society had been formed[11]

> for the purpose of advancing Chemistry and Pharmacy and promoting a uniform system of Education of those who should practise the same and also for the protection of those who carry on the business of Chemists and Druggists . . . [and] to provide a Fund for the relief of the distressed Members and Associates of the Society and of their Widows and Orphans.

By 1843 the Pharmaceutical Society had become a typical professionalising association. It aimed to unite under its auspices all the chemists and druggists in Britain; it would be active in promoting the solidarity and professional consciousness of its members; it would represent its members to the public, to other professions, and to the government. It would protect the interests of the profession and guard it against interference and encroachment. It would ensure that the profession was self-governing and self-regulating: it would secure its members' professional autonomy. The ignorant, incompetent, and unscrupulous would be excluded by a system of education, qualification and registration. Educated practitioners would be protected against unfair and unethical competition and their status and remuneration would be enhanced. The progress of chemistry and pharmacy would be promoted. The victims of circumstance would be relieved by an occupational welfare scheme.

Why did Jacob Bell and his friends feel the need to set up the Pharmaceutical Society in 1841? What did they hope to achieve? What problems in the practice of pharmacy did they identify? What opportunities for progress did they hope to seize?

The fear that the Medical Reform Bill of 1841 aroused in the chemist and druggist was reinforced by the activity of the Society of Apothecaries. In the same year, the Society of Apothecaries took its first case against a chemist, a Mr Greenough of Liverpool, who admitted attending, advising, and furnishing medicines to patients without obtaining the society's licence. On 25 May 1841 the Court of Queen's Bench, on appeal by the Society of Apothecaries, ruled that if a chemist not only sold but also administered medicines in the course of attending patients, he was practising as an apothecary, and as such was not protected by section 28 of the 1815 Act.[12] The *Lancet*, the self-appointed spokesman of the general practitioner, lost little time in ramming home the significance of this decision. From September to November it went through the case, week by week, exalting in this victory of the apothecaries over their rivals, and vividly exaggerating the dangers to the public of unqualified prescribing.[13] The resulting anxiety and sense of foreboding among chemists and druggists was skilfully exploited by Jacob Bell. 'The "Medical Reformers" have not abandoned their design. They are only waiting for an opportunity to carry it into execution, and they are likely to persevere until an alteration of some kind is effected.' Since 'Chemists must and will be included in the scheme of "reform", it remains for them to decide whether they will allow measures . . . to be forced upon them by persons who are indifferent or opposed to their interest, or whether they will maintain their independence under such regulations as shall conduce to their own welfare.' The setting-up of the Pharmaceutical Society is 'the only step which . . . can remedy existing evils and prevent the crisis of a destructive revolution by promoting a wholesome and desirable reform.' 'The daily papers and medical periodicals teem with gross and offensive attacks on Chemists and Druggists, which they are *not in a position* to refute; and charges are made against them which they are unable to controvert or to obviate.' 'They must, in their present position, submit to any indignity because they have no power to resist it.' Hence, 'the Chemists have no safe alternative but to take the government of their Body into their own hands'.[14]

Jacob Bell and his small coterie of London druggists intended to do exactly that; 'to take the government of their Body into their own hands'. To justify their action they used familiar arguments. Unless we set our own house in order, others, much less benevolently disposed, will intervene. The public image of the profession can only be improved if the ignorant and unscrupulous members are rooted out. It is this 'minority of the worst' which is dragging down the whole body, destroying the profession's credibility, undermining public confidence by its disreputable, unethical behaviour. The strictures of outsiders are made plausible by the actions of this small minority.

As long as Chemists and Druggists *collectively* neglect to take those means which are within their reach for rectifying these evils, the stigma, which ought to be confined to some individuals among them, is extended to all — as long as they continue to be subject to no educational regulations, they are exposed to the imputation of ignorance — as long as they are disjointed, unrecognized, and indifferent, the influence which they would possess as an organized body, is lost in the confusion of inoperative individual efforts.

The Pharmaceutical Society, under the leadership of the leading London druggists, would transform group disgrace into collective virtue. Instead of the tone of the profession being determined by 'the minority of the worst', it would be set by 'the minority of the best'. Bell and his clique set themselves up as exemplars of good practice, as men 'solicitous of maintaining an unblemished reputation'. To them it was peculiarly galling that 'the want of a uniform education among Druggists, and the variable quality of the drugs which are found in the market (whether from adulteration, defects in the preparation, or the loss of their properties from keeping), are continually brought before the public'. There must be 'a systematic regulation' of chemists and druggists; the righteous must supervise the wicked:[15]

The difficulty which exists in a majority of cases in estimating, with any degree of precision, the qualities of drugs, increases very much the responsibility of the Druggist by placing the Public in a great measure at his mercy. The chief ground therefore on which he can hope for success in his business is, *the confidence of the Public in his integrity and experience*; and any circumstance which could tend to increase that confidence must necessarily be of great importance.

Once more Jacob Bell draws on a familiar line of argument. As principles of commercial activity, laissez-faire and *caveat emptor* are perfectly acceptable: it is taken for granted that the customer can satisfy himself as to the suitability of the goods he proposes to buy by preliminary inspection. The customer knows what he wants and can recognise it when he sees it. In the case of professional services, however, neither of these assumptions can be made. The relationship between the professional and the public is dominated by the fact that the former's services cannot be judged by the layman who is obliged to take them on trust. The ignorance of the layman makes it possible for the expert to exploit the market either by overcharging or by rendering inadequate service. In time this will lead to the profession falling into disrepute. It is, therefore, in every member's long-term interest to ensure that the public receives only efficient and ethical service from his colleagues. The function of a professional association is, therefore, to provide an acceptable substitute for the market relationship by guaranteeing in its members both competence and integrity, the two requirements without which the market for professional services would rapidly become reduced to chaos.[16] The Pharmaceutical Society would carry out this function by rooting out the incompetent and unscrupulous, by exercising surveillance over the activities of its members, by drawing up a code of ethics, and by controlling the entry, education and registration of future members:[17]

The organisation of a Body of Chemists into a Society, the chief objects of which are avowedly to raise the character of the Profession of Pharmacy, and to ensure a uniform and efficient administration of medicine, will confer upon every Member that public confidence to which he is entitled. It will be in the power of the Society to inculcate the impolicy of adulterations, to enlighten the public mind as to the mischief of cheap medicines, and thus to overcome to a great extent the prejudice which exists amongst too many of us in favour of a mistaken economy, and also to disseminate the advantages of that scientific knowledge which every Druggist ought to possess.

138 *The Orthodox Fringe*

The society would have a moral influence on its members which would enhance professional status, for 'there is, perhaps, no avocation in which *character* is of more importance than that of a Chemist and Druggist'.[18]

> That which the law of the land or the laws of an association cannot effect, may be brought about by the moral influence of a code of ethics voluntarily subscribed to, and recommended for general adoption. The Chemists having until lately been disunited, and ranked rather with the trades than the professions, have not had the advantage of that discipline which is the natural result of organization and professional intercourse.[19]

From the outset, the Pharmaceutical Society laid great stress on education as a means of raising the status of its members: 'Professional character *prima facie* is supposed to result from liberal and scientific education.'[20] The experience of the great London drug houses revealed for Jacob Bell both the deficiencies of existing educational provision and the model for its reform. The London druggists, he wrote, have great difficulty in obtaining competent assistants:[21]

> Young men from the Country constantly present themselves as candidates for that office, who are found to be entirely ignorant of the elements of Chemistry, and unqualified for ordinary dispensing business. Some London houses, which have been long established, keep up a communication with Assistants whom they have educated, and who have afterwards settled in different towns in the country, and by taking their Apprentices, complete the education which has been commenced on their own principles. This arrangement may be compared to a private school of Pharmacy, as it is evident that men who have learned their business in a well regulated establishment are able to supply it in rotation with better qualified Assistants than those who have not had this advantage. As this system is found to be successful when adopted by individuals, it cannot fail to be much more so if extended to the Body at large . . . The School of Pharmacy . . . will also be a place of reference; and a mutual benefit will be enjoyed by Members who want Assistants, and Associates requiring situations.

The educational activities of the Pharmaceutical Society began in a modest way. The pharmaceutical tea-parties of March 1841 gave way in May to a series of monthly scientific meetings at Jacob Bell's house,[22] and as the new society had now been founded, these were ostensibly meetings of the society, to which the members, together with medical and other scientific men who took an interest . . . were invited for the purpose of reading and discussing papers relating to the practice of pharmacy . . . Although instituted and conducted by Mr Bell on his sole responsibility and at his own expense, these meetings were designed . . . for the purpose of illustrating the advantage of scientific discussion, and, as a starting point for meetings of a similar description which it was hoped the Pharmaceutical Society would carry out . . . But the question arose, what was to be done with the papers read at these meetings? There was no journal devoted to pharmacy in which they could be published, . . . [so] Mr Bell started a monthly publication, the first number of which appeared in July 1841 . . . Mr Bell was not only the proprietor of this publication, but took the position of editor.

In January 1842 the scientific meetings were transferred to the newly acquired premises of the society at 17 Bloomsbury Square. It was here that the School of Pharmacy was opened with a series of evening lectures in the spring of 1842: the first systematic courses commenced that autumn. In 1844 the school became the first in Britain to supplement lectures in chemistry and pharmacy with practical instruction in its own laboratory. A new laboratory with accommodation for twenty-one students was opened the following year: it later became the model used in the setting-up of the Birkbeck laboratory at University College, London. Pharmacy students were 'to "walk the laboratory" as medical students "walk the hospitals" '.[23] A museum of *materia medica* and a library were established and the Bloomsbury Square premises provided facilities for evening scientific meetings, conversaziones, and research groups. The examinations for the admission of members and associates did not come into full operation until February 1844. In 1848 Jacob Bell wrote:[24]

> The Pharmaceutical Society was designed as a means of raising the qualifications of pharmaceutical chemists, and placing between them and unqualified persons a line of demarcation. The diploma was intended as a distinctive mark for the information of the public . . . precautions were taken from the beginning to exclude all persons known to be disreputable or unworthy of being classed with the general body of Chemists and Druggists and . . . the certificate may be taken generally as a test of respectability. It also denotes that the possessor

is one of those who has united with others in the endeavour to raise the qualifications of his class.

Behind the educational and examining activities of the Pharmaceutical Society lay the aim of making pharmacy a distinctive branch of the medical profession. In 1842 Jacob Bell wrote a historical survey of the healing arts which led him 'to the consideration of the position which Pharmacy occupies, or ought to occupy, as a branch of the medical profession'. He gave lengthy consideration to the way in which the traditional pharmaceutical practitioners — the apothecaries — had become general medical practitioners, while retaining their right to dispense and sell drugs:[25]

> Our predecessors, the original Apothecaries, who were merely compounders of medicine, possessed very limited advantages in respect to education, and in proportion as they advanced in intelligence and knowledge they encroached on the Physicians, until they became to all intents and purposes medical men. When they established a Hall, and laid down a regular course of study for their apprentices, they were not content with instructing them in those sciences which relate to the compounding of drugs, but included in their curriculum surgery, physiology, anatomy, the practice of medicine and midwifery. By this means they supplied the public with a very useful class of medical practitioners . . . But, by the same course, they left a gap to be filled up by another class of compounders of medicine.

The art and science of pharmacy, claimed Bell, had in Britain been degraded 'to the level of mere trade'. This had led to the idea that a necessary consequence of improving the character and education of the chemist and druggist would be to convert him into a medical practitioner. The apothecaries adopted a system of education which was medical and surgical rather than pharmaceutical: 'the odium which rested on Pharmacy as a *trade*, induced them to aspire to medical practice as a *profession*'. But pharmacy was now 'deserving of a separate and distinct place in the arrangement of the medical profession'.[26] A need had emerged for specialist practitioners of pharmacy to assimilate and put into practice the changes in *materia medica* and improvements in dispensing which had been created by the advances in chemistry and botany:[27]

> Pharmacy in the present day embraces so many sciences, and has become so complicated from the discoveries which have recently

been made, especially in Chemistry, that a complete knowledge of the subject can only be acquired by those who devote their exclusive attention to the pursuit. The science of Chemistry is alone sufficiently comprehensive to engage the whole time of those who are desirous of becoming acquainted with all its details . . . These revolutions in chemical science give rise to changes in nomenclature, and improvements in the processes of the laboratory, which innovations involve the study of Pharmacy in increasing difficulty, and confer on the pursuit the character of a philosophical profession. It is the province of the Pharmaceutical Chemist to apply the various discoveries which are made in this science to his own peculiar department . . . the principles of Chemistry should be understood by every person who undertakes to prepare a prescription, and in many of the daily operations of Pharmacy a profound knowledge of the science is indispensable.

The range of the Materia Medica is too extensive to be embraced in the mind without a systematic study of all its minutiae in the first instance, followed up by constant application. The variations in the quality of drugs, and the sophistications to which they are liable, increase the responsibility of the Druggist . . . The detection of adulterations is, therefore, one of the most onerous duties of the Pharmaceutical Chemist, and it is one which requires, beside chemical knowledge, a practical acquaintance with the sensible properties of all the substances used in medicine; . . . and even that amount of knowledge which every Chemist ought to possess of the plants which are used in medicine cannot be acquired without many years of study . . .

[Pharmacy] is not likely to advance as a science, and keep pace with other sciences, unless it be followed by a class of persons who devote themselves exclusively to it . . .

But if proper encouragement were given to the followers of pure Pharmacy; if this pursuit were held in the estimation which it deserves, and which it enjoys in other countries; if the same professional credit were attainable in this field of labour which is within the reach of the members of other professions, the inducement which now exists to encroach on the medical practitioner would be greatly diminished, or cease altogether, and the science of Pharmacy might be expected to flourish.

Jacob Bell's vision of the future becomes clear in these passages. His argument is unequivocal: a scientific revolution is creating a new division of labour within the medical profession. The Pharmaceutical Society is required to organise the practice of pharmacy in the way the Royal Colleges already organise the practice of physic and surgery. The Fellows of the Royal College of Physicians confine themselves to the practice of 'pure' medicine: membership of the council of the Royal College of Surgeons is restricted to those who practise 'pure' surgery. The founder of the Pharmaceutical Society proclaims the virtues of 'pure' pharmacy. Although justified by reference to innovations in knowledge, Jacob Bell's vision is securely tethered to the past. The medical profession is seen as having its ranks and orders, each with its own function and sphere of usefulness, and each regulated by its own corporate body. The time has come for pharmacy to take its place, separate but equal, alongside the other orders.[28] 'We look forward to the time,' declared the *Pharmaceutical Journal* in 1845, 'when it will be considered as much beneath the dignity of a Pharmaceutical Chemist to become an irregular Medical Practitioner, as it would be derogatory to a Physician to practice Pharmacy.'[29] The daily activities of the great majority of chemists and druggists throughout the country are condemned as undignified: attending patients and prescribing over the counter by chemists are as much anathema to the Pharmaceutical Society as they are to the Society of Apothecaries. The key to professionalism is greater specialisation. A medical profession founded on a rational division of scientific labour would be characterised by interdependence and co-operation instead of the present antagonism and competition. Strong fences make good neighbours. Jacob Bell concluded his survey of the progress of pharmacy with these words:[30]

> Those who are sincere in the desire for the advancement of our own legitimate profession, which is pure Pharmacy, will perceive the importance of confining our attention as much as possible to that pursuit, by which course we shall not only be more likely to attain the object in view, but shall also conciliate the other branches of the profession, and establish an amicable and harmonious relation among all parties.

Pure pharmacy meant scientific pharmacy. The elite group of London druggists who founded the Pharmaceutical Society saw themselves as the carriers of the seeds of a new scientific discipline. They proclaimed the gospel according to Magendie, Pelletier and Liebig. For them, the analysis and synthesis of drugs and chemicals, the discovery and manufacture of new and effective medicines 'for the relief of human suffering' were the only areas within the true domain of the pharmaceutical chemist.[31] This belief in the authenticity and utility of science informed their plans for the reform of the profession. The emphasis on education, examination, qualification and registration coincided with their commitment to the canons of orthodox science. The 1840s were a time of great excitement and opportunity: the work and ideas of Magendie, Pelletier and Liebig were transforming the practice and prospects of scientific pharmacy.

The beginning of modern pharmacy can be traced to the work of François Magendie (1783-1855) and Pierre-Joseph Pelletier (1788-1842). In 1809 Magendie carried out a series of ingenious experiments on various animals to study the toxic action of several drugs of vegetable origin, such as upas and nux vomica. For the first time an experimental comparison was made of the similar effects produced by drugs of different botanical origin. Magendie held that the toxic or medicinal action of natural drugs depends on the chemical substances they contain, and that it should be possible to obtain these substances in the pure state. As early as 1809 he suspected the existence of strychnine, isolated ten years later, in accord with Magendie's predictions, by Pelletier. Pelletier, who spent his adult life investigating drugs at the Ecole de Pharmacie in Paris, achieved his first major success in 1817 when he discovered the emetic substance in ipecacuanha root, which he named emetine. By pioneering the use of mild solvents, Pelletier successfully isolated a whole range of important biologically active compounds from plants, thus founding the chemistry of the alkaloids. For over twenty years Pelletier continued his alkaloid and phytochemical research. He discovered brucine, caffeine, cinchonine, colchicine, narceine, strychnine, veratrine and, most important of all, quinine. Quinine, the chief alkaloid in cinchona bark, became for the next 100 years the only effective treatment for malaria and represents the first successful use of a chemical compound in combating an infectious disease. Pelletier's isolation of active constituents from crude drugs was a major development in pharmacy, but it was Magendie who was responsible for introducing the recently discovered alkaloids into medical practice. In 1821 he published the first edition of his *Formulaire pour la préparation et l'emploi de plusieurs nouveaux médicaments*, a revolutionary therapeutic manual which led to the use of strychnine, morphine, brucine, codeine, veratrine and quinine by physicians. Magendie also generalised the therapeutic applications of iodine and bromine salts, and indicated the use of hydrocyanic acid in therapeutics.

The work of Magendie and Pelletier not only introduced a new level of precision into the practice of pharmacy but created a need for educated and skilful practitioners. Gone were the days of crude drugs of unknown and variable composition, of imprecise plant extracts and mixtures. If pure compounds were used, accurate dosage could be prescribed and the toxic effects due to impurities in crude drugs could be eliminated. The growing use of experiments to investigate the action of such substances on the animal body led to the determination of doses and detailed descriptions of the properties of drugs. With the entry into medicine of pure, toxic, chemical substances, a premium was placed on their standardisation and purity and the administration of precise doses. This in turn required practitioners whose integrity and reliability, technical skill, and knowledge of the theory and practice of chemistry, could be guaranteed.[32]

The other great influence on early-nineteenth-century pharmacy was Justus Liebig (1803-73), who, as J.R. Partington reminds us, 'was unquestionably the greatest chemist of his time'.[33] His achievement, which involved the isolation, analysis and synthesis of new compounds, and includes his work on ethyl and benzoyl radicals, on the hydrogen theory of acids, and in agricultural chemistry, cannot be examined here. But that achievement bears witness to the fact that it was Liebig who was largely responsible for transforming animal and vegetable chemistry into organic chemistry and biochemistry. It is, however, for the perfecting of the chemical laboratory as a teaching instrument and for his theory of the disease process that Liebig is important for our inquiry.

The opening of Liebig's chemistry laboratory at the University of Giessen in 1824 was, as J.B. Morrell has convincingly argued, a critical event in the history of nineteenth-century science. Liebig's was the first institutional laboratory in which students underwent systematic preparation for chemical research. After an initial course of qualitative and quantitative analysis using known compounds, each student was required to produce pure substances in good yield from raw materials. Once this preliminary training had been satisfactorily completed, the student was allowed to pursue original research under Liebig's general supervision. The combination of the most rigorous practical training and its incredibly low cost proved irresistible to students from all over Europe. The success of Liebig's laboratory depended on his invention of relatively simple, fast and reliable experimental techniques. With practice, any determined student could obtain reliable results using Liebig's combustion apparatus for analysing organic compounds. The use of this apparatus and its relatives permitted both brilliant and mediocre students to produce knowledge in the emerging field of organic chemistry in a systematic way and on a large scale. Liebig codified and systematised both the research techniques employed and the preliminary training he gave his students. Two of his pupils, H. Will and C.R. Fresenius, published books on the methods of qualitative and quantitative analysis used at Giessen, and these were rapidly translated into English.[34]

From its foundation the Pharmaceutical Society placed great emphasis on practical chemistry. The early volumes of the *Pharmaceutical Journal* contain many articles on pharmaceutical chemistry: Richard Phillips, the editor and translator of the 1836 edition of the *Pharmacopoeia Londinensis*, contributed a series of reports on pharmacopoeial preparations, incorporating tests for adulteration.[35] An attempt was made to keep journal readers abreast of the most important continental research. A knowledge of chemistry was expected of examinees for both the minor and major examinations.[36] The society's laboratory was modelled on that at Giessen, and when Liebig visited it 'two or three of the processes usually conducted by students in the laboratory were modified at his suggestion'.[37] The emphasis on practical chemistry in the society's curriculum is obvious from the comments of the director of the laboratory, John Attfield, and from the complaints of examinees that too much weight was placed on this part of the syllabus.[38] The case for training pharmacists in chemistry, however, was eloquently stated by the first vice-president of the society, Charles James Payne, in 1842:[39]

Without some knowledge of Chemistry a man is working in the dark, he can know nothing correctly of the results of, or the reasons for the operations he constantly performs — he can never properly judge the accuracy and quality of his preparations, he can neither detect any error that may occur nor rectify any untoward circumstance that may arise — he has no established data to reason upon — no fixed principles to guide him; but is like a mariner without a compass, exposed to endless confusion and mishap.

If Liebig's laboratory was a model for pharmaceutical education, his theory of disease was a prospectus for pharmaceutical imperialism. Liebig explained the disease process in terms of fermentation; fermentation, putrefaction and decay were elucidated in terms of a mode of change characteristic of organic molecules.[40] He sought to explain these organic processes in terms of the basic properties of matter. By asserting the continuity in real chemical terms of organic matter, he hoped to demolish explanations which referred to the supposed peculiar properties of living matter. His account of how the food of animals was elaborated from elementary constituents by plants seemed a convincing demonstration of this basic premiss. For full value, the processes of excretion and decomposition were added to complete the cycle. Liebig's theory was particularly attractive to pharmaceutical chemists. His law of contagious molecular action substituted physico-chemical for specific biological explanations and simultaneously suggested an idea of process common to all epidemic, endemic and contagious diseases. It provided an intellectual umbrella to shelter the views of both sanitarians and medical men: the universality of contagious molecular action made questions of the specificity or contagiousness of various diseases irrelevant. For Liebig, effects were not to be referred merely to like causes, but rather to laws covering a wide range of phenomena. Explanation in 'covering law' terms was welcome to those who hoped that medicine would thus find a firm foundation in the properties of matter and the methods used to arrive at these. Liebig's theories constituted their ideal of rational scientific knowledge: beneath the great maze of unending complexity, the uniform operations of nature could be discerned. Liebig's theory implied a reversal of the traditional relationship of chemistry to medicine. Not only was chemistry emerging from its former position of dependency on medicine and claiming to be a science in its own right, it was even threatening to usurp the leading role. Not surprisingly, physicians' reactions to Liebig's ideas reveal a marked concern for professional prerogatives. They resented any attempt to derive principles of treatment from his laws. They claimed that chemistry had nothing to say of the vital functions of the organised tissues. Chemists should stick to nutrition: vital laws were the province of the physiologist. Although the *Lancet* published Henry Ancell's exposition of Liebig's views and declared that 'there is far more chemistry in medicine, . . . there is far more of exact science in medicine, than physicians are inclined to believe,' the medical press generally was hostile.[41] The prevalent view was that of Dr Golding Bird: 'a more melancholy error can scarcely be committed than that of explaining the phenomena of the animal organism too exclusively on chemical principles'.[42]

In 1837 Liebig travelled to England to deliver an address to the British Association for the Advancement of Science. In it he urged English men of science to participate in advancing the frontiers of organic chemistry 'and unite their efforts to those of the chemists of the Continent':[43]

> We live in a time when the slightest exertion leads to valuable results, and, if we consider the immense influence which organic chemistry exercises over medicine, manufactures, and over common life, we

must be sensible that there is no problem more important to mankind than the prosecution of the objects which organic chemistry contemplates.

The chemists who founded the Pharmaceutical Society in 1841 were eager to participate in Liebig's enterprise. Although Liebig himself claimed to be 'a man of science and not of Commerce', he could not resist the temptation to be lured into business. In 1866 he assumed the directorship of the scientific department of Liebig's Extract of Meat Company. The famous meat extract made use of the wasted meat of the Rio de la Plata cattle, slaughtered for their leather, to provide the 'plastic food' required to produce blood, build organs and replenish muscles. Within a few years the successful company was supplying the British army in Abyssinia.[44]

Liebig and his followers saw no contradiction between profit and *Wissenschaft*. The search for scientific truth is paramount, but since all knowledge is practical, it is science which gives nourishment to industry. The profits of industry provide an index of the validity of science. One of Liebig's most striking phrases, 'Intelligence in union with Capital',[45] epitomises the founders of the Pharmaceutical Society. They were a small band of the wealthiest and most enterprising chemists and druggists in London. They were men who had been quick to exploit the commercial opportunities presented by scientific progress. They combined scientific conviction with business acumen.

The names of the men who created and controlled the Pharmaceutical Society in its first decade constitute a directory of the leading chemical and drug brokers, wholesalers and manufacturers of London in the 1840s. Theophilus Redwood referred to them as 'the most influential members of the drug trade, representing every department of the business'.[46] Two of the firms associated with the birth of the society had been trading in drugs and chemicals since the seventeenth century. One of these was Corbyn & Co., which claimed to have been established before the Great Fire of 1666.[47] By the eighteenth century the company had developed an extensive trade with North America. Another seventeenth-century firm, still in business as drug merchants in the 1890s, was Horner & Sons. It was said that this company had started as spicers and grocers in the thirteenth century. Edward Horner was a member of the original committee of the Pharmaceutical Society. The connection between overseas trade and scientific pharmacy was recognised by the society when it set up 'a scientific committee for the promotion of pharmacological knowledge' in 1845. The idea came from Dr Jonathan Pereira, a good friend of Jacob Bell and an authority on *materia medica*. No country in the world, he argued, was as well placed as Great Britain for carrying out scientific inquiries into the properties of drugs:[48]

> Her numerous and important colonies in all parts of the world, and her extensive commercial relations, particularly fit her for taking the lead in investigations of this kind . . . From her extensive possessions in different parts of the world, we draw a very large portion of the substances now used in medicine. By the establishment of a committee on pharmacology in the mother country, an opportunity would be obtained of bringing into notice the various medicinal substances produced in the different portions of this great empire. In this way substances now unknown to, or little employed by us might be brought into use, and in some instances, perhaps, the produce of our own colonies might be advantageously substituted for that of other countries . . . In these and other ways . . . such a committee would prove useful in a commercial as well as scientific point of view.

William Allen, Hanburys & Barry was another old-established firm, with a continuous history at 2 Plough Court in the City of London since 1715.[49] William Allen FRS was the first president of the Pharmaceutical Society, and both John Barry and Daniel Hanbury served on the first committee. William Allen (1770-1843) was a Quaker, scientist and philanthropist.[50] He served an apprenticeship in the pharmaceutical establishment of Joseph Gurney Bevan in Plough Court and later succeeded to the business. He was then joined by another Quaker, Luke Howard FRS (1772-1864),[51] and the firm became Allen & Howard. In addition to the retail business, Allen & Howard established a laboratory at Plaistow for the manufacture of chemicals. From 1802 to 1826 Allen lectured on chemistry and experimental philosophy at Guy's Hospital and for several years he held the chair of experimental philosophy at the Royal Institution. He was elected a Fellow of the Royal Society in 1807. In the same year Luke Howard, who became a Fellow of the Royal Society in 1821, decided to sever his partnership with Allen to concentrate on the manufacture of chemicals instead of galenical preparations which were then Allen's main concern. The Howard family provided both capital and scientific expertise. In the 1830s Howard concentrated on the production of the new substance quinine, and demonstrated a flair for devising improved methods of producing pharmaceutical chemicals. By the 1860s the old corn mills that housed his works in the East End of London were known as Howards' Quinine, Borax and Tartaric Acid

Works, and employed some 200 people. Meanwhile, Allen journeyed far in the cause of 'promoting and extending religion, charity, education and civil liberty',[52] wisely leaving his business interests in the hands of his confidential clerk, John Thomas Barry (1789-1864), who joined him as a partner. Allen's activities fostered business with overseas customers, especially those in North America and the West Indies: Barry developed the manufacturing side.[53] Once described as a 'neat and exact experimentalist', Barry evolved, in 1819, a method of preparing extracts by evaporation *in vacuo*, using a temperature of 100°F instead of 212°F. By this means he obtained extracts three times as strong as those prepared by boiling in open pans. Not only were these extracts more uniform in strength but could also be produced at lower cost. When cod liver oil came into prominence in 1847 as a remedy for consumption, Allen, Hanbury & Barry began to process it in quantity, later setting up its own factories in Newfoundland and in the Lofoten Islands.[54]

The wealth of the majority of the founders of the Pharmaceutical Society was of a more recent origin. The first half of the nineteenth century offered great opportunities for the medium-sized well-run retail business. The demand for drugs from the growing middle class and from the hospitals and dispensaries for the sick poor was the spur to the development of the wholesale trade and of chemical and drug production. Even in the eighteenth century some chemists made up their own remedies and some of these enjoyed a local celebrity and were sold to other retailers. In the nineteenth century this became common in London. The retail chemists in the City and West End developed laboratories and manufactories where they made up their own preparations for wider distribution. The names of two of the founding fathers of the society became known to a wide public by their association with a proprietary medicine: Charles Dinneford (Fluid Magnesia) and Thomas Keating (Keating's Powder). When Jacob Bell's father, John, opened his shop in Oxford Street in 1798 he was so dissatisfied with the quality of the drugs he could purchase that he set up his own laboratory for their manufacture. He began to supply others in the trade and the wholesale business became so important that Jacob took into partnership Thomas Hyde Hill, in order to assist in its expansion.[55]

Many of the leading pharmaceutical manufacturing companies of the years following the Second World War trace their own origins back to the businesses set up by founding members of the Pharmaceutical Society. J.S. Lescher was a partner in the wholesale firm of Evans & Lescher, which specialised in supplying galenical and chemical preparations to hospitals and dispensaries. Evans & Lescher became Evans Medical

Ltd. Barron, Harvey & Barron formed part of the group that became British Drug Houses Ltd. Samuel Foulger & Son of Wapping and Herring Brothers were both later absorbed by Willows Francis Ltd. Thomas Morson & Son was amalgamated in the late 1950s with Merck, Sharp & Dohme Ltd. Charles Barron, Samuel Foulger and J.S. Lescher were members of the first committee and both Thomas Herring and Thomas Morson served as presidents of the society.

Thomas Herring (1785-1864) and his brother Thrower Buckle Herring were wholesale druggists who moved in 1815 to extensive premises at 40 Aldersgate Street. The firm produced on a large scale vegetable and other powders of superior quality by means of a powerful and efficient drug-mill which they installed on the premises. Such work had invariably been done in the past by a class of men called 'drug-grinders', who were not noted for the production of good and genuine powders. Herring's vegetable powders — such as rhubarb, jalap, bark and ipecacuanha — 'were fine, soft, impalpable, bright-looking powders, such as could not be produced with the pestle and mortar'.[56] Thomas Newborn Robert Morson (1799-1874) acquired an interest in scientific chemistry during his apprenticeship to an apothecary in the old Fleet Market in the City. Morson succeeded to that business in 1821 but before doing so, he lived for three years in the establishment of M. Planche, a *pharmacien* of Paris. Here he came under the influence of Magendie and Pelletier and learned about the new processes being developed for manufacturing chemicals and the newly discovered alkaloids. Morson was quick to realise the commercial potential of the alkaloids: in his Fleet Market laboratory he made the first morphine and the first quinine sulphate produced in Britain. These premises proved to be too restrictive and he moved in 1826 to Southampton Row and two years later purchased premises in Hornsey Road to build a laboratory for the manufacture of drugs and chemicals. Creosote, another recent discovery, was produced there in large quantities. Morson's linguistic ability, scientific interests and considerable wealth enabled him to develop contacts with distinguished European scientists. Among the many famous visitors to his 'Science Sunday Evenings' was Baron Liebig.[57]

Richard Hotham Pigeon (1789-1851) was the chairman of the inaugural meeting of the Pharmaceutical Society on 15 April 1841, and became the first treasurer of the society. He was a prominent member of the Wholesale Druggists' Club and ran a very prosperous business from the house in Throgmorton Street which he had first entered as an apprentice at the age of 16. In 1835 he was elected treasurer of Christ's Hospital and was instrumental in increasing the number of children educated there, widening the curriculum and persuading Queen Victoria, Prince Albert, the Prince of Wales and the Duke of Cambridge to become patrons. The early meetings of the Pharmaceutical Society took place in his house, and his contacts proved invaluable in obtaining the society's Royal Charter in 1843.[58] Another chemist whose influence was important in this respect was Peter Squire (1798-1884), the owner since 1831 of a notable pharmacy in Oxford Street. In 1837 he had become the first chemist to replace an apothecary in holding the Royal Warrant for supplying medicine. He played a prominent part in the founding of the society in 1841 and was elected president in 1849-50 and again during the years 1861-3. He made the ether inhaler used in 1846 by Robert Liston in the first surgical operation under ether to be performed in Britain. By his many papers on the practice of pharmacy and the publication of *The Three Pharmacopoeias* (1851), *The Pharmacopoeias of the London Hospitals* (1863) and *A Companion to the British Pharmacopoeia* (1864) he greatly improved the processes for making pharmaceutical preparations and stressed the need for uniformity in formulas. He retained his connection with the Oxford Street pharmacy for almost fifty years.[59]

Robert Alsop (1803-76), like so many of the leading lights in the Pharmaceutical Society, was a Quaker. After an apprenticeship and assistantship with John Bell, he established himself in 1826 as a chemist and druggist in an 'old-fashioned shop at the corner of Sloane Square, Chelsea, with its palms, ferns, and tree-frogs in the window'.[60] He made several important contributions to practical pharmacy: he introduced an infusion jug and a minim measure. His methods for preparing mercuric nitrate ointment and spirit of nitrous ether were used for many years. But it was the production of soda and mineral water which brought the prosperity that enabled him to give up the practice of pharmacy in 1855 to devote himself to philanthropic and religious causes.[61] Richard Battley (1770-1856) was a very active and zealous supporter of the Pharmaceutical Society and the first of a line of distinguished pharmacognosists. About 1800, after serving as an assistant surgeon in the navy, he bought an apothecary's business in St Paul's Churchyard. In 1812 he moved to Fore Street, where he carried out many improvements in pharmaceutical processing. Like Alsop, he made significant contributions to pharmaceutical practice. He has a good claim to introducing the cold-water process for making infusions and extracts, particularly of opium and cinchona. His liquor cinchonae was made official in the London *pharmacopoeia*. He became a highly regarded lecturer in *materia medica* at several London hospitals, as well as holding classes at his own *materia medica* museum. His wealth, however, was created by the wholesale business he established under the name of Battley & Watts.[62]

It is no disparagement of Jacob Bell's achievement in creating the Pharmaceutical Society to be reminded of the strength of bonds which already existed among the leading London chemists and druggists. Prior to 1841 they were enmeshed in a network of cross-cutting ties: the Quaker faith, the ordeal of apprenticeship, mutual involvement in business endeavour and a commitment to rational science united them. Above all, they were linked by the experience of success: the combination of enterprise and expertise had made them wealthy men. Yet trade jealousies, suspicion and distrust prevailed, in spite of the bedrock of common interests. As Theophilus Redwood reminds us: 'It required a man of independent means, disinterestedly devoted to the work, with tact, temper and powers of persuasion, to overcome the difficulties of the undertaking, and such a man was Jacob Bell.'[63] Once formed, the Pharmaceutical Society took on the character of a crusade, a drive for higher standards of performance and greater recognition by other professions and the public. The moral and social status of recruits would be raised and educational standards enforced. Specialisation in pure pharmacy would lead to co-operation with other branches of the medical profession. Commitment to science, research and development would enhance economic rewards and social prestige. The professionalising strategy of the society was designed to make the extraordinary occupational behaviour of the metropolitan elite the criterion for evaluating the work of the common-and-garden variety chemist and druggist. The programme of reform was a reflection of the activities of wholesalers and manufacturers and derived from a belief in the authenticity and utility of science. It was clearly not designed to meet the needs of the great majority of British chemists and druggists.

The most important fact about the creation of the Pharmaceutical Society is that it was not a response to the demands of the profession. Jacob Bell and his friends in London were not bombarded with *cahiers* and lists of grievances, with cries of anguish and outrage from their colleagues in the provinces. The dog, as Sherlock Holmes once observed, did not bark in the night. Nor did it occur to anyone to discover why. No attempt was made to gather information about the problems and difficulties, the hopes and aspirations of Britain's chemists and druggists. A series of articles in the *Pharmaceutical Journal* entitled 'Illustrations of the Present State of Pharmacy in England' was not an inquiry into the profession's requirements, but an exposé of its shortcomings.[64] Not that the policy was to let sleeping dogs lie. The founding fathers developed a strong sense of mission: the sinners to be converted were the potential members of the society. They were branded as thoroughly unprofessional:[65]

> The majority of those who called themselves chemists and druggists had no just claim to the former of these appellations, nor could they in the full sense of the term be called pharmacists; they were dealers in drugs and chemicals just as grocers are dealers in tea, sugar, and vinegar, without knowing anything of the real nature of the articles in which they dealt.

They were ignorant, uneducated adulterators of drugs, pandering to the ill-informed public demand for cheap medicines, indiscriminately retailing all manner of goods and services, motivated solely by the desire for profit, and thus antagonising the apothecaries by advising patients and prescribing over the counter:[66]

> The indiscriminate sale of drugs by unqualified persons would produce much less injury to the credit and interests of the regular Druggists, if the public had the means of forming a correct estimate of the value of the articles they purchase, and of the qualifications of the parties concerned. But, unfortunately, in most country towns, not only is every Grocer and Oilman a Druggist, but also every Druggist is a Grocer and Oilman. The Druggist has no badge or credentials to designate his superior qualification; in fact, he is not *of necessity* more qualified than the Grocer. The blue and red bottles in the windows are common to all; and this is the criterion understood by the public as indicating what is called 'a doctor's shop'.

The foundation of the Pharmaceutical Society was an act of aggression against the ordinary chemist and druggist. It was an attempt by an influential and closely knit sector to regulate and control the other segments. The great mass of chemists and druggists had no desire to become 'professional men'. They were not eager to acquire commercially irrelevant educational qualifications, nor to pay an annual levy to a remote London corporation. Above all, they did not welcome the prospect of having their work subjected to inspection and surveillance. They wanted to be left alone. Nor is this surprising: the chemist and druggist was thriving. There were, of course, many levels of prosperity and many divisions within the ranks. A great gulf stretched between the established, substantial manufacturer-cum-retailer and the corner shopkeeper scraping a living little better than that of his working-class customers. A series of gradations between these extremes reflected the character of the neighbourhood and the status of the clientele. The occupation was already regulated by the mechanisms of the market economy. Entry at any level was restricted by the requirement of capital. Breaking into the better-class market was certainly not easy. Extensive premises were needed for storage and safekeeping of materials, for workshops and laboratory, and for living quarters for assistants, apprentices and servants. The purchase or renting of such places in fashionable town centres, the cost of equipping them, purchasing stock and materials, paying rates, all necessitated a hefty initial capital outlay. Only by satisfying the demands of his clients could the retail chemist and druggist secure an adequate return on his investment. What was the nature of this demand? Why was the retail chemist and druggist prospering? What was the basis of his success?

It was clearly not the practice of pure pharmacy and the dispensing of physicians' prescriptions. Once more, the experience of the London elite and the rest of the profession stood in marked contrast. In the elegant streets of the City and West End were to be found those great dispensing establishments to which physicians were in the habit of recommending their patients; but most chemists and druggists rarely saw a physician's prescription and had little occasion to dispense. Before the introduction of the 1911 National Insurance scheme, 90 per cent of all dispensing took place in doctors' surgeries.[67] In the first half of the nineteenth century the rank-and-file chemist and druggist was scarcely a part of the system of orthodox professional medicine. He was a product of another, older, more deeply rooted practice — the tradition of family self-medication. Up to the present century, folk medicine was an integral part of popular culture. It was used more frequently and regarded more highly by the mass of the population than the advice of the medical profession. It is misleading to think of family self-medication as something employed by the poor for the want of better means or as merely residuary to the activities of the medical profession. Pre-industrial beliefs and traditions survived the rapid urbanisation of the nineteenth century. Migrants from the countryside brought their folk practices and herbal remedies with them. The rise of the chemist and druggist is an aspect of the adaptation of folk medicine to industrial, urban society. In Elizabeth Gaskell's novel *Mary Barton* (1848), Alice Wilson was able 'on fine days, when no more profitable occupation offered itself' to ramble in the fields around Manchester, gathering wild herbs from the hedgerow, ditch and field, 'for drinks and medicine'. But for most people the local chemist and druggist became the source of supply. Dr J.K. Crellin has drawn our attention to the evidence of the many domestic medicine chests that have survived and to the fact that chemists and druggists generally advertised their services for the dispensing of family recipes: 'Many customers certainly came in to have family prescriptions dispensed and for the purchase of the refilling of home medicine chests . . . The home medicine chests seem to have become popular during the second half of the eighteenth century, a time when many Family Recipe Books were still widely used.' The extent of self-medication in early Victorian England is suggested by the continued popularity of the relevant literature. In 1847 Buchan's *Domestic Medicine* was still being republished, and at least six new or reprinted editions of Wesley's *Primitive Physic* appeared in the 1840s, while the edition of *Cox's Companion to the Family Medicine Chest and Compendium of Domestic Medicine* published in 1846 was described as the thirty-fourth.[68]

The continuity of folk medicine was more than the precarious survival of old habits, for it involved a strain of determined opposition to expertise and professionalism. It was an assertion of the right of 'every man of common sense', as John Wesley put it in his *Primitive Physic* (1747), to 'prescribe either to himself or his neighbour'.[69] It was a form of popular resistance against the cultural aggression of the professionalisation of medicine. Folk medicine was, of course, anathema to the founders of the Pharmaceutical Society. In their minds it was associated with superstition, magic and astrology: it was irrational and unscientific.[70] The society's founding fathers saw themselves engaged in a militant struggle against the vernacular tradition of self-medication. Their drive for professionalism was intended to vindicate the claims of the medical expert against the freedom of the consumer.

The elite fringe, those who occupied the centre of the pharmaceutical arena, believed that scientific rationalism was the modern orthodoxy, and were rash enough to label the established beliefs of the many as 'fringe' medicine.

Notes

1. Leslie G. Matthews, *History of Pharmacy in Britain* (Edinburgh, E. & S. Livingstone, 1962), 117-25.
2. J.K. Crellin, 'Pharmaceutical History and its Sources in the Wellcome Collections', *Medical History*, 11 (1967), 216-17.
3. Jacob Bell and Theophilus Redwood, *Historical Sketch of the Progress of Pharmacy in Great Britain* The Pharmaceutical Society of Great Britain, London, (1880), 40-107. The first part of this *Historical Sketch* was written by Jacob Bell in 1842 as an introduction

to the *Pharmaceutical Journal*.
  4. Bell and Redwood (note 3), 40-71.
  5. Crellin (note 2), 216.
  6. Bell and Redwood (note 3), 73-4.
  7. *Pharmaceutical Journal*, 11 (1851/2), 46-7.
  8. Bell and Redwood (note 3), 96-7.
  9. *Ibid.*, 110-11.
  10. *Ibid.*, 98, 101, 109-10.
  11. W.S. Glyn-Jones, *The Law Relating to Poisons and Pharmacy* (London, Butterworth & Co., 1909), 254-5.
  12. *Apothecaries' Company* v. *Greenough*, 11 L.J.Q.B. 156 and 1 Q.B.799.
  13. *Lancet* (1840-1, 2; and 1841-2, 1), *passim*.
  14. Jacob Bell, *Observations Addressed to the Chemists and Druggists of Great Britain on the Pharmaceutical Society* (London, 1841), 4-6.
  15. *Ibid.*, 5-7.
  16. R.H. Tawney, *The Acquisitive Society* (London, G. Bell, 1945), 108.
  17. Bell (note 14), 7-8.
  18. *Ibid.*, 7.
  19. *Pharmaceutical Journal*, 12 (1852-3), 369.
  20. *Pharmaceutical Journal*, 9 (1849-50), 345.
  21. Bell (note 14), 9-10.
  22. Bell and Redwood (note 3), 149-51.
  23. Bell (note 14), 10.
  24. *Pharmaceutical Journal*, 7 (1847-8), 156.
  25. Bell and Redwood (note 3), 115.
  26. *Ibid.*, 118.
  27. Bell and Redwood (note 3), 116-19;
  28. S.W.F. Holloway, 'Medical Education in England, 1830-1858: A Sociological Analysis', *History*, 49 (1964), 299-324.
  29. *Pharmaceutical Journal*, 4 (1844-5), 251.
  30. Bell and Redwood (note 3), 143. See I.S.L. Loudon, 'A Doctor's Cash Book: The Economy of General Practice in the 1830s', *Medical History*, 27 (1983), 249-68.
  31. Bell and Redwood (note 3), 118.
  32. J.M.D. Olmsted, *François Magendie: Pioneer in Experimental Physiology and Scientific Medicine in XIX Century France* (New York, Schuman's, 1944); M.P. Earles, 'Early Theories of Mode of Action of Drugs and Poisons', *Annals of Science*, 17 (1961), 97-110.
  33. J.R. Partington, *A History of Chemistry* (London, Macmillan 1963), 4, 300.
  34. J.B. Morrell, 'The Chemist Breeders: The Research Schools of Liebig and Thomas Thomson', *Ambix*, 19 (1972), 1-46.
  35. Richard Phillips, 'Illustrations of the Present State of Pharmacy in England', *Pharmaceutical Journal*, 2 (1842-3), 315-20, 396-9, 528-32, 651-2; and *Pharmaceutical Journal*, 3 (1843-4), 108-11, 244-7.
  36. *Pharmaceutical Journal*, 3 (1843-4), 339.
  37. Bell and Redwood (note 3), 193.
  38. John Attfield, *A Pamphlet on the Relation to Each Other of Education and Examination, especially with Regard to Pharmacy in Great Britain* (London, McCorquodale 1882).
  39. *Pharmaceutical Journal*, 2 (1842-3), 323.
  40. For this see Margaret Pelling's authoritative study, *Cholera, Fever and English Medicine 1825-1865* (Oxford University Press, 1978), especially ch. 4, 113-45.
  41. Henry Ancell (1802-63) was an active member of the General Association of Chemists and Druggists of Great Britain in 1829 (see Bell and Redwood (note 3), 103) but, by 1852, was very hostile to the Pharmaceutical Society (see *Report from the Select*

Committee on Pharmacy Bill, 1852 (387) XIII).
    42. Quotations from Pelling (note 40), 130 and 132.
    43. Quoted in Robert H. Kargon, *Science in Victorian Manchester* (Manchester University Press, 1977), 103.
    44. *Ibid.*, 105.
    45. *Ibid.*, 106.
    46. Bell and Redwood (note 3), 148. Their names and the names of their firms can be found on pp. 90, 92, 101-2.
    47. Matthews (note 1) is a mine of information about the leading London druggists and their companies.
    48. Bell and Redwood (note 3), 170-1.
    49. E.C. Cripps, *Plough Court, the Story of a Notable Pharmacy* (London, Allen & Hanburys, 1927).
    50. *Dictionary of National Biography*, 1, 322.
    51. *Ibid.*, 28, 51.
    52. Bell and Redwood (note 3), 164-6.
    53. *Ibid.*, 330-1.
    54. Cripps (note 49), 55-6.
    55. The firm became John Bell, Hills & Lucas Ltd. See Matthews (note 1), 220.
    56. Bell and Redwood (note 3), 330.
    57. *Ibid.*, 192-3; and *Pharmaceutical Journal*, 3rd series, 4 (1873-4), 726-7.
    58. *Pharmaceutical Journal*, 11 (1851-2), 46-7; and Bell and Redwood (note 3), 212.
    59. Bell and Redwood (note 3), 176, 205-6, 236, 276, 329; and Crellin (note 2), 219-20.
    60. *Pharmaceutical Journal*, 3rd series, 6 (1875-6), 620.
    61. Crellin (note 2), 219.
    62. Matthews (note 1), 246.
    63. Bell and Redwood (note 3), 148-9.
    64. *Pharmaceutical Journal*, 2 (1842-3) and 3 (1843-4); and Bell and Redwood (note 3), 157.
    65. Bell and Redwood (note 3), 163.
    66. *Pharmaceutical Journal*, 3 (1843-4), 101.
    67. *Pharmaceutical Journal*, 189 (1962), 33-5.
    68. Crellin (note 2), 226; and P.S. Brown, 'The Providers of Medical Treatment in Mid-nineteenth-century Bristol', *Medical History*, 24 (1980), 297-314.
    69. See Stanley Chapman, *Jesse Boot of Boots the Chemists* (London, Hodder & Stoughton, 1974), ch. 1, 11-30.
    70. See, for example, Jacob Bell's comments on Culpeper's translation of the *Pharmacopoeia* (1653), in Bell and Redwood (note 3), 7-9.

8 BONES OF CONTENTION? ORTHODOX MEDICINE AND THE MYSTERY OF THE BONE-SETTER'S CRAFT

Roger Cooter

Many reasons might be assigned for why the subject of this paper has hardly figured in historical discussion of the relations between 'regular' and 'irregular' medicine. Not least of these is that little is known of the history of the practice of bone-setting, either ancient or modern. Indeed, the very nature of bone-setting is unclear, since at different times and places it was an area evidently more concerned with manipulative therapeutic techniques than with the mending of fractures.[1] The fact, too, that bone-setting was a practical craft and not a theory-laden medical system has obviously not encouraged its historical pursuit; nor has the fact that bone-setting was never an organised medical, or alternative medical, cult (unlike its descendants, osteopathy and chiropractic). Although the absence of similar epistemological and sociological engagements has not deterred the historical pursuit of the bone-setter's near neighbour in popular culture, the untrained midwife, bone-setting clearly lacks the compensating feature of the medical politics of gender.

Not unrelated to these factors, but probably more central in accounting for the historical neglect of bone-setting, is the subject's failure to supply what most history of 'irregular' medicine tends to draw from and rest upon: a clear profile of confrontation with orthodox medicine. Although it is possible to cite evidence as early as the seventeenth century to support the view that bone-setting was perceived as a popular antiestablishment form of healing, it is also possible to bring forward other evidence to show that orthodoxy was largely untroubled by bone-setting and able, simply, to accommodate it. The latter view has been suggested by George Rosen, one of the few historians ever to refer to the subject. In his classic work on medical specialisation, Rosen remarked of bone-setting that it affords an interesting and impressive example of 'primitive specialism' 'merging with modern surgical practice'. In order to illustrate his point, Rosen drew attention to the fact that modern fracture therapy began with the work of Hugh Owen Thomas, of Liverpool (1843-91), a qualified practitioner who came from a long line of traditional Welsh bone-setters. Thus Rosen gave weight, if inadvertently, to an essentially uncontentious version of both the history of bone-setting and the rise of modern orthopaedics. Had it not been that his main concern was with ophthalmology, Rosen might well have added that the major ambassador of the modern orthopaedic specialism, Sir Robert Jones (1857-1933), was nephew, as well as apprentice, partner and successor, to Hugh Owen Thomas.[2]

This paper looks more closely at 'the merger' of bone-setting with orthodox medicine during the latter part of the nineteenth century, and questions the extent to which bone-setting can be exempted from the framework of conflict common to the analysis of the relations between 'regular' and 'irregular' medical practice. But the purpose is not simply to fit bone-setting into a conventional historiography — least of all to characterise its relations with orthodoxy in terms of manifest confrontation. The object, rather, is to broaden understanding of the relations between 'regular' and 'irregular' medicine by drawing attention to what has been subjected to least historical scrutiny: on the one hand, the means by which an 'irregular' practice could survive despite the extension of the professional and legal hegemony of orthodox medicine and, on the other hand, the way in which orthodoxy could contend with and profit from 'irregular' competition, not necessarily by protesting, dismissing, denying and closing ranks, but by granting a certain legitimacy to the practice in order to appropriate it.

In an otherwise misty historical landscape, James Paget's clinical lecture 'On the Cases that Bone-setters Cure' stands as a welcome signpost. Published in the *British Medical Journal* in 1867, and reprinted in 1875 and 1902, it marks what in retrospect can be seen as the beginning of the end of traditional bone-setting.[3] Though not directly responsible for the wave of interest in the subject that followed its publication, it signifies a shift in the relations between orthodox medicine and bone-setting, and thus serves as an organising principle for the discussion of those relations.

Before Paget's work, though there is evidence here and there of regular practitioners taking an interest in bone-setting in order to learn from it,[4] the general picture is one of mutually exclusive spheres of practice. How these separate spheres of practice evolved is not clear. Fragmentary evidence suggests that bone-setting may have obtained some moorings in hospital surgery towards the end of the sixteenth century, but that thereafter it was let slip — the manipulative part of the craft being wholly abandoned, while fracture treatment was absorbed into general surgery.[5] Surgeon Richard Wiseman's complaint against 'the wickedness of those who pretend to the reducing of luxated joints by the peculiar name of *Bone-setters*', suggests that by then (1676) bone-setting was a world apart from that of elite medicine, at least in London.[6] From Robert Turner's *The Compleat Bone-setter* (1656), it further appears that bone-setting had come to have a popular anti-orthodox significance. Turner, an astrologer, confessed no faith in 'Sutarian or Scissarium doctors' (those too fond of suturing and scissoring), and dedicated his book to a woman 'who bounds [sic] the wounds of her poor neighbours'.[7]

Since bone-setting, like midwifery, seems often to have been pursued only as a sideline, the extent of the practice at any one time is impossible to tell.[8] All that is certain is that the practice was carried on and that its mysteries were acquired not through any learned tradition, but rather through informal apprenticeship. Most commonly, the skills were learned either at sea, in the merchant service or in the Royal Navy, or else within a family — the skills passing from fathers to sons and, sometimes, to daughters.[9] By the nineteenth century, a dozen or so of the latter 'hereditary' or 'natural' bone-setting families had acquired great reputations and practices in Britain; in addition, there was an extensive population of itinerant bone-setters.[10] But the fact that all these bone-setters tended to be situated in rural areas, away from large towns, and away from London in particular, suggests that the continuance of bone-setting depended to a large extent on its geographical separation from both the authority and the provisions of orthodox medicine. In London there were few reports of bone-setters; indeed, the perception of a London surgeon writing on quackery in 1837 was that 'happily in this country [in contrast to America] we have few, if any, of these *natural bone-setters* ... such is the improved state of scientific attainment among us, and such is the state of our public surgical establishments'.[11]

It is difficult to say whether the geographical distribution of bone-setters was the result of aggression from orthodox practitioners in urban centres, or whether it was simply the consequence of the continuation of the practice in rural agricultural areas (where bone-setting is said to have arisen from the method of treating farm animals). The available evidence points to the latter explanation, though obviously there were disincentives against bone-setters migrating to those urban places where accident hospitals and hospital outpatient departments had come to exist and where, at least as far as fracture treatment was concerned, there would have been direct rivalry with orthodoxy. The bone-setter Evan Thomas, who moved from Anglesey to Liverpool in 1831, experienced considerable hostility from the local medical profession, and there is evidence that at least one of the four prosecutions brought against him for malpractice between 1840 and 1860 — that of 1854 — was indeed a 'miserable attempt at persecution ... got up against him by certain members of the medical profession'.[12] Since Thomas ran what amounted to his own accident hospital, where he treated daily between forty and eighty patients mostly for fractures and dislocations (charging 5s. or more per patient), not only was the physical territory of his practice in proximate contact and conflict with orthodoxy, but so too was a large part of his therapeutic territory. Of course it did not make for smoother relations with orthodoxy that Thomas's skills were held in such high esteem by laypersons as for it to be suggested on one occasion that he be put in charge of a ward or two in the Liverpool Northern Hospital.[13] Nor did it help that Thomas was regarded popularly as the medical underdog who dared to stand up against the medical monopolists. Carried from the court on the shoulders of a crowd after his trial of 1854, Thomas was given a hero's dinner and presented with testimonials of his fame as it 'resounded through the lower classes of Liverpool'. Like some other bone-setters, Thomas could capitalise not only on the popular custom of referral to bone-setters and on the popular fear of hospitals (where injured limbs stood a good chance of being amputated, and the amputation of causing death),[14] but also on the popular political distaste of medical institutions and the hauteur of those who governed and worked within them.

Outside of urban medical centres, however, among the scattered populations of labouring poor, the bone-setter's trade might be perceived by orthodoxy more as a source of amusement and incredulity than as a serious threat to professional reputations and incomes. In 1806, a medical man reported the case of a Dorset bone-setter supposedly earning 'between two and three hundred pounds per annum by selling small bags, containing the web of a frog's foot, at two shillings and sixpence each, as a charm for the cure of scrophula'. In the same year another reported from Perthshire:[15]

> Besides a number of itinerant quacks and *pill doctors*, there is an old man, who has practised many years in this circuit as a *bone-setter* and curer of all diseases; . . . he attempts to instruct others in the mysteries of his inspired abilities. Perhaps you will hardly believe me, when I inform you that this self-taught medicaster cannot read English even tolerably, and the little he can read, he does not understand; yet the lower classes of people are so convinced of his superior medical skill, that he is held as a divinity amongst them.

Yet other examples indicate that the survival of bone-setting could as readily obtain through a separate sphere of operations granted openly by orthodoxy itself. For instance, a case of manslaughter in 1856, brought against an unqualified bone-setter in Ffestiniog, Wales, reveals that for over twenty years the accused had been employed by the local slateworks expressly for the purpose of attending broken bones, and that in this capacity he had been accepted by the regular practitioners as one of the three 'doctors' to the quarrymen: 'He attends to the bone-setting generally, and we perform more the parts of physicians,' stated one of his qualified colleagues, who was also the surgeon to the Ffestiniog hospital.[16] In this case the bone-setter seems to have acted more or less as the medical officer to the quarry, presumably thus serving the convenience of the employers as much as of the qualified practitioners by referring to the latter only those cases of serious injury which could not adequately be dealt with on the spot.

A similar kind of 'paramedical' niche for bone-setters may have come into existence in parts of the industrial North of England towards the end of the nineteenth century. Evidence from Medical Officers of Health to the parliamentary *Report as to the Practice of Medicine and Surgery by Unqualified Persons in the United Kingdom* (1910) indicates that over the previous few decades the numbers of bone-setters had increased (as much as 40 per cent in Sunderland), and that this was partly attributable to the introduction of the Employers' Liability Acts (1880 and after). Since there are also suggestions that many members of this new tribe of bone-setters were persons who had obtained certificates of training from St John Ambulance courses, their function in factories (as well as at football matches and in Friendly Society 'sick clubs', where they were also reported) may have been primarily to administer first aid, referring all but minor injuries to local infirmaries and qualified practitioners. Whether or not this was the main role of these bone-setters, the fact that they can be seen to have moved into spaces where orthodox medicine had not yet established itself further indicates how the practice was able to survive by maintaining a division of medical labour which did not threaten orthodoxy, either socio-economically or therapeutically.

Broadly speaking, the publication of Paget's lecture on bone-setting in 1867, can be understood in terms of a response to an evident breakdown in the maintenance of these separate spheres of practice. Only two months before its appearance a social stir had been created when the bone-setter Richard Hutton successfully relieved the longstanding suffering of the Hon. Spencer Ponsonby.[17] Hitherto, as noted above, there had been little evidence of bone-setting in London, and certainly no evidence of any upper-class or middle-class custom for the practice. Hutton (1801-71), whose family had practised bone-setting in

Westmorland for over two centuries, had emigrated to London many years before, but apparently turned to bone-setting only in the 1860s, after he retired from his trade as an upholsterer. It was then, according to Wharton P. Hood (the general practitioner who succeeded to the practice) that Hutton was[18]

> induced . . . to try his hand at the work of restoring a crippled joint to usefulness. One case led to another, and his successes among the poor, to whom his services were always freely given, led to their being frequently sought and remunerated by the rich.

Since the latter invariably praised Hutton at the same time as they condemned 'the distinguished hospital surgeons by whom they had originally been treated', it is not surprising that Paget opened his lecture with the remark that 'Few of you are likely to practise without having a bone-setter for an enemy, and if he can cure a case which you have failed to cure, his fortune may be made and yours marred.' Thus we might think of Paget as responding to Hutton's cure of Ponsonby with the same sense of professional indignation that Percivall Pott had felt in the 1730s when the celebrated bone-setter Sally Mapp was reputed to have cured the niece of Sir Hans Sloane.[19] Like Pott, Paget was among the London medical elite and keen to defend its reputation and territory.

But it would be historically short-sighted to offer this as the whole explanation for Paget's interest in bone-setting. After all, identifying the bone-setter as 'the enemy' was really the least of his concerns; more central was his attempt to invade the therapeutic territory of the bone-setter and to appropriate to orthodox medicine specifically those manipulative techniques whereby bone-setters managed to give speedy relief to stiff and anchylosed joints, dislocations and sprains (fractures, Paget maintained, were 'as well, or better done by regular surgical rules'). To understand this concern it has to be recalled that at the same time that Hutton was making a name for himself, there was developing within orthodox medicine an interest in the use of physical therapeutic agents in the treatment of musculo-skeletal disorders — in particular, medical gymnastics, massage, and mechano-, electro-, galvanic- and hydro-therapy.[20] Although all of these therapies were prone to use by medically unqualified persons and were, therefore, of concern to orthodoxy for social and professional reasons, they were also the subject of a more purely technical therapeutic interest. On the continent, and in Germany especially, the use of these agents in orthodox practice was becoming routine. That Paget's publication appeared shortly after its author's return from a tour of Germany and is thus possibly of as much significance as its temporal proximity to the Ponsonby case.[21]

Similarly, the fact that Wharton Hood was busy learning the secrets of Hutton's bone-setting *before* Paget's lecture was published, strongly confirms a medical context of emerging interest in physiotherapeutic and manipulative techniques. Further, before Hood undertook his apprenticeship with Hutton, he sought and obtained the approval of the distinguished surgeon Sir William Fergusson, who had recently become the great advocate of 'conservative' surgery. Since Fergusson also had homoeopathic interests (as did other early advocates of physical medicine),[22] it may not be unwarranted to suggest that orthodoxy's interest in this area of medicine partly reflects its learning from homoeopathy; at the very least, the interest in bone-setting reflects a medical profession sufficiently confident in itself to be able to pursue and appreciate other than invasive surgical techniques. Hood's demystification of the bone-setter's craft in his *A Treatise on Bone-setting* (1871) was, at any rate, warmly received by the profession as a contribution to what the *Lancet* declared to be 'a neglected corner of the domain of surgery'.[23]

But if Hood's treatise fully legitimated orthodox medicine's growth of interest in bone-setting,[24] it was far from fulfilling the *Lancet*'s hope of rendering bone-setters extinct. Indeed, in 1878 — the year that Samuel Smiles and William Chambers did much publicly to vindicate and legitimate recourse to bone-setters[25] — the surgeon Howard Marsh, writing 'On Manipulation . . . as a Means of Surgical Treatment', could ask[26]

> how it is that while herbalists, who hold about the same relation to medicine that bone-setters hold to surgery, have fallen into the background, bone-setters have rather gained than lost in popularity?

Because others in medicine at this time made similar observations, it is tempting to argue that orthodoxy had been hoist by its own petard: that the more it sought to follow Paget and 'imitate what is good . . . in the practice of bone-setters', the more it elevated bone-setters in the public's estimation; at the same time, orthodoxy cast doubt on its own probity through its attempt to burgle the bone-setter's skills after having previously ignored them or denounced them as quackery.

But such an argument appears to have little basis in fact, despite the support for bone-setters among popular writers, and despite the fact that orthodoxy's growth of interest in bone-setting coincided with the late-nineteenth-century popular challenge to the authority of materialist science and medicine. The only evidence of bone-setting being enlisted in the rhetoric against 'medical popery' appears to be that contained in *Medical Specialism* (c. 1890), by homoeopath, anti-vivisectionist, anti-vaccinator and all-round medical heretic J.J. Garth Wilkinson MRCS. Not unlike Robert Turner's *The Compleat Bone-setter*, Wilkinson's work (which was first published in the *Homoeopathic World*) celebrated the uneducated and unlicensed bone-setter as an earthy democratic symbol of protest against the arrogance of the orthodox medical specialists. The latter, with their bloody surgery and fragmented gaze, were wholly lacking what Wilkinson saw as the bone-setter's 'profound intuition, not formalized'. Like generations of common people before him, Wilkinson claimed to have 'seen what relief [the bone-setter] gives, and had decisive evidence of his cures'.[27]

But Wilkinson's comments on bone-setters, aside from being fleeting and intentionally homoeopathic, seem to have had little resonance in the late nineteenth century. Possibly this is because the popular image and meaning of the bone-setter had changed. The rugged and venerated bone-setter, 'Dr' Jabez Mortimer, depicted in Francis Brett Young's novel *Dr Bradley Remembers* (1938) was, after all, a distant memory of a rural healer who was supposedly 'a very old man' even in 1850.[28] Though doubtless in some corners of Britain in 1900 there were still bone-setters of Mortimer's sort travelling the country with their herbs and splints, on the whole the post-1870 evidence tends to an impression of bone-setters as figures whose outlook and whose popular regard was mostly commercial, whether they worked up-market or down.[29] Bone-setters charged as much or more than regular practitioners and (although there were bone-setters and bone-setters) many people probably regarded them no differently from other medical specialists.[30] 'Bone-setter', 'bloodless surgeon', 'manipulating surgeon', 'osteopath', 'orthopaedist' — all must often have seemed much of a muchness to the general public: Liverpudlians, for example, knew of their townsman and orthopaedic specialist Sir Robert Jones, only as a 'bone-setter', long after his bone-setting ancestors had passed into obscurity.[31] And the fact that the sons of bone-setters often took a medical qualification (e.g. Evan Thomas's three sons; and James Taylor, the last of the bone-setting Taylors of Lancashire[32]) must further have blurred any meaningful distinctions in the public mind between the 'heterodoxy' of the one and the 'orthodoxy' of the other. If, as some orthopaedists were still complaining in the 1930s, 'the bone-setter holds in the estimation of the wage-earning classes a place . . . unduly elevated',[33] this may have had little to do with any strong sense of social rapport with bone-setters; it may have been simply because bone-setters (like osteopaths and chiropractors today) continued to attend to the common aches and sprains for which orthodox medicine, then as now, had little time. Crucially, for a working person, such attention might make the difference between earning or not earning.

Certainly, there was little either to endorse or to encourage Wilkinson's regard of bone-setters in the popular middle-class vindications of the craft by Smiles, Chambers and the naturalist Charles Waterton in the late 1870s.[34] Though Waterton and Smiles did something to enhance the image of the bone-setter as rugged and 'self-made', and Chambers acclaimed the bone-setter's intuitive 'gift of touch', there was in these writings scarcely a glimmer of recognition of the bone-setter as a possible bastion of laissez-faire principles in medicine (as previously the middle class had buttressed its faith in homoeopathy). Rather, by praising the bone-setter's manipulative skills (and these alone), such writers essentially endorsed orthodox medicine's appropriation of those skills. For Chambers (before becoming aware of Hood's treatise) it was the first duty of 'intelligent inquiry' to acknowledge the bone-setter's latent ability in order that humanity should profit from it. Once aware of Hood's treatise, however, he declared: 'Now that the subject has been scientifically looked into, any discussion regarding it may be allowed to drop'.[35] Even W.T. Stead's defence in 1910 of the 'bloodless surgery' of the fashionable bone-setter Herbert Barker — a defence directed against 'the aboriginal instincts of the Faculty' — was ultimately a call to end the situation in which manipulative practices existed only in 'the hinterland of surgery'.[36] Indirectly, by leading bone-setters themselves to publish rational, scientist vindications of their craft,[37] the popular middle-class writers on bone-setting helped to undermine whatever meaningful 'alternative' status bone-setting may have had in popular culture.

What seems more certain than the generation of any populist or counter-cultural regard for bone-setting towards the end of the century is, rather, the cultivation and exploitation of any signs of popularity by those in orthodox medicine in the general area of orthopaedics. Such practitioners were hoping thereby to legitimate new professional space for themselves. This partly applies to Paget himself who, it is worth recalling, had formerly been a dresser to the founder of the Royal Orthopaedic Hospital in London, and several of whose publications in the 1860s and 1870s were on diseases of the bones ('Paget's Disease', for instance, being identified by him in 1870). However, the trend is most marked in the case of Howard Marsh, a disciple of Paget, who began advocating the appropriation of the bone-setter's craft in 1878, the same year in which he was appointed demonstrator of orthopaedics at St Bartholomew's Hospital.[38] By drawing attention to the popularity of bone-setting and, at one and the same time, praising certain of the bone-setter's skills while deprecating others, Marsh can be seen as endeavouring to do more than merely 'occupy the place and receive the fees of the ousted Bone-setters' (as claimed by the bone-setter G.M. Bennett).[39] He can also be seen as attempting to seize hold of a body of practice whose proven efficacy commanded both popular and professional respect, but which could at the same time be shown to be in need of control by those specially trained in anatomy and in the care of musculo-skeletal disorders. As orthopaedics was still a minor branch of surgery mostly dealing with the treatment of chronic deformities by use of mechanical appliances, such a tactic had an authority and status-raising potential.[40] On the one hand, it exploited orthodox medicine's fear of unqualified practice; while, on the other, it held out the promise of therapeutic advance. Significantly, it was only later in the century, when orthopaedics had become better established within general surgery, through the practice of antiseptic osteotomy (bone surgery) and other operative techniques, that the claim was to be made (by a member of the British Orthopaedic Society (est. 1894)) that 'the progress [of orthopaedics] was due to what had been taught them by Lister, not to what they had learned from bone-setters'.[41]

Such a thesis is confused, however, (though not refuted) by reference to the pioneer orthopaedist, Hugh Owen Thomas (the qualified son of Evan Thomas). Contrary to what might be supposed from Rosen's reference to him, Hugh Owen Thomas contended 'that in the practice of bone-setting nothing is to be found that can be added to our present knowledge, yet discussing the matter will show us our ignorance'. Concerning diseases of joints, in particular, Thomas maintained (in 1883), that he had 'never met with the slightest evidence that any of them [bone-setters] had any knowledge of the subject or a method of treatment which was not utterly wrong'.[42] However, Thomas was responding here not to popular celebrations of bone-setters, but rather to the professionalisers in orthopaedics (in particular, Paget and Marsh) who had made bone-setting 'the topic of debate in medical societies'. Capitalising only on the latter interest in bone-setting, Thomas endeavoured to expose the interest as 'ill-advised' because it inclined to a practice of active manipulation which was at odds with his own therapeutic principle of enforced and prolonged rest.[43]

Yet Hugh Owen Thomas's position on bone-setting was in all respects unique and his views remained remote from the medicine and surgery of the London establishment. Having inherited the bone-setting skills and much of the practice of his unqualified father, and having built up his own fully equipped private clinic for the treatment of acute and chronic deformities, Thomas needed neither to vie for the bone-setter's custom, nor to pursue for purposes of professional aggrandisement the rhetoric of a popular bone-setter posing a threat to orthodox medicine. A fiercely independent general practitioner, Thomas was far more interested in taking the medical elite down a peg than in helping them to carve out and enter into a specialist niche. Thus he can hardly be spoken of in the same breath as Paget or Marsh, or even of his nephew Robert Jones; more like the unqualified bone-setter of old, Hugh Owen Thomas was a practitioner in a self-contained, separate sphere.

It was Robert Jones who broke that isolation and established Hugh Owen Thomas as the pioneer of 'modern orthopaedics' — a specialism concerned with the treatment of both chronic disorders and acute injuries, especially fractures, by means of manipulative and invasive surgery. But Jones — in part because he was fully aware of how much of his uncle's and his own expertise derived from their unqualified bone-setting ancestors — never sought to make capital for the embattled specialism of orthopaedics by referring to bone-setters. He was hardly in a position to do so, since those contesting his specialist claims for orthopaedics were only too anxious to dismiss him as a provincial 'bone-setter'. Thus veering away from his uncle in this respect and tending towards Paget, he called for the incorporation into orthopaedics of the useful manipulative practices 'that go by the name of bone-setting'.[44] During the First World War, while Herbert Barker was puffing his skills to the middle and upper classes (in order to earn for himself a knighthood), Jones set about acquiring the physiotherapeutic equipment that had belonged to Wharton Hood; he also began to instruct a new generation of orthopaedists partly from the pages of Hood's *Treatise on Bone-setting*.[45]

Although lack of evidence must leave the full history of bone-setting as much a mystery as the craft itself, it is more than merely a want of evidence that renders bone-setting in late-nineteenth-century Britain an odd and awkward contributor to the history of the relations between 'regular' and 'irregular' medicine. The problem is not just that bone-setting was not an area for gladiatorial combat between medical heretics and medical monopolists, and hence fails to live up to conventional expectations of what the past relations between 'regular' and 'irregular' medicine *ought* to have been. Further, bone-setting is a case of a body of practice neither withering passively in the face of modern medicine, nor being simply incorporated into it. Bone-setting was a hardy survivor well into the twentieth century, partly because it continued to shift its sphere of operations to wherever the influence of orthodox medicine was weakest, but, above all, because it continued to provide a therapeutic for which the greater part of regular practice had neither the time nor the aptitude. On the other hand, though, to the extent that bone-setting skills were taken up by orthodox medicine, this has to be understood not as some inevitable consequence of disinterested medical insight into the value of those skills, but rather as the result of active appropriation — which inevitably involved contest and the assertion of hegemonic interests. Yet this invasion of the bone-setter's therapeutic space by those whose professionalisation could be served by it, relied to only a limited extent on popular support for bone-setters and seems not to have generated any popular resistance.

The history of the relations between bone-setting and orthodox medicine thus fails to offer a satisfying, straightforward picture of the relations between 'regular' and 'irregular' medicine. Neither simplistic models of conflict and confrontation nor ideas of uncontentious 'mergers' accurately depict the reality of those relations. But to say merely that the relations were complex is hardly an adequate conclusion. 'Complexity' here surely stems purely from our failure as historians sufficiently to appreciate not only that hegemony in medicine (as in politics and culture) is never all-embracing, but also that 'regular' medicine is no more monolithic and single-minded than 'irregular' medicine. Both spheres — to the extent that they remain separate at all — are obviously compounds of interest with different ways and means of attempting to secure their survival. Nineteenth-century bone-setting, as an unincorporated and unprotected practice, was as protean in its survival techniques as it was open to raids by maurauders from orthodoxy. As such, like 'irregular' medicine as a whole, it would be absurd to expect that bone-setting should evince one or other tidy and symmetrical set of relations with 'regular' medicine.

Acknowledgement

I am grateful to John Pickstone for his comments on an earlier version of this paper, and to Bill Luckin for his various suggestions.

Notes

1. See J. Cyriax and E.H. Schiotz, *Manipulation, Past and Present* (London, Heinemann, 1975), 29-31; cf. R. Dacre Fox, 'On Bone-setting (So-called)', *Lancet* ii (1882), 843-5.

2. George Rosen, *The Specialization of Medicine, with Particular Reference to Ophthalmology* (New York, Froben Press, 1944), 10-11. On Thomas and Jones see, respectively, D. Le Vay, *The Life of Hugh Owen Thomas* (Edinburgh, E. & S. Livingstone, 1956), and F. Watson, *The Life of Sir Robert Jones* (London, Hodder & Stoughton, 1934). Among the few works in the history of medicine to refer to bone-setting are F.B. Smith, *The People's Health, 1830-1910* (London, Croom Helm, 1979), 284-7, and F. Cartwright, *The Development of Modern Surgery from 1830* (London, Barker, 1967), ch. 7.

3. *British Medical Journal*, 5 January 1867, 1-4; reprinted in S. Paget, *Clinical Lectures and Essays* (London, Longmans, 1875), and in S. Paget (ed.), *Selected Essays and Addresses* (London, Longmans, 1902).

4. Notably William Cheselden, as revealed in his *The Anatomy of the Human Body*, 6th edn (London, W. Bowyer, 1741), 37-8. For other examples, see Cyriax and Schiotz (note 1), 59ff.

5. See J.L. Thornton, 'Orthopaedic Surgeons at St. Bartholomew's Hospital, London', *St Bartholomew's Hospital Journal*, 59 (1955), 195-204 at p. 195; and R.T. Anderson, 'On Doctors and Bonesetters in the 16th and 17th Centuries', *Chiropractic History*, 3 (1983), 11-15. Cf. W.A. Clark, 'History of Fracture Treatment Up to the Sixteenth Century', *Journal of Bone and Joint Surgery*, 19 (1937), 47-63.

6. Richard Wiseman, *Severall Chirurgicall Treatises* (London, R. Norton & J. Macock, 1676), as quoted in Cyriax and Schiotz (note 1), 29.

7. *The Compleat Bone-Setter, Wherein the Method of Curing Broken Bones, and Strains, and Dislocated Joynts, to-gether with Ruptures, vulgarly called 'Broken Bellyes,' is fully demonstrated* (London, Lamb, 1656). Turner claimed this to be an 'Englished and Enlarged' edition of the hugely popular sixteenth-century work, *This is the Myrrour or Glasse of Helthe*, by Friar Thomas Moulton, but there is little resemblance in fact. Only a few pages of Turner's work actually deal with bone-setting.

8. Thus, nineteenth-century trade directories and census surveys are an imperfect guide; E.M. Sigsworth and P. Swan, surveying the Census Enumerators' Notebooks for the West Riding of Yorkshire for 1841 to 1881, were able to trace only three bone-setters: 'Para-medical Provision in the West Riding', *Society for the Social History of Medicine Bulletin*, 29 (1981), 37-9.

9. See Cartwright (note 2), 146. Among female bone-setters were Ann Thomas, daughter of Welsh bone-setter, Richard Evan Thomas, who carried the art to Wisconsin (ibid., 147); and Sarah Mapp ('Crazy Sally'), the daughter of a bone-setter of Hindon, Wiltshire, on whom see James Caulfield, *Portraits, Memoirs and Characters of Remarkable Persons* (London, T.H.Whitely, 1820), vol. 4, pp. 70-7; W. Wadd, *Mems., Maxims, and Memoirs* (London, Callow & Wilson, 1827), 168-70; and C.J.S. Thompson, *Quacks of Old London* (London, Brentano's, 1928), 299-307.

10. Among the best-known British bone-setting families were the Thomases of Anglesey, the Taylors of Lancashire, the Maltbys of Nottingham, the Masons of Lincolnshire, the Huttons of Westmorland (subsequently of London), the Crowthers of Yorkshire, and the Matthews of the Midlands. References to the less famous are hard to find; unique is the source cited in note 15 below. See also R.G. Hodgkinson, *The Origins of the National Health Service* (London, Wellcome Institute for the History of Medicine, 1967), 137.

11. William Wright (Surgeon-aurist) in his notes to 'Of Natural Bone-Setters — Natural Fools . . . etc. , in anon., *An Exposition of Quackery and Imposture in Medicine* (London, J.S. Hodson, 1839), 192n. On bone-setting in America, see R.J.T. Joy, 'The Natural Bonesetters with Special Reference to the Sweet Family of Rhode Island', *Bulletin of*

the History of Medicine, 28 (1954), 416-40.

12. 'Presentation of a Testimonial to Mr. Evan Thomas, Bone-setter, Liverpool', *North Wales Chronicle*, 2 September 1854. See also, *Verbatim Report of the Trial, Crowley versus Thomas, in the Liverpool Court of Passage . . . February 8, 1854 . . . from the Short-hand Notes of Speeches, Evidence, etc., of Mr. T.A. Humphries, Reporter* (Liverpool, C. Ratcliffe, 1854).

13. Letter to editor, *Liverpool Albion*, 26 February 1844, in 'Letter Book of Evan Thomas and Hugh Owen Thomas' (MS, Liverpool Medical Institute).

14. For an example of concern over amputations see, Roy Porter, 'Laymen, Doctors and Medical Knowledge in the Eighteenth Century: The Evidence of the *Gentleman's Magazine*', in Roy Porter (ed.), *Patients and Practitioners* (Cambridge, Cambridge University Press, 1985), 283-314 at pp. 305-6. The mortality rate for amputations in British hospitals prior to the 1870s varied between 25 and 50 per cent (see R.B. Fisher, *Joseph Lister, 1827-1912* (London, Macdonald & Jane's, 1977), 124); thereafter, amputations for fractures declined significantly. See G. Callender, 'Seven Years of Hospital Practice', *St Bartholomew's Hospital Reports*, 14 (1878), 183-95 at p. 192. See also F.C. Skey, 'On Fractures', in his *Operative Surgery* (London, Churchill, 1850), 137-73; and O.H. and S.D. Wangensteen, *The Rise of Surgery* (Folkestone, Dawson, 1978), 48-51.

15. Replies to Dr Edward Harrison's questionnaire on irregular medical practice: *Medical and Chirurgical Review*, 13 (1806), pp.clxxix and lii. I am grateful to Irvine Loudon for drawing my attention to this source.

16. 'The Charge of Manslaughter at Festiniog', *Carnarvon Herald*, 27 July 1856.

17. See Wharton P. Hood, *The Treatment of Injuries by Friction and Movement* (London, Macmillan, 1902), ch. 1: 'Introductory and Personal', p. 5; and G. Matthews Bennett, *The Art of the Bonesetter: A Testimony and a Vindication* (London, T. Murby, 1884), reprinted with an introduction by P. Hawkins (Isleworth, Middlesex, 1981), 47-50. On Hutton, see also the entry in the *Dictionary of National Biography* on his nephew, Robert Hutton (1840-87), the fashionable London bone-setter.

18. Hood (note 17), 7-8.

19. See Wadd (note 9), 169-70.

20. See, for example, Mathias Roth, *Notes on the Movement-Cure, or Rational Medical Gymnastics* (London, Groombridge, 1850); and F. Busch, *General Orthopaedics, Gymnastics, and Massage*, trans. Noble Smith (London, F.C.W. Vogel, 1886). See also, V. Putti, 'The Cripple in Italy', *Cripples' Journal*, 2 (1926), 258-62; and M. Rowbottom and C. Susskind, *Electricity and Medicine, History of their Interaction* (London, Macmillan, 1984)., Cyriax and Schiotz (note 1), 60, refer to a Dutch doctor, Johnn Mezger, whose manipulative treatments were drawing large numbers of patients and medical visitors from all over Europe in the 1860s and 1870s. Special hospitals and wards for the treatment of deformities, in which many of these therapies were tried out, were only just beginning to be established in this period. The Hospital for the Ruptured and Crippled was established in New York in 1863; Liverpool's Royal Southern Hospital installed gymnastic equipment in 1858: see V.P. Gibney, 'Reminiscences of the Orthopaedic Surgeons of the Latter Half of the Nineteenth Century', *New York Medical Journal*, 4 May 1912, 913-15; and C. Macalister, *The Origin and History of the Liverpool Royal Southern Hospital* (Liverpool, W.B. Jones, 1936), 69-72. For the pre-history see R.J. Cyriax, 'A Short History of Mechano-therapeutics in Europe until the Time of Ling [i.e. to 1813]', *Janus*, 19 (1914), 178-240. See also, A. Bryce, 'Remarks on Mechano-therapy in Disease', *British Medical Journal*, 3 September 1910, 581-4, and the editorial, ' "Undeveloped Land" of Medicine', *British Medical Journal*, 3 September 1910, 638-9.

21. See S. Paget (ed.), *Memoirs and Letters of Sir James Paget*, 3rd edn (London, Longmans, 1903), 234-5.

22. Notably Roth (1819-91), note 20. On Fergusson (1808-77), see entry in *Dictionary of National Biography*.

23. *Lancet* (editorial), 1 April 1871, 451-2.

24. There were special sessions on bone-setting at the Abernethian Society in 1878 and at the Clinical Society of London in 1880: see *St Bartholomew's Hospital Reports*, 14 (1878), 339-46; and Bennett (note 17), 90ff.

25. Smiles, *George Moore, Merchant and Philanthropist* (London, Routledge, 1878), revealed how Richard Hutton in 1867 had successfully relieved Moore of longstanding pain and distress. Chambers, through his review of this work, extended the vindication: *Chambers' Journal*, 6 July 1878, 417-21; and 'The Bone-setter's Mystery', *Chambers' Journal*, 22 February 1879, 113-15.

26. *St Bartholomew's Hospital Reports*, 14 (1878), 205-19 at p. 206.

27. As quoted in Logie Barrow, 'An Imponderable Liberator: J.J. Garth Wilkinson', in R. Cooter (ed.), *Alternatives: Essays in the Social History of Irregular Medicine* (London, Macmillan, forthcoming).

28. Francis Brett Young, *Dr. Bradley Remembers* (London, Heinemann 1938), 68-89.

29. See, for example, the interview with Herbert Barker in *Spy*, 25 August 1894, 9. Barker, to be knighted in 1922 for his bone-setting among the upper classes, was then struggling for work in Manchester; see his autobiography *Leaves From My Life* (London, Hutchinson, 1927).

30. On fees, see Smith (note 2); for an example of a consultation with a bone-setter, see J.E. Phythian, 'Reminiscences of Whitworth and its Doctors Fifty Years Ago', *Transactions of the Rochdale Literary and Scientific Society*, 12 (1914-16), 55-66.

31. As discovered by the American orthopaedic surgeons when they arrived in Liverpool in 1916: see, J. Goldthwait, *The Division of Orthopaedic Surgery in the A.E.F.* (Norwood, Mass., Plimpton Press, 1941), 9.

32. See LeVay (note 2) p. 14; and J. West, *The Taylors of Lancashire: Bonesetters and Doctors, 1750-1890* (Worsley, H. Duffy, 1977), appendix C, 115-21.

33. E.M. Little, 'Mrs Mapp and Others', *Cripples' Journal*, 5 (1929), 183-5; see also, R.C. Elmslie, 'Quacks'., *Cripples' Journal*, 4 (1928), 284-9; and R. Ollerenshaw, 'The Present Attitude toward Bone-setting and Manipulation', *British Medical Journal*, 7 June 1930, 1056-7. (All three authors were senior orthopaedic surgeons.)

34. For Smiles and Chambers, see note 25; Waterton's comments (on the bone-setter Crowther) from his *Wanderings and Essays in Natural History*, new edn (London, Longmans, 1879), are quoted in Bennett (note 17), 4-6.

35. *Chambers' Journal*, 22 February 1879, 115.

36. W.T. Stead, 'The Hinterland of Surgery', *Review of Reviews* (1910), quoted in Barker (note 30), 88.

37. Notably those by Bennett (note 17) and J.M. Jackson, '*The Bone-setter's Mystery': An Explanation* (Boston, Lincs, J.M. Newcomb, 1882).

38. On Paget and Marsh, see Thornton (note 5).

39. Bennett (note 17), 90. See also, Mr. Bruce-Clarke, 'The Rationale of Bone-setting', *St Bartholomew's Hospital Reports*, 14 (1878), 339.

40. See B. Valentin, *Geschichte der Orthopädie* (Stuttgart, Thieme, 1961); and R. Whitman, 'The Emancipation of Orthopaedic Surgery', *Proceedings of the Royal Society of Medicine*, 36 (1942-3), 327-9.

41. C.B. Keetley, *Transactions of the British Orthopaedic Society*, 3 (1899), 35. For the orthopaedists' perception of Lister's place in the history of their specialism, see, A. Rocyn Jones, 'Lister'. *Journal of Bone and Joint Surgery*, 30B (1948), 196-9.

42. Thomas, *Principles of the Treatment of Diseased Joints* (London, H.K. Lewis, 1883), 63-4.

43. See A.G. Timbrell Fisher, *Treatment by Manipulation in General and Consulting Practice* (London, H.K. Lewis, 1925), 'Historical Introduction', especially pp. 8-9.

44. Jones, 'Remarks on Orthopaedic Surgery in Relation to Hospital Training', reprinted from *British Medical Journal*. 20 November 1920, 2.

45. See: G.M. Levick *et al.*, 'Organisation for Orthopaedic Treatment of War Injuries', in *Medical Services in the History of the Great War: Surgery of War* (London, H.M.S.O., vol. 2, 1923), 381-408 at p. 397; and H. Osmond-Clarke, 'Half a Century of Orthopaedic Progress in Great Britain', *Journal of Bone and Joint Surgery*, 32B (1950) 620-75 at pp. 642-3.

9 PHYSICAL PURITANISM AND SANITARY SCIENCE: MATERIAL AND IMMATERIAL BELIEFS IN POPULAR PHYSIOLOGY, 1650-1840

Virginia Smith

When the literary critic Samuel Brown described what he meant by the term 'physical puritanism' in his *Westminster Review* article of 1852, he announced:[1]

> nobody can deny that this is pre-eminently the age of physiological reformers. A new sort of puritanism has arisen in our times, and its influence is as extensive as its origin is various. In some of its features it is as ancient as history, in others as modern as yesterday, and in all not inexpressive of certain of the wants and aspirations of society. It is the puritanism of the body; but the common purpose of all its manifestations is the healing, cleansing, and restoration of the animal man.

According to Brown, 'physical puritanism' referred to a cluster of therapies which all in their way related to ascetic belief, but which historians have tended to treat as separate entities. He listed them as vegetarianism, hydropathy, mesmerism, phrenology, teetotalism, homoeopathy and popular physiology. Without in any way discounting those features which were 'as modern as yesterday', more particularly mesmerism, phrenology and homoeopathy, a great deal more has to be said about the features which were 'as ancient as history' — the 'popular physiology' held as part of a communal psyche and inherited 'lore' relating to the body. In this essay I shall examine some of the primary characteristics of the corpus of popular physiology between 1650 and 1840, in relation to certain 'core' beliefs connected with the philosophy of hygiene.

The theoretical and practical problems surrounding the body have been a neglected subject: medical historians have been content to take academic texts as given, and a rather limited number of texts at that. The social history of cleanliness has proved to be a vantage-point for the narrower history of hygiene, the long-term demographic and economic implications of which have yet to be disinterred as part of the medical history of daily life.[2] I am more concerned here, however, with the lengthy pay-off between the social realities and the rich and coherent social fantasies that surround hygiene; there is a strong argument for suggesting that 'pollution fears' represent a spiritual or 'immaterialist' or psychic constant which has always to be satisfactorily resolved within the utilitarian medical framework. Perhaps precisely because of these materialist/immaterialist tendencies, the *problem* of cleanliness as a social virtue and a physical necessity has been a central theme in medicine and an open arena of debate. This longer history of the *mentalité* of cleanliness further tends to make the nineteenth-century preoccupations appear highly specific.

The Democratic Polemic

If we are to arrive at a better understanding of the structure and content of nineteenth-century 'physical puritanism' — how far it was 'fringe', how far it was 'orthodox' — we have to acquire a working knowledge of the *ancien régime* of medicine, the physical cosmology which was available to all social classes during the long retreat of classical civilisation, and throughout the period of Christian feudalism up to the so-called 'High' Middle Ages. As an all-embracing and constantly shifting cosmology, it provided a great body of 'lore' on all the technical procedures of medicine as understood and/or recorded — on surgery, pharmacy and dietetics. In addition, there was a central core of classical metaphysics which did not change markedly, and provided for the immaterialist or 'occult' tendencies via the holistic paradigm of the elements and the humours. Written *practica, consilia*, herbals and regimens were widely used to give succinct medical advice in the absence of professional consultation.[3]

Passing beyond the sources, we also need to define some of the main features of the democratic polemic with which regimens especially were associated. In the league table of European *incunabula* between 1450 and 1500, the early publishing trade in England was characterised by a comparatively low output but an exceptionally strong vernacular tradition — some 60 per cent of all works.[4] The vernacular output that dealt with medical advice was above all concerned with utility and the necessities of life: 'how' to preserve life as well as 'why'. Most vernacular advice was as much concerned with well-tried practices of traditional medical lore as it was with the exploration of new and useful skills, and giving advice about the ingestion of food, drink and drugs was by no means the exclusive prerogative of the physician. These 'lay' rights were especially strongly protected and upheld with regard to drugging practices. The new Paracelsian chemistry introduced in the sixteenth century, for example, did not supplant rural drug lore. Not only did Paracelcianism tend to intensify expert drugging practices, but because of the reductivist alchemical cosmology of mineral elements, it could also be construed as denying the purificatory and humoral processes of 'in-go' and 'out-go'. In the advice books, the 'straw man' was not the mild Galenist but the professionally aggressive 'chymical' doctor.[5] By contrast, however, the work of sixteenth-century experimenters on the 'mechanisms' of diet and longevity was quickly assimilated into the regimen tradition. The method of Sanctorious (1561-1636), proving the mechanical action of the invisible evacuations of perspiration, marked the beginning of an era of continental and British spa balneology.[6] Balneology was an early and successful example of the reinterpretation of medical science on the mechanical model, a part of the experimental programme advocated by Francis Bacon as the only way out of the well-worn sophistry and contradictions of medieval lore.

If utility was one strand of the democratic polemic, immaterialist thought was definitely another: the right to manage the body for personal salvation was a special preoccupation closely associated with classical and Christian philosophic traditions and earlier magical practices. How far later philosophic refinements overlapped with earlier practices is difficult to judge; we can, however, posit a common holistic cosmology which upheld the rights of individual experience in relation to the natural as well as to the supernatural cosmos. One of these experiences was purification, and it was the purification of the 'immanent' world — the cosmos held in common — that Greek hygienic physiology sought to rationalise.[7]

It is premature to give an explanation of the popular usage of a hot-cold cosmological polarity found within the advice book tradition, especially from the mid-seventeenth century, but it is clear that the polarisation of hot and cool elements was laden with a religio-mystic symbolism, that was structurally built into the Greek scheme. Thus the hot-cold polarity was one of the crucial diagnostic axes of humoralism. It is, moreover, one that is known to have ethnographic roots which transcend the European experience.[8] It would be easy to label certain seventeenth-century vernacular authors as isolated examples, were it not for the wide and long-lived diffusion of hot-cold symbolism, in which coldness remained a primary guarantor of godly ascetic life. The historian's problem is how to expose the breadth and depth of the 'cool regimen', while the trace elements of associated beliefs and practices are well concealed behind the doors of the private household. The 'elemental' cold-air and cold-water bathing are relatively easily tracked down outside the household; the 'cool vegetable system' is the best concealed domestic practice of all.

Physically Cool Puritanism and the *Vis Medicatrix Naturae*

Although the principle of coolness may at first sight appear tangential to physiology, on closer inspection it becomes more thoroughly complementary. The nineteenth-century evidence suggests that the use of 'cool' and clean foods and drinks (i.e. a diet of vegetables and water — a form of fasting), may be regarded as the most radical form of the philosophy of asceticism. By contrast with seventeenth-century balneology, seventeenth-century vegetarianism was derived from earlier humoralism and the purgative or anti-pollutory action of the fluids, translated via the philosophy of temperance. It could also frequently be combined with a commitment to occult herbalism and the use of vegetable simples; a hatred of mineral drugs; and a semi-monastic physical seclusion that was the mark of sect-membership such as that advocated by lapsed Anabaptist vegetarian Thomas Tryon.[9] Those with vegetarian leanings were often later called Pythagoreans, but this was a loose use of a term with wider philosophical implications; the 'philosophic regimen', if not actually practised, may have been commonly understood among classically educated groups. Thus Henry More (1614-87), the Cambridge neo-Platonist, adhered to the hierarchical philosophy of Plotinus, in which the threefold 'Triad' described the levels of spiritual purification which lay between the One and the Good, and brute matter; or, Platonically, 'The Platonists doe chiefly take notice of Three kindes of Vehicles, Aetherial, Aerial, and Terrestrial, in every one whereof there may be several degrees of purity and impurity.' More's biographer Richard Ward noted a passage in More ['which I take to belong much to himself':][10]

> Temperance and Devotion, and a Chearful Dependence on God's Blessing, even, with Mean Diet, must contribute much to Health and Beauty, and a quick and delicate Air in the Countenance. This is what the Pythagoreans called Philosophical Temperance, the Mother of that Wisdom which makes the Face to Shine, and nourisheth the Soul's Luciform Vehicle.

More felt 'quick and delicate', Thomas Tryon felt 'nimble, brisk, and eesie' on the 'Mean Diet'; while to both the body was a 'Vehicle', a 'Temple', for the 'Plastick faculty of the Soul'. Not that More, a lifelong Fellow of Christ's College, Cambridge, was likely to have been vegetarian; however, he did aver that it was the duty of one who by nature 'came into a body undefiled' to 'endeavour after the Highest Purity'. Some indication of the comparative rarity of serious vegetable-eating was given by the courtier and horticulturalist John Evelyn (1620-1706) who, through 'sallets' and vegetables, 'would recall the World, if not altogether to their Pristine Diet, yet to a much more wholesome and temperate one than is now in fashion ' — adding, 'the Product of them is come unto more Request and Use amongst us, than heretofore'.[11]

There is a good case for saying that there were two major outbreaks of 'serious' vegetarianism at the beginning and at the end of the eighteenth century bringing vegetable-eating into fashion in Britain and then percolating downwards as the temperate mixed meat and vegetable diet. But it may be an error to limit the 'philosophic regimen' to current findings. In the iconography of nineteenth-century vegetarianism, claims are made for practising individuals as diverse as Isaac Newton (1642-1727), Alexander Pope (1688-1744), Philip Stanhope, Lord Chesterfield (1694-1773), James Thomson (1700-48), David Hartley (1705-57), William Cullen (1710-90), John Howard (1726?-90), Oliver Goldsmith (1728-74), William Paley (1743-1805) and John Sinclair (1754-1835).[12]

Two mystic neo-Platonic phases can at present be identified. The first, in the 1720s and 1730s, was that surrounding the quietist natural philosophers George Cheyne (1671-1743) and William Law (1686-1761). While Law and his admirers such as John Byrom and John Wesley were conducting philosophic vegetarian experiments, Cheyne's influential advice book *Essay of Health and Long Life* (1724) laid the basis for the popular acceptance of the vegetable-based diet.[13] Antonio Cocchi's treatise on *The Pythagorean Diet* (1745) was written 'to render those more cautious, who (tho' otherwise ingenious) call the Doctrines of Pythagoras by the names of Dreams and Follies'.[14] The second phase, at the end of the eighteenth century, was that of the evangelical and Romantic enthusiasts, with their 'clerk' Thomas Taylor 'The Platonist' (1758-1835). The vegetarian works of John Oswald (1791), Joseph Ritson (1802) and J.F. Newton (1811) were addressed to the serious evangelical reader, rather than to the aristocrat or the philosopher. The philosophical roots, however, are more clearly evident in the classically trained late-eighteenth-century Romantic poets, epitomised by Samuel Taylor

Coleridge's deep appreciation of British and European transcendentalism.[15] Coleridge (1772-1834) appears to have been idolised by a generation of nineteenth-century universalists and aesthetes as

> a shining representative of those transcendental divines of the Platonic, Aesthetic, and metaphysical school, who not only raise their own soul to God as the supreme good, but likewise raise the souls of all around them . . . Would to heaven that we may also resemble Coleridge!

Shelley, however, was the more devout vegetarian.[16]

The late-eighteenth-century medical advice books show the vegetable diet in ascendance, judiciously interpreted in the light of anti-sepsis and the 'low' cooling regimen; William Buchan's *Domestic Medicine* gave a lead in 1769, and thereafter there was a general empirical acceptance of its utility, as well as its prevalence in non-European cultures. The advice books also show vegetable-eating as a fashionable 'quackery' in the hands of the nature doctor James Graham; or as a mark of piety in the Methodist vegetable drug-vendor Joshua Webster.[17]

Pursuing the philosophy of coolness a little further into the cold-water therapy of balneology, it is fairly evident that there were few, if any, examples of shining transcendentalism. In other words, balneology was more decidedly 'terrestrial' and utilitarian — and less 'aetherial' — than vegetarianism; it is not possible to suggest, even in outline, a common bank of philosophic inheritance on a par with neo-Pythagoreanism and neo-Platonism. Balneology was, as noted, one of the practical applications of medicine on the mechanical model, and remained so — the cold-water empiric John Hancocke (d. 1728) made a point of wishing 'the Mechanical Men good success; for no body would be more glad to see Physick, both in Theory and in Practice, reduced to Demonstration, than I would be'.[18] Nevertheless, it was associated with an ascetic anti-materialism of a type that was considerably more dispersed than the select 'high' mysteries of the cool vegetarian spiritualist. Balneologists, for example, included the use of air (air-bathing) as a necessary part of the ascetic hardening process; and the virtue and necessity of cool sweet air was deeply rooted in medieval lore. We are familiar with the regulated ascetic cold-water and air 'training' of John Locke's *Some Thoughts Concerning Education* (1697); but the balneologist John Floyer's polemic on the corrupted customs of 'hot regimen' (1697) was the text of a Protestant sermon:[19]

> Brandy, spirits, strong wines, smoking Tobacco, strong Ale, Hot

Baths, wearing flannel and many clothes, keeping in the House, warming of Beds, sitting by great fires, drinking continually of Tea and Coffee, want of due exercise of body, by too much study or Passion of the Mind, by marrying too young, or by too much venery (which injures Eyes, Digestion, Perspiration, and breeds Wind and Crudities); and for all the Effeminacy and Niceness and weakness of Spirits that is produced in the Hysterical and Hypochondriacal.

The iatro-mechanical (and iatro-chemical) foundation should have been enough to have given balneology the honourable professional position it held on the continent. In the North of England, however, it became associated with Presbyterianism; and in the South with the work of empirics who gave popularised versions of the virtues of 'cool regimen'. In the 1720s cold water was often associated with the fasting of 'Spare Diet'. The cold-water enthusiast, John Smith, gave an appendix of rules on the use of cool air and the 'Spare Diet' — which was an appeal to longevity and the primitive diet if not to the extreme purity of vegetarianism. Fasting, 'with the assistance of common water' was explicitly recommended. John Hancocke saw in Sydenham's 'new and cooler regimen in the Cure of Fevers' confirmation of 'Things that agree with our own notions'. John Wesley's *Primitive Physic* (1747) could be said to have built the cold-water therapy, with the Spare Diet, into the foundations of new Dissent.[20]

In addition to its democratic, ascetic and utilitarian appeal, water had further cosmological implications; there was a venerable tradition of religious ritualism surrounding the old holy-wells which, to some extent, also helps to account for the ease with which cold-water bathing and 'dipping' became a renowned British pastime and its efficacy a cherished national belief. As with vegetarianism, evidence of 'serious' domestic use is at present limited to the occasional reference — such as John Howard's daily use of the cold-water sheet; or the cold-water nurse who 'would not dry a child's skin lest it should destroy the effects of the water'. Strictly speaking, all that was needed was cold water and the tub; and the advice books were strongly in favour of cold water as a tonic regimen for the debilitated or dissipated; for the hardening of children; or for the perfection of 'natural' bloom and beauty. Equally significantly, they were highly suspicious of the use of hot water. These moral scruples were soon to be moderated by new physiological explanations.[21]

What, then, was the status of hygiene towards the end of the eighteenth century? The humanist debates among educated physicians and laymen had helped force change on to medieval therapeutics in the cause of empirical truth and utility — and, indeed, without the type of political compromise that this represented, the seventeenth-century 'bourgeois revolution' in civil politics and medical science could not have been carried through. The great liberal figure of the late seventeenth/early eighteenth century in this humanist tradition, was Hermann Boerhaave (1668-1738).[22] There were in the eighteenth century — as there were to be in the nineteenth century — professional practitioners from all classes who were caught between post-Paracelsian 'heroic' chemotherapy, and the broadly democratic coalition of interests in favour of the humoralist/mechanist paradigm of bodily harmony, the cool *vis medicatrix naturae*. Beyond the charmed circles of medical power and prestige — the working majority of barber-surgeons and apothecaries, well- and semi-educated householders, public and commercial 'quacks' and empirics — traditional remedies were often combined with the moral self-help therapies (herbalism, vegetarianism, balneology) in a rejection of polypharmacy on a scale that the profession could not and did not ignore. The eighteenth-century medical profession could thus be said to have been divided over therapeutics on pious grounds: since the profession was also, by virtue of its Baconianism, constitutionally eclectic and pragmatic, it was — as monopolists complained — wide open. The high plateau of the empirical practices of cool regimen ran from *c.* 1730 to *c.* 1790. Between 1790 and 1840, there was detectable social, professional and scientific change; the mounting costs of the long American and Napoleonic wars disrupted the flourishing eighteenth-century domestic economy, diverted the profits away from the needs of the growing urban centres, and revived the old issues of political rights which led to political compromise in the shape of the Reform Act of 1832. All of these disturbances, divisions and compromises were reflected in the medical world of *c.* 1790-1840, which exhibited all the signs of having become highly politicised and socially aware, certainly in comparison with the politically quiescent, private and local world of eighteenth-century medicine.

Progress of the Polemic: Popular Physiologies in the Nineteenth Century

One of the first signs to the medical historian of the social changes that were taking place is not only the qualitative but the quantitative change in the literature itself. In the nineteenth century, all of the traditional forms of hygienic information were expanded so greatly by technological change and a new wave of literacy, that it is by no means obvious whether or not it is possible to compare the new sources with the old. Public interest in medical affairs was expressed through a plethora of organised voluntary societies, public events and social experiments which, as reported, often had little to do with 'book learning' — though they frequently had a great deal to do with the self-advertisement of short, cheap, easily produced and transitory magazines. Thus it is extremely pertinent to ask whether the idea of a health 'genre' can be maintained in the face of this type of evidence. Or should we, perhaps more accurately, suggest that a 'genre' is only a superficial classificatory device which should not be allowed to obscure the actual structures of beliefs, with all their formal and informal social groupings? In this latter sense the nineteenth century is a salutory reminder of all the evidence on health and hygiene that has been lost to view in the previous centuries.

If, however, one regards the continued production of books on the art of preserving health as an inescapable fact, then the nineteenth-century examples force a reconsideration of their function at that time. The first noticeable change to have occurred in the genre between 1790 and 1830 is that the grip of the profession had tightened. Over 75 per cent of a random sample of books on general health advice in the 1830s were by authors who were careful to indicate that they were qualified professionals; in the 1790s the proportion of lay or unaccredited works was more like 50 per cent. Some of these changes can be illustrated by comparing the works of two bestselling authors: William Buchan in the 1770s and Andrew Combe in the 1830s. A.F.M. Willich in the 1800s stands between the older Buchanite view in which the lay public was seen both as consumers of healthcare and as active proponents; and what was more obviously the view of Combe, that professional training was (and should be) both diverging from and out-stripping, traditional methods of voluntary lay education. To this extent lay interest and representation declined in the early nineteenth century; but in fact, though the self-perceptions of particular groups had changed, there was no clean break in the internal dynamics of cure and care. There were few initiatives, but the authors of the 1820s and 1830s were also well aware of the traditions within which they were writing, and were able to supply material which apparently met specific public demands.

The 1820s

In view of the better-known revival of 'popular physiology' in the 1830s, it is important to note the immediate antecedents. After the Napoleonic wars, the advice book market began to lift to its prewar levels, and was dominated by a new generation of aspiring middle- and lower-range surgeon/general practitioners. Judging from the strength of surgeon authorships in the eighteenth century (and at earlier periods), surgeons as a group seem to have been strong supporters of regimen throughout — more consistently so than their humorally based colleagues, the chemist-apothecaries. The blurring of professional boundaries in the early nineteenth century showed that the concerns of the chemist had slipped painlessly into the realm of the surgeon-general practitioner, many of whom had little hesitation in recommending calomel alongside temperance and a little exercise, in a way that would have been unthinkable to a concerned Hippocratic surgeon of the late eighteenth century. Cool, non-natural regimen had slipped and fluidic humoralism, so it appears, flourished.

Some part of the explanation of this changing professional era can be found in the elevation of the surgeon's clinical role as an echo of the Paris hospital movement of this period, with its accompanying flood of commentary, such as that of the Parisian surgeon François Joseph Victor Broussais (1772-1838) and his many followers. The equivalent figure in London was undoubtedly John Abernethy (1764-1831), whose name was raised sufficiently frequently in the advice books to indicate that there was indeed an Abernethian school of 'localism' and gastric disorders, with its case work Bible, Abernethy's *Surgical Observations on the Constitutional Treatment of Local Diseases* (1809, seven editions by 1824). According to the popularised 'Abernethian Creed', the 'golden rules of health' consisted solely in:[23]

> an attention to the *due regulation* of the *Stomach* and *Bowels*, the *grand Elaboratory* by which the *Blood*, the source of *Vitality*, is prepared and transmitted to every part for the purposes of life, or, in fact, by simply promoting the *processes* of *Digestion* and the *natural* and *free* Secretion of all the *organs*.

Abernethy's preferred digestive strengthener was the mercurial 'blue pill'.

There seems no doubt that drug-taking was restored to a higher therapeutic status in the 1820s as a result of this reductivist theory and humoral therapy of blood-purging. By the 1830s it was noted that the dosage of calomel (mercurous chloride) was often 'fifteen or twenty times' what it used to be — even though hardly anyone actually died of 'venous congestion' or a 'bilious liver'. As a sign of the times, the 'quack' James

Morison ('The Hygieist') appeared in 1821 with his Universal Vegetable Medicine to combat calomel. A thorough anti-professional and a physical puritan, Morison's hygiene movement retained public support well into the 1860s under the slogan: 'Blood of Man is the Life — Diseases arise from impurities in the blood — Cleanse the Blood, and you banish disease.'[24]

At the same time, the debates surrounding food-taking and indigestion amounted to a public obsession which cannot be laid exclusively at the door of the profession. Gluttony emerged as the chief scapegoat of the 'nouveau riche' urban life, and fast living was single-mindedly condemned in a way reminiscent of sixteenth-century dietetics. Appeals to temperance were continuous: whole texts, such as those by J. Tweed (1820) or J.S. Forsyth (1827), were devoted to diet alone. One result of throwing out the liberal therapies of the immediate past was the derision accorded by the new professionals to vegetarians and vegetarianism. Satirical gibes against vegetarian circles peppered the *Family Oracle of Health* (1824), and the *Medical Adviser* (1824), confirming the vegetable diet as an eccentricity or, if possible, a quackery. The lay author 'Hortator' thought that vegetarianism could not be followed 'either with propriety or safety . . . those who attempt to emancipate themselves from [society's] trammels are generally rewarded for their pains, by being set down as eccentric or "queer" fellows'.[25]

The intensive observations of the chronic symptoms of dyspepsia had produced a working definition of 'quality and quantity' which relegated the issue of quality — 'with regard to the quality and quantity of food, excess in the latter is by far more prejudicial and dangerous than any defect in the former'. The new 'dyspeptic' invalid was fed on a scale of 'digestibility', also a feature of Willich's macrobiotic diets of the 1800s; there was a consensus on the advisability of the mixed diet, and a new appreciation of the digestive usefulness of bread and grains.

The condemnation of the 'vegetable system', however, was by no means complete; J.S. Forsyth conceded that the pure vegetable diet was suitable for hot climates if not for cold, and that animal food had its dangers. Joel Pinney, the democratic temperance author, while noting that Ovid, Pythagoras, and 'most eminent historians, physicians, philosophers, and poets of antiquity' agreed that man did not eat flesh in the 'golden age' of temperance, nevertheless felt that modern life usually required a 'union of animal and vegetable food'.[26] A small but significant precursor of later sectarianism was a tract on *A New System of Vegetable Cookery* (1821) by a member of the Society of Bible Christians at Salford, Manchester.

Interest in diet was to some extent made up by the somewhat conscience-stricken efforts of certain populist general practitioner authors to redress the balance towards mechanist therapy — with the use of balneology, but above all with the newly rediscovered principle of physical exercise. T.J. Graham highlighted exercise not only because of its 'general neglect' and 'uncommon utility', but also because[27]

> a third reason with much propriety might be added, viz. the unusual stress laid on *diet* . . . In the directions now given by physicians for the preservation of health, and the cure of disease, so much stress is laid on diet that regimen (of which exercise is the chief branch) is too often overlooked.

The therapeutic revival and development of physical training in the nineteenth century was comparable to that of balneology in the eighteenth century. Although it had always been technically a part of non-natural regimen and featured in the cool hardening system (which highlighted the exercise of bathing), Francis Fuller's *Medicina Gymnastica* (1777) had been no more than an isolated eighteenth-century text. Early-nineteenth-century texts — such as those by C.G. Salzman or Sir John Sinclair — paved the way for the detailed textbooks of Peter H. Clias (1825), Signor Voarino (1827) and Gustavus Hamilton (1827).[28]

Most of the techniques involved were those which had been laid down between the sixteenth and eighteenth centuries — walking, riding, friction with a flesh brush, fencing, sports and games, the use of dumbbells. In addition, there was the celebrated Captain Barclay's special mode of 'jogging' ('bend forward the body, to throw the weight upon the knees. [The] step is short, and [the] feet are raised only a few inches from the ground. Any person who will try this plan, will find that his pace be quickened'); and the programmes of gymnastic exercises ('Make prolonged inspirations, sitting . . . movement of feet upon the ground, the patient sitting . . . beating time, with both hands fixed to the horizontal pole . . . Lying down horizontally, to raise the body without assistance of the arms').[29] The solidly professional authors gave case studies of exercise used as physiotherapy in order to advertise the medical 'product'; but exercise was also seen more broadly as both the cure and preventive of indigestion, and as the steadying discipline of a daily moral routine. Consequently, it was much taken up by authors who placed their faith in longevity through temperance.

T.J. Graham demonstrated his appreciation of traditional longevity studies in a work published anonymously in 1829 — familiar names included Cornaro, John Wesley, and the recently deceased evangelical educationalist Mrs Sarah Trimmer. Joel Pinney started his series of works on temperance in 1830, and both Pinney and J. Harrison Curtis were actively involved in the newly formed Temperance Societies.[30] It was undoubtedly this revival of temperance, together with the self-disciplinary aspects of regimen — abstinence and the importance of daily routine — that gave the cholera advice books of 1831-2 their overwhelmingly admonitory character, as well as their simplified insistence on the rules of regimen. Cleanliness, temperance and regularity was the message repeated *ad nauseam* in the pages of A.B. Granville's *Catechism of Health*, with its precise hourly instructions. The same is true of the earnest physiological laws put forward in John Conolly's *Working Man's Companion*, or the emergency advice of Dr Challice of Bermondsey. In many other ways, however, the cholera epidemic exposed the unreformed — or undirected — nature of health advice in the 1820s, with its humoral concerns and partisan physiology. There had been changes proposed by 'enlightened' liberal and radical authors in the 1800s which together constituted a science of 'vital physiology'; and following the hygienic miasmatist triumph of 1831-2, when pressure of public opinion forced the government to moderate the ancient 'contagion' regulations of quarantine, certain groups within the profession evidently believed that the time was ripe for its renewal.

The 1830s

The critical shift of therapeutics in the 1790s appears to have provided a considerable part of the scientific rationale for the 'popular physiology' movement of the 1830s. By the 1790s, the modified hygienic humoralism and mechanism of the mid-eighteenth century had become outdated; it no longer provided an adequate terminology for the late-eighteenth-century physiology of the nervous system and sense impressions, set within late-eighteenth-century physics. A.F.M. Willich, and contemporary academics such as William Cullen, Thomas Beddoes or Christian Struve (whose works were translated from German) favoured the moderate control of all the vital forces as the basis of normal 'healthy' physiological functioning, the harmonising and conserving of bodily functions in the natural progress of the organism towards death.[31] Thus the new criteria employed in the 1800s were under-stimulation (as with a low, or cool, or asthenic regimen) and over-stimulation (as with a high, or hot, or sthenic regimen). This reinterpretation was enough to bring the precise management of preventive and nursing care back into the professional orbit — the new professional vitalist on a par with the old professional Galenist. Both concerned with the measurement of exact 'degrees'. Moreover, the German physiology employed the empirical findings of a later generation of balneologists with regard to the 'sensible' effects of the warm cosmetic bath. As a disciple of the German hygienist C.W. Hufeland, Willich placed the sense impressions of the skin in a central therapeutic position.[32] Moderate diet and moderate exercise preserved the 'vital' tone of the body; but dirty, flabby skin was the chief cause of nervous irritation and a range of debilitating diseases. The European vitalists had also taken it upon themselves to uncover a species of 'national debility' in urban populations, which could be corrected, among other things, by the use of the domestic bath. But there was little equivalent appreciation in Britain that national 'police' measures were either necessary or desirable, or that chronic urban diseases (even the traditional concerns with fever) were in any way abnormal.[33] It took cholera to force the government machinery into unaccustomed action and to revive public health reform movements — of which public health education was one.

Although Andrew Combe's *The Art of Preserving Health* (1833) may be presumed to be a companion volume to his brother George Combe's *oeuvre* on the mental science of phrenology — a 'physiology of mind as well as of body' — this best-selling hygienic work succeeded on its own terms in re-establishing the liberal/progressive vital physiology.[34] It is notable that the arrangement of the work corresponded closely to that of the earlier vitalists such as Willich — except in one revealing particular. Thus Combe at first omitted a section on 'Physiology of Digestion' on the grounds, he said, of the 'treatises of the digestive organs already in extensive circulation'; he may also have wished to disassociate himself from these works. The missing section on diet and dietetics was provided separately in a later work.[35] Skin physiology was put at the top of the list in two short chapters on the management of the organs and the organic systems. From the skin it was a short step to the muscular system and the rules of muscular exercises: the lungs and the use of air; the nervous system and mental exercise.

Throughout the work Combe took a line which neatly side-stepped the contemporary academic and clinical preoccupation with secretions and which treated the modern physiological material (such as that by Xavier Bichat) respectfully but eclectically — caring less about the probable action of tissues than the known action of organs. Like the vitalists, he was sensitive to holistic bodily dynamics, and to the moral and utilitarian interaction between the physical and psychic (or mental) forces. This put him well within the advice book tradition, and he consciously used the physiological corpus of the eighteenth century to underpin his arguments. It was work which was judiciously pitched both high and low — like Willich's and, it might be said, Buchan's — and it was this moderate synthesis that ensured its great public success. It became common for the authors of the 'popular physiology', which followed Combe's model in the late 1830s, to conflate cheerfully the old physiology with the new, without any damage to their own underlying beliefs. As the Quaker author J. Harrison Curtis commented:[36]

> Long recognised principles become truisms; but as such, instead of being disregarded, they should be more highly valued. In the present advanced state of physiological knowledge there is little left to the writer on this subject, but to shew the practical applications of these truisms to the actual state of society, and how their tendency may be most beneficially worked out for mankind at large.

The 1830s can be seen as a triumphant return to utilitarian mechanism. The prominence given to the physiology of the skin, and the brain, underscored the relative decline of exclusive interest in humoral dietetics. There was now an easily acceptable consensus on diet and it was accepted that there could (and in some cases, *should*) be a choice in the matter. The new 'general rule' was flexibility — 'we ought not to observe a rigid uniformity, at least not for any considerable time'.[37] Moreover, the rules for the mental exercise of the brain, now heavily emphasised, virtually overrode the fluidic gastric demands of the stomach: 'hence the important rule, never to enter upon continued mental exertion, or to rouse deep feeling, immediately after a full meal, as the activity of the brain is sure to interfere with that of the stomach, and disorder its functions'. The demands of mental health involved repose (under the old non-natural category of sleep), exercise (also a non-natural), and regularity (implicit in regimen). The old category of the passions was refined almost beyond recognition by the simple expedient of presuming passions to be organic. Melancholy, for example, had always been known as a wasting disease in adults; but even Locke would not have considered it feasible to eradicate it by physical training alone. As Combe argued with direct reference to the Lockean training of the sense impressions, 'in improving the *external* senses, we admit this principle readily enough; but whenever we come to the *internal* faculties of thought and feeling, it is either denied or neglected'. Internal mental health and external physical health were part of the same physical organisation:[38]

Were a general acquaintance with the laws of organisation to be held as an indispensable part of a liberal education, we would then be able to inculcate, with ten-fold force and success, the necessity of actively exercising every faculty, whether of thought, feeling, or motion, directly *on its own* objects, and at once explode the mistake of supposing that . . . it is sufficient to address ourselves to intellect alone.

There is no doubt that the utility of the 'practical applications' of modern medicine enhanced the reputation of the new physiology, and that the reformers' gradual displacement of the older 'heroic' cold regimen was a great public success: happiness and animal pleasures were allowable, even necessary. Perhaps nothing symbolised this more than the 'luxuriance' of the cosmetic warm bath, subsumed under the rhetoric of cleanliness. Earlier generations of lower-rank surgeons and apothecaries knew by long experience the efficacy of warm water for beautification, for sexual diseases and diseases of the skin — even though the physicians fought shy of some of these 'marginal' practices. Virtually all the techniques of bathing were in place by the 1800s — dipping, swimming, strip-washing, showering — and it only remained to add the hot-water technique of vapour baths to the art. A significant number of the 1820s authors were keen to display the new cosmetic knowledge — even though others were clearly devotees of cold water. By the 1830s, warm bathing was the new universal remedy. The longstanding Sanctorian doctrine of insensible perspiration remained the all-important channel for the evacuation of vaporous excreta, and retained its position as a truism readily understood by all. The vitalists had added precise temperatures from Fahrenheit's thermometer, and these could be displayed as well — from 98° for a young child to a 'safe' 75°-85° for the normal adult. The family health magazines and domestic economy writers quickly took the 'domestic bathing place' on board as the status symbol of healthy living — 'there is no part of the household arrangement so important to the domestic economy as cheap convenience for personal ablution'.[39] For those who could not afford the bath, the shower was an acceptable alternative. The obvious conclusion arrived at from whatever physiological viewpoint, or perfunctory physiological paragraph, was that uncleanliness was physically bad for you:[40]

> It results from this that personal cleanliness is a matter of first-rate importance. The entire body ought frequently to undergo ablution, and tepid bathing is perhaps the best mode of performing it. It is gratifying to observe the attention that is now beginning to be paid to this

subject, and the facilities that are afforded to every one for taking care of his health in this direction.

It had been the cholera which had crystallised the public dogma on personal cleanliness, and had given hygiene a political edge. The radical free-trader, utilitarian and educationalist A. Kilgour regarded physiology as a political tool to analyse the physical needs of 'masses and nations'. In *Lectures of the Ordinary Agents of Life* (1834) he eulogised cosmetic baths and public bathing in the form of factory baths (recently introduced as a philanthropic use of the waste hot water from steam engines) and above all hoped that 'the time is not far distant when the British government will take stronger measures with respect to the police of towns and villages. As yet all improvement in this department has come from without government.'[41] Legislation on public baths, the soap tax, parks, libraries and food adulteration was gradually introduced to accompany the Chadwickian emergency sanitary measures as part of a long-term parliamentary public health programme. There should have been an immediate gain for the hygienic professional in the proposed transfer of public resources, but for the longstanding professional ambiguity concerning hygiene. Both Combe and Kilgour repeated what John Roberton had said before them — namely, that the solution to public health was not simply to educate the public and the politicians, but to tackle the thorny problem of internal standards of training in hygiene.

Moreover, they and others — such as the President of the Royal College of Surgeons, Sir Anthony Carlisle — were aware that public confidence in the profession had dropped to an alarmingly low point due to the 'heroic' drugging practices of an inexperienced younger generation of practitioners; this problem was not apparently so extreme as it was in America, where state medical registration laws were toppling in the face of a massive switch of public allegiance to sectarian 'irregulars'.[42] In Britain, progressive public opinion was all on the side of 'enlightened empiricism so long as it served the public interest, as it had in the past, by reducing the number of drugs swallowed and the size of bills paid', the lay watchdog Joel Pinney, indeed, hoped that the medical state would 'wither away' and confine itself to emergency alleviation — the idealistic civic philosophy of later sanitarianism. But practical considerations also prevailed: 'That there should be so little ground for confidence in the medical profession', commented Pinney, 'is a circumstance sufficient to alarm any reflecting mind.'[43]

Hand in hand with the recent professional disdain for empirical hygiene went the lack of hygienic research and development, already well below levels commonplace on the continent. The first specialist periodicals appeared in Britain in the late 1830s, some ten to twenty years after the first French and German publications; hygiene as a specialist field did not appear on an academic curriculum in Britain until 1864.[44] The fact that the popular press still had to be used by liberal professionals as a main forum of debate on hygienic physiology was in clear contrast to the old hardline professional view (such as that suffered by William Buchan or John Roberton) that young physiological demagogues brought the profession into disrepute.[45] By European professional standards, therefore, British hygienic physiology was academically backward, professionally divided and socially constrained; by American standards, it was relatively socially secure; by British standards, it was definitely 'marginal'.

From 1650 to 1840 — Dialectic and Synthesis?

The increasing quantities of evidence on health affairs in the 1830s tells its own tale; in the 1840s, the situation becomes even more rampant, diverse and impossible to contain within the parameters of the advice books — or of this paper. In a real sense, what we know as a national political venture, 'sanitarianism' so-called, was also a common intellectual resource — the point at which a number of therapies, when brought together under the rubric of 'regimen', formed a common framework of inherited physiological 'truisms'. In the 1830s and 1840s there were Quaker sanitarians, democrat sanitarians, even 'quack' Morisonian sanitarians, who regarded the term as their own. All were very different from the high-profile Benthamite Utilitarians — and different again from the local level, where every sanitarian battle was fought out over decades by shifting alliances of local interest groups. Just how intricate a task it will be to define sanitarianism has been demonstrated by Roger Cooter's lengthy study of the phrenology movement, with extensive lists of participants who span the political spectrum, opt in and out of the movement at different times of their lives, and act as self-appointed missionaries to convert the population. The same could undoubtedly be said of the cluster of hygienic movements which Brown identified as 'physical puritanism'.[46]

Enough evidence has been given in bare outline to suggest that the new term 'physical puritanism' was linked to a very old set of beliefs: the ascetic moral cosmology connected with the prudent purification of the body and the bodily processes. It was the contemporary view, from the seventeenth to the nineteenth century, that 'physical puritanism' was inevitably opposed to narrower monopolistic amibitions. It was also implied by medical 'regulars' that there was a continuum of belief linking all therapies that were alternative to professional care and drugging practices — a 'quackery' which descended from the overarching 'truisms' of popular physiology to the specific metaphysical 'universals' of sectarian health beliefs.[47] The radical sectarian theorists of hygienic therapy in the 1840s tended to seal each physical therapy off in the search for perfect bodily purity and/or moral consistency; it was this universalism which set them apart from the synthetic and pragmatic analysis of the sanitarians.

It could be said that the 'organicism' of the physiological demogogues in the 1830s — from Combe to the socialist Robert Owen — was a principle that was built into the philosophic rationale of vegetarianism, with the 'Plastick faculty of the Soul'; or into balneology, with its cure for the 'niceness and weakness of the spirits'. The localised, anatomised, materialism of the new physiology, however, contrived to *assume* a holistic and vitalistic centre, but effectively sheared away the old threads of immaterialist philosophy. Gone were the extremist ascetic practices which had more or less loosely accompanied the *vis medicatrix naturae* since the seventeenth century. What was left was the materialist principle of utility which so affronted the sectarians, but gave utopian hopes to the 'philanthropic' and 'socialist' sanitarians. The wider revival of 'popular physiology' displayed the temperate 'mean' — the liberal, middle stratum of health belief, which had itself emerged from, and had continuously assimilated, the radical extremes and minorities. In short, by the early nineteenth century, more people had come to value the hygienic therapies for their 'comforts' and 'relief', than for their metaphysical benefit.

The science of physiology, from the amalgam of medieval lore onwards, was integral to the dialectical discourse of popular health; and it is quite legitimate to argue that physiology remained public property in the first half of the nineteenth century, into the early years of the sectarian and sanitarian movements. If we accept that the terms 'fringe' and 'orthodoxy' (like 'regular' and 'irregular') are primarily related to a defensive professional strategy that is intended to deny the common ownership of medical knowledge, there remains a question yet to be resolved. Just how successful was this defence after the medical state had been publicly re-instated? In short, what happened to the populist physiological polemic between 1850 and 1950?

Notes

1. 'Physical Puritanism', *Westminster Review*, 2 (1852), 409. I am indebted to J.F.C. Harrison and Roger Cooter for this reference, and for identifying Samuel Brown as the anonymous author. Further thanks to John Harley Warner, John Henry, Vivian Nutton, Mike Barfoot, David Harley, and Leo Gerulaitis for discussions and information.

2. Further reference to the arguments outlined in this article can be found in Virginia Smith, 'Cleanliness: The Development of Idea and Practice in Britain, 1770-1850' (unpublished PhD thesis, University of London, 1985); and in Ginnie Smith, 'Prescribing the Rules of Health: Self-help and Advice in the Late Eighteenth Century', in Roy Porter (ed.), *Patients and Practitioners* (Cambridge, Cambridge University Press, 1985), 249-82. For the use of different sources on the medical history of daily life, see Françoise Loux, *Traditions et soins d'aujordhui* (Paris, Inter Editions, 1983).

3. Owsei Temkin, *Galenism: The Rise and Decline of a Medical Philosophy* (Ithaca, New York, Cornell University Press, 1973); W. Burkert, *Lore and Science in Ancient Pythagoreanism*, trans. E.L. Minar, Jnr (Cambridge, Mass., Harvard University Press, 1972); for a closer study of the late medieval milieu, see N.G. Siraisi, *Taddeo Alderotti and His Pupils* (Princeton, Princeton University Press, 1981). On popular sources in Europe, see Miriam U. Chrisman, *Lay Culture, Learned Culture: Books and Social Change in Strasbourg* (New Haven, Yale U.P. 1982); L.V. Gerulaitis, *Printing and Publishing in Fifteenth-century Venice* (Chicago/London, Mansell Publishing Ltd, 1976). For England, see Paul Slack, 'Mirrors of Health and Treasures of Poor Men: The Use of Vernacular Medical Literature in Tudor England', in Charles Webster (ed.), *Health Medicine and Mortality in the Sixteenth Century* (Cambridge, Cambridge University Press, 1979), 237-73.

4. Gerulaitis (note 3), 60-3.

5. The interaction between 'knowledge as power' and 'knowledge as service' has been picked up by Aant Elzinga and Andrew Jamison, 'Making Dreams Come True — An Essay on the Role of Practical Utopias in Science', in E. Mendelsohn and H. Nowotny (eds), *Nineteen Eighty-four: Science between Utopia and Dystopia* (Dordrecht/Boston, D. Reidel Publishing Co., 1984). On iatro-chemistry, see Allen G. Debus, 'Paracelsian Doctrine in English Medicine', in F.N.L. Poynter (ed.), *Chemistry in the Service of Medicine* (London, Pitman, 1963), 5-26; Charles Webster, *The Great Instauration. Science, Medicine, and Reform, 1626-1660* (London, Duckworth, 1975). Paracelsianism was not only an attack on humoral pharmacy; if we take humoral regimen as the point of departure, the picture appears rather different. For one opponent of Paracelsianism, see Ginnie Smith, 'Thomas Tryon's Regimen for Women: Sectarian Health in the Seventeenth Century', in London Feminist History Group (eds), *The Sexual Dynamics of History* (London, Pluto Press, 1983), 47-65. On the commercialisation of iatro-chemistry in the seventeenth and eighteenth centuries, see Roger A. Hambridge, 'Empiricomany, or an Infatuation in Favour of Empiricism, or Quackery: the Socio-Economics of Eighteenth-century Quackery', in S. Soupel and R.A. Hambridge (eds), *Literature and Science and Medicine* (Los Angeles, W.A. Clark Memorial Library, University of California, 1982), 76, 96-7.

6. Sanctorius, *Medicina Statica: or, Rules of Health, in Eight Sections of Aphorisms. English'd by J.D.* (London, J. Starkey 1676); Tobias Venner's *Via Recta ad Vitam Longan* (London, E. Griffin 1620), the definitive, second-generation, humanist treatise on the nonnaturals and the principle of longevity, was published with a new edition of the first-generation humanist — William Turner, *A Booke of the Natures and Properties of Baths in England* (Cologne, A. Birkman, 1568 edn), seven editions by 1633.

7. Keith Thomas, *Religion and the Decline of Magic* (Harmondsworth, Penguin, 1973); Frank Bottomley, *Attitudes to the Body in Western Christendom* (London, Lepus Books, 1979). The classic anthropological study of purity rules is Mary Douglas, *Purity and Danger: An Analysis of the Concepts of Pollution and Taboo* (Harmondsworth, Penguin, 1970); and in medical history, the concept of pollution defined as the basis of Greek hygiene

by Owsei Temkin, 'An Historical Analysis of the Concept of Infection', *Studies in Intellectual History* (Baltimore, John Hopkins Press, 1953), 123-47.

8. The ideological content of humoralism has received more attention from European medievalists — see, for example, collected essays in D. Buschinger and A. Crepin (eds), *Les Quatre Elements dans la culture médiévale* (Kummerle, Verlag for the Université de Picardie, Centre d'Etudes Médiévales, 1983). The ethnographic axis is well illustrated in R.L. Currier, 'The Hot-Cold Syndrome and Symbolic Balance in Mexican and Spanish-American Folk Medicine', *Ethnology* (1966), 251-63; the Chinese five-element system is described in Colin A. Ronan (ed.), *The Shorter Science and Civilisation in China. An Abridgement of Joseph Needham's Original Text*, 2 vols (Cambridge/London, Cambridge University Press, 1978), vol. 1: *The Fundamental Ideas of Chinese Science*, 127-90; see also Smith, 'Prescribing the Rules of Health' (note 2), 249-82.

9. For a detailed analysis of closed sectarian beliefs, designed to keep the believer free from the pollutions of the material world, see Smith, 'Thomas Tryon' (note 5), 47-65. The lack of evidence relating to puritanism and domestic habits causes problems in Stephen Mennell's *All Manners of Food, Eating and Taste in England and France from the Middle Ages to the Present* (Oxford, Basil Blackwell, 1985).

10. Henry More, *The Immortality of the Soul, So Farre Forth as is Demonstrable from the Knowledge of Nature and the Light of Reason* (London, J. Flesher, 1659) 258; Richard Ward, *The Life of the Learned and Pious Henry More* (London, Joseph Downing, 1710), 229-30. Ward's quotation comes from More's translated *Opera Omnia, The Theological Works of H. More etc.* (London, 1708), Preface General, 'Temper of Body and Mind'; the British Library copy has MS notes by S.T. Coleridge.

11. John Evelyn, *Acetaria. A Discourse of Sallets*, 2nd edn (London, B. Tooke, 1706), Preface.

12. A total of three poets, two philosophers, two philanthropists, one aristocrat, a physician, and a divine. See Howard Williams, *The Ethics of Diet. A Biographical History of the Literature of Humane Dietetics, from the Earliest Period to the Present Day* (London, Ideal Publishing Union Ltd, 1896); *The New Age and Concordium Gazette. A Journal of Human Physiology, Education, and Association*, (1844), 149. Confirmation will have to be laboriously assembled; I am indebted to Mike Barfoot for reference to Cullen's 'vegetality' and indication of a possible vegetarian social grouping within the Edinburgh Royal Infirmary. See W. Cullen, *A Treatise on the Materia Medica*, 2 vols (Edinburgh, Charles Elliot, 1789), vol. 1, pt 1, ch. 2, 333-70.

13. George Cheyne, *An Essay of Health and Long Life* (London, G. Strahan, 1724). On Law's circle, see S. Lee (ed.), *Dictionary of National Biography* (London, Smith Elder, & Co, 1909), vol. 11, 677-81; and R. Parkinson (ed.), *The Private Journal and Literary Remains of John Byrom*, 2 vols (printed for the Chetham Society, 1854-7). I am indebted to David Harley for reference to Byrom's vegetarian experiments. John Wesley was converted to water-drinking and the vegetable diet by Cheyne — see Bryan S. Turner, 'The Government of the Body: Medical Regimens and the Rationalization of Diet', *British Journal of Sociology*, 33 (June 1982), 254-69. Turner emphasises Cheyne's mechanistic provision of exact dietary quantities for the 'human machine'; but has little to say about religion, or dietary 'quality', concluding that the Cheynian diet 'may . . . have reached an audience in the middle or lower middle class, but it is still very doubtful that the full medical regimen had any relevance for the working class' (pp. 265-6).

14. Antonio Cocchi, *The Pythagorean Diet of Vegetables Only, Conducive to the Preservation of Health, and the Cure of Diseases* (London, R. Dodsley, 1745), 7.

15. Thomas Taylor, usher and secretary, dedicated his life to translating all of Plato not originally translated by Thomas Sydenham; see W.E. Axon, *Thomas Taylor the Platonist. A Biographical and Bibliographical Sketch* (London, reprinted from *The Library*, 1890). The English view of Plato (and of Thomas Taylor) was reported by Ralph Waldo Emerson in conversation with Wordsworth: 'I told him it was not creditable that no one in all the country knew anything of Thomas Taylor, the Platonist, whilst in every

American library his translations were found. I said, "If *Plato's Republic* were published in England, as a new book, to-day, do you think it would find any readers?'' He confessed it would not; "and yet" he added, after a pause, with that complacency which never deserts the true-born Englishman, "and yet we have embodied it all" ' (quoted in ibid., 2, from R.W. Emerson, *Representative Men* (London, The Catholic Series, 1850), 39). John Oswald, *The Cry of Nature, or an Appeal to Mercy and Justice, on Behalf of the Persecuted Animals* (London, 1791); Joseph Ritson, *An Essay on Abstinence from Animal Food as a Moral Duty* (London, R. Phillips, 1802); J.F. Newton, *The Return to Nature, or, a Defence of the Vegetable Regimen* (London, 1811).

16. A.F. Barham, *An Odd Medley of Literary Curiosities* (London, The Author, 1845), 'Lecturing', 33-48. Barham placed Coleridge with the nineteenth-century 'transcendental' lecturer and vegetarian James Pierrepont Greaves. On Coleridge, see David Pym, *The Religious Thought of Samuel Taylor Coleridge* (Gerrards Cross, Colin Smythe, 1978); T.H. Levere, *Poetry Realised in Nature. Samuel Taylor Coleridge and Early Nineteenth Century Science* (Cambridge, Cambridge University Press, 1981). David Bloor, 'Coleridge's Moral Copula', *Social Studies of Science*, (November 1983), 605-19, criticises Levere (p. 616) for failing to bring out Coleridge's religio-political opposition to the 'selfish and sensual character and immediate utility' of science.

17. Smith 'Cleanliness', (note 21), 81-92.

18. John Hancocke, *Febrifugum Magnum: or, Common Water the Best Cure for Fevers, and Probably the Plague* (London, R. Walsey & J. Roberts, 1723/4), 10.

19. John Floyer, *An Enquiry into the Right Use and Abuses of the Hot, Cold and Temperate BATHS in England* (London, R. Clavel, 1697), Preface; John Locke, *Some Thoughts Concerning Education* (London, A. & J. Churchill, 1693). On air, see Smith, 'Cleanliness' (note 2), 114-32.

20. David Harley, 'Religion and Professional Interests in Northern Spa Literature, 1625-1775', *Bulletin of the Social History of Medicine*, 35 (1984), 14-16; Jon Eklund, 'Of a Spirit in the Water: Some Early Ideas on the Aerial Dimension', *Isis*, 67 (1976), 527-50. John Smith, *The Curiosities of Common Water: or the Advantages thereof in Preventing and Curing many Distempers . . . to which are added Some Rules of Preserving Health by Diet*, 6th edn (London, J. & B. Clark, 1724), 67-80; Hancocke (note 18), 17; J. Wesley, *Primitive Physic* (London, T. Trye, 1747).

21. See Smith, 'Cleanliness' (note 2), 99-113, 241-58. The domestic life of Howard was taken from the *Ladies' Magazine* (1792), reprinted in the *New Age and Concordium Gazette*, (1 December 1843).

22. And see Elzinga and Jamison (note 5), 165.

23. Anon. *The Abernethian Code of Health and Longevity* (London, J. Williams, 1829), 3; J. Abernethy, *Surgical Observations on the Constitutional Origin and Treatment of Local Diseases; and of Aneurisms*, 7th edn (London, Longman, Hurst, Rees, Orme, Brown, & Green, 1824);Erwin Ackerknecht, 'Broussais, or a Forgotten Medical Revolution', *Bulletin of the History of Medicine*, 27 (1953), 320-43.

24. T.J. Graham, *A Treatise on Indigestion: with Observations on Some Painful Complaints Originating in Indigestion, Especially Mental Aberration*, 3rd edn (London, Simkin & Marshall, 1833), 119; James Morison, *The Hygiest. A Monthly Publication Intended to Establish Unity and Certainty in Medicine upon Rational Principles*, 3 (1 December 1851), 216. On levels of drug prescribing in the United States, see John Harley Warner, 'Professional Power, Sectarian Conflict, and Orthodox Identity, in Mid-nineteenth-century Medicine: Therapeutic Change at the Commercial Hospital in Cincinatti' (forthcoming).

25. J. Tweed, *Popular Observations on Regimen and Diet: in which the Nature and Qualities of our Common Food are Pointed Out and Explained* (Chelmsford, Meggy & Chalk, 1820); J.S. Forsyth, *Practical Advice on Diet and Regimen; Comprising Natural and Medical Rules for Eating, Drinking, and Preserving Health, on Principles of Easy Digestion* (London, Sherwood, Gilbert, & Piper, 1827); Hortator, *Simplicity of Health* (London, Effingham Wilson, 1829), 8-9, 115.

26. Joel Pinney, *An Exposure of the Present Deteriorated Condition of Health, and Diminished Duration of Human Life, Compared to that which is Attainable by Nature . . . Forming a Code of Health and Long Life* (London, Longman, Rees, Orme, Brown & Green 1830), 107-9.

27. T.J. Graham, *Sure Methods of Improving Health, and Prolonging Life . . . by Regulating Diet and Regimen . . . to which is Added, the Art of Training for Health*, 2nd edn (London, Simpkin & Marshall, 1827), vi-vii.

28. Peter H. Clias, *An Elementary Course of Gymnastic Exercises Intended to Develop and Improve the Physical Powers of Man . . . a Treatise on the Art of Swimming* (London, Sherwood, Jones & Co., 1823), 4 edns by 1825; Signor Voarino, *A Treatise on Calisthenic Exercises. Arranged for the Private Tuition of Ladies* (London, J. Ridgeway, 1827); idem, *A Second Course of Calisthenic Exercises . . . with a Private Course of Gymnastic Exercises for Gentlemen* (London, J. Ridgeway, 1828); Gustavus Hamilton, *The Elements of Gymnastics for Boys, and of Calisthenics for Young Ladies* (London, R. Phillips, 1827).

29. Graham (note 27), 219, 197-8.

30. T.J. Graham, *An Account of Persons Remarkable for their Longevity . . .* (London, Simkin & Marshall, 1829); see also James Easton, *Health and Longevity, as Exemplified by the Lives of 623 Persons . . . Remarks on Longevity from Buffon, Fothergill, etc . . .* (Salisbury, The Compiler, 1823); J. Harrison Curtis, *Observations on the Preservation of Health* (London, H. Renshaw 1837), p 64; Joel Pinney, *The Alternative: disease or premature death, or, health and long life: being an exposure of the prevailing misconception of their respective sources*, (London, S. Highley, 1838), pp 21-33.

31. A.F.M. Willich, *Lectures on Diet and Regimen* (London, Longman & Rees 1799); C.A. Struve, *Asthenology, or the Art of Preserving a Feeble Life*, (London, J. Murray & S. Highley 1801); Thomas Beddoes, *Hygeia: or Essays Moral and Medical on the Causes Affecting the Personal State of our Middling and Affluent Classes*, 3 vols, (Bristol, Mills 1802-3). See C.J. Lawrence, 'The Nervous System and Society in the Scottish Enlightenment', in B. Barnes and S. Shapin (eds), *Natural Order: Historical Studies of Scientific Culture*, (Beverley Hills/London, Sage, 1979) 19-40; on the post-Enlightenment development of 'the norm', see G. Canguilhem, *On the Normal and the Pathological*, trans. C.R. Fawcett, 2nd edn, (D. Reidel, Dordrecht/Boston, 1978).

32. British appreciation of dermatology was forshadowed by W. Falconer, *An Essay on the Bath Waters, in four parts*, 2 vols, (Bath/London, T. Lowndes 1772). The warm bath for children was accepted in the 1790s by amongst others, M. Underwood, *A Treatise on the Diseases of Children* (London, J. Matthews 1795); W. Buchan, *Advice to Mothers*, (London, T. Cadell & W. Davies 1803); see Smith, 'Cleanliness', 180-85.

33. The major full-length British work on medical police was John Roberton, *Treatise on Medical Police, and on Diet, Regimen, etc* (Edinburgh/London, J. Muir for T. Bryce, 1809). Other medical advice book authors compiled lists: Walker Keighley, *A New System of Family Medicine, for the Use of Midwives, Mothers, and Nurses* (London, B. Crosby, 1806); Sir John Sinclair, *The Code of Health and Longevity; or a Concise View of the Principles Calculated for the Preservation of Health and the Attainment of Long Life*, 4 vols (Edinburgh, A. Constable & Co., 1807-8).

34. Andrew Combe, *The Principles of Physiology Applied to the Preservation of Health, and to the Improvement of Physical and Mental Education* (Edinburgh, Maclachlan & Stewart, 1833). On physiology, phrenology, and the Combes, see Roger Cooter, *The Cultural Meaning of Popular Science. Phrenology and the Organisation of Consent in Nineteenth-century Britain* (Cambridge/London, Cambridge University Press, 1984.) While it seems clear that phrenology provided 'a channel for the easy flow of phrenphysiological literature', it is not enough to take phrenologists' claims for the appropriation of physiology at face value, i.e. that 'hitherto, it often seemed, that no one else had made the effort to extend this knowledge outside medical circles', or, 'phrenology succeeded in breaking through the prudery barrier'; or in the case of Andrew Combe, 'the supposed laws of

general health . . . were made to seem as if they were as immutable as the laws of mechanics, and as if in a like manner they had just been discovered. This was specifically the task of Andrew Combe's *Principles of Physiology* . . .'*ibid.*, 177-9).

35. Combe (note 34), Preface, 1-2; Andrew Combe, *The Physiology of Digestion, Considered in Relation to the Principle of Dietetics* (Edinburgh, Maclachlan & Stewart, 1836).

36. Curtis (note 30), iv-v.

37. Pinney (note 30), 99.

38. Combe (note 34), 306, 316-17.

39. Mrs W. Parkes, *A New System of Practical Domestic Economy* (London, 1823), 148; C. Struve, *A Familiar Treatise on the Physical Education of Children* (London, Murray & Highley, 1801), 353-54; R. Reece, *A Practical Dictionary of Domestic Medicine* (London, Longman, 1808), under 'Baths', no page no.; see also the works of Sir Arthur Clarke, as *An Essay on Warm, Cold, Vapour Bathing, with Practical Observations on Sea-bathing*, 4th edn (London, Henry Colburn, 1819).

40. Curtis (note 30), 13.

41. A. Kilgour, *Lectures on the Ordinary Agents of Life, as Applicable to Therapeutics and Hygiene; or, the Uses of the Atmosphere, Habitations, Baths, Clothing, Climate, Exercise, Foods, Drinks, and etc. in the Treatment and Prevention of Disease* . . . (Edinburgh, The Author, 1834), 65.

42. R. Shryock. 'Public Relations of the Medical Profession in Great Britain and the United States, 1600-1870', *Annals of Medical History*, new series, 2 (1930), 308-39; John Harley Warner, *The Therapeutic Perspective: Medical Practice, Knowledge, and Professional Identity in America, 1820-1885* (Cambridge, Mass., Harvard University Press, 1986; and see Warner in this volume, ch. 12. On professional problems, see Roberton (note 33), xl-xliii; Kilgour (note 41), xix; Combe (note 34), 3-5.

43. Pinney (note 26), 177, 161-98; on the later sanitarians and the 'withering away' of the medical state, see Lloyd G. Stevenson, 'Science Down the Drain. On the Hostility of Certain Sanitarians to Animal Experimentation, Bacteriology, and Immunology', *Bulletin of the History of Medicine*, 29 (1955), 1-26.

44. The international comparison can be traced in H.C. Bolton, *A Catalogue of Scientific and Technical Periodicals, 1665-1882, Together with Chronological Tables*, 2nd edn (Washington, Smithsonian Miscellaneous Collection, 40, 1897); details of Edmund Parkes's curriculum at the Army Medical School from 1861 in his *Manual of Practical Hygiene* (London, Churchill, 1864); see D. Watkins, 'The English Revolution in Social Medicine, 1889-1911' (unpublished PhD thesis, University of London, 1984).

45. Roberton (note 33), xxxvii-xxxix: 'if he attempt to shew the weakness of the fashionable system, or to introduce any alteration in practice, the whole faculty are alarmed; their vanity is piqued, in having opinions, which they thought perfectly established, brought into question, and exposed by a young man; and their interest is to crush him as soon as possible'. Buchan was also exposed to 'many prejudices', *Advice to Mothers*, (note 32), 139.

46. See especially Cooter (note 34), Conclusion, 194-214, on the social descent of phrenology; also Julia Twigg, 'The Vegetarian Movement in England 1847-1981: A Study in the Structure of its Ideology' (unpublished PhD thesis, University of London, 1981), 113-15, on the changing class membership of the Vegetarian Society (founded 1847.)

47. Samuel Brown's 1852 *Westminster Review* list of moral therapies was virtually identical to those picked out for satire by a medical 'regular' in 1850, popular physiology included; see *The Hygeist*, 3 (1 August 1850), 82, reprinted from 'a Medical Journal of July 20th, 1850'.

10 EARLY VICTORIAN RADICALS AND THE MEDICAL FRINGE

J.F.C. Harrison

In the further study of the medical fringe there is a need to locate it in the wider context of Victorian social and intellectual history. Did fringe movements, for instance, relate in some way to the problems of continuity and disruption which marked the first industrial society? Did they contribute to or reflect the post-1848 stabilisation of Victorian England? To what degree was their ideology an expression or extension of more general social attitudes and concerns? We are unlikely to be able to answer such questions with assurance until more monographic work has been done. But in the meantime, it may be possible to probe a little way into the subject by considering the evidence from one particular group, the radical reformers of the early and mid-Victorian period. They were people who, for one reason or another, were critical of the world in which they found themselves and wished to change it. In pursuit of this aim they resorted to various measures, looked for a variety of allies, and adopted several different intellectual positions.

The starting-point of this essay is the observation that a number of Owenites and Chartists were, or later became, spiritualists, mesmerists, phrenologists, herbalists, vegetarians and homoeopaths.[1] A preliminary check shows at least ninety individuals who can be traced as having associations with both social reform and fringe medical movements. They range from well-known examples like Robert Owen, who converted to spiritualism in the 1850s, or William Lovett, who approved of phrenology, to the lesser-known cases of the Chartist R.G. Gammage and his enthusiasm for vegetarianism or Frederick Hollick, who undertook an odyssey from Owenism and atheism to neuropathy and popular sexual reform. Further delving would no doubt uncover many more. If the search were extended to include, on the one hand, involvement in education, temperance, co-operation, trade unionism, secularism, Friendly Societies and freemasonry, and, on the other, anti-vaccination and physical puritanism in general, the numbers would be even larger. Why should Owenites and Chartists become spiritualists and mesmerists? The short answer, of course, is that the majority did not; but the minority who did so identify themselves is sufficiently large to raise questions of significance.

A problem that faced many Victorian working men in middle age was how to come to terms with the apparent failure or defeat of the ideals and hopes and programmes that had inspired them until c. 1848, when Chartism and Owenism died away. What were they to put in place of their earlier beliefs, having given so much of themselves to the cause? Was there a failure mechanism of some sort? How did they fit into the new society? Did they adapt or merely conform? In such a probing of the mental world or some Victorian artisans and reformers, the medical fringe may provide a few clues. The following observations are preliminary, tentative and empirical, and lack any theoretical or conceptual sophistication. They simply document the links between political and cultural radicalism. Themes which were present among Owenites and Chartists are also found in the medical fringe.

First and foremost, there was a common commitment to democratic doctrines and assumptions. The medical fringe, like Owenism and Chartism, aimed to secure the active involvement of ordinary people in its organisations and institutions. Although firm evidence is scanty, it would seem likely that the social composition of membership was similar: a mixture of labouring people, artisans, tradesmen, some of the lower middle classes, and a sprinkling of professionals. Some of the plebeian elements in spiritualism (which was very much a religion of healing) have been explored recently.[2] The point to be made here is that the democratic sensibilities of reformers could find comfort or confirmation in the doctrines and practices of the spiritualists: 'spiritualism is democratic, it can be demonstrated to everyone'.[3] Similarly, herbal medicine was regarded by its practitioners as a movement of the people.[4] John Stevens, advocating the Thomsonian system of botanic medicine in 1849, argued that[5]

> however lofty Medical Science has appeared when clothed in mystery, or flaunting in the false airs of pedantic learning, it is not, if stripped of that mystery, higher than the reach of the ordinary mind, or beyond the attainment of common sense . . . the common sense of the people, when in possession of a *true theory* of medicine, will be found quite capable of curing all diseases to which they are subject.

Stevens claimed to have helped over 10,000 patients, 'chiefly consisting of those who had sought relief in vain by all other means.'

To one old Chartist it was quite clear that herbal medicine was a true reform movement. John Skelton, a London shoemaker, had been one of the signatories to the People's Charter in 1838 and throughout the

1840s was a leading Chartist in the metropolis. In the 1850s he left London and practised as a medical botanist in Leeds and later in Manchester. According to his own account, Skelton studied medical botany under Isaiah Coffin in Manchester during the spring of 1848, and thence 'commenced our mission in the smaller towns; our first essay being at Rotherham, next Sheffield, then Blackburn, Bacup, Ramsbottom, Oldham, Wakefield, Barnsley, Stockport, Birmingham, Manchester, Derby, Nottingham, Leicester, and others of smaller note'.[6] Skelton had apparently met Coffin some years previously when Skelton's wife had been one of Coffin's first London patients. In the pages of his monthly journal, *Botanic Record and Family Herbal* (1852-5), Skelton describes the progress of medical botany as a reform movement. A spirit of mission, of spreading 'the truth', is constantly invoked; and there are reports of lectures, tea parties and branch organisations very similar to those in the Owenite *New Moral World*. Skelton's 'Six Propositions' of vegetable medicine are reminiscent of the six points of the Charter; and in the first number of the *Botanic Record and Family Herbal* he states that 'the ranks of Medical Botanists [are] generally of the working class'. *Coffin's Botanical Journal and Medical Reformer* (1849-59) is similar in tone; and Coffin himself was described in 1840 as 'botanic physician and socialist lecturer' in a local directory.[7] The genre to which these journals belong is that small group of magazines published in the later 1840s which were devoted to the 'progress of the people' and encompassed a variety of humanitarian and social reform causes.[8] As with most popular reform in the 1830s and 1840s, their roots were in philosophic radicalism, but they were not as a rule overtly political. In a typical report from the Nottingham Medico-Botanic Society in 1853, the lecturer D.W. Heath, after commending Skelton's *Plea for the Botanic Practice of Medicine*, concluded:[9]

> Despite irregularities, social disadvantage, educational drawbacks, the working men in many places have made a noble stand in defence of their rights, duties and privileges, and not a few of the wealthy have given the helping hand. The truth is becoming general 'that all men are of one blood', differing only in degree . . . The poor and despised of our land are rising over circumstances.

The means of effecting this transformation of the working class was self-help. In Victorian England this method of social advance took two forms, individual and collective. Both modes were advocated by reformers, and herbal medicine provided splendid opportunities for their practice. First, the do-it-yourself element was always strongly emphasised: 'there is now actually in existence a *complete system of medical treatment* which each individual can take into his own hands with little trouble, and almost without expense — a system at once embracing all that is safe and good in all others known,' claimed Stevens.[10] Similarly, through the discovery and practice of mesmeric trance, or communication with the spirit world and the use of healing mediums, or the adoption of a vegetarian diet, or the reading of phrenological bumps, individuals could make their own decisions. But collective or mutual self-help (of the type exemplified by a Friendly Society, a co-operative store, or a trade union) was also part of fringe medicine. Stevens, Coffin and Skelton all urged their followers to establish local botanic societies, 'that the people may mutually assist each other in the study of Medical Botany'.[11] From his Leeds headquarters in March 1853 Skelton launched the Friendly United Medico-Botanic Sick and Burial Society, with a complete set of rules and officers. The botanic medical journals carried details of the activities of the local societies, much as the Chartist and Owenite branches were reported in the *Northern Star* and the *New Moral World*.

Self-help was frequently posed as an alternative to professionalism. Among working people there was a rejection of the elitism of those in authority, and a distrust of the services of professionals which was manifested in various spheres. Anti-professionalism is observable, for example, in the preference for old-style unqualified women midwives over professionals; in the continuance of working-class private venture (dames') schools long after provision of elementary education by the churches and the state; and in the numbers of adults who attended humble mutual improvement societies rather than the civically approved Mechanics' Institutes. Local preachers and an unpaid ministry were felt to be nearer to the people than the 'hireling priests' of the Church of England. When on trial, radicals such as Thomas Cooper preferred to conduct their own defence rather than hand over their case to a barrister. Fringe medicine, with its slogan 'The People their Own Physicians' and its demands for reform of the medical profession, harmonised well with such anti-professional attitudes.[12]

In their conflict with orthodox medicine, herbalists, mesmerists and homoeopaths saw themselves, and could be perceived by others, as persecuted minorities struggling against the monopoly of a privileged and legally entrenched profession. The parallel with religious dissenters opposed to a priesthood and established church was not lost upon some nonconformists. Edward Miall, middle-class radical and editor of the

Nonconformist ('The dissidence of Dissent and the protestantism of the Protestant religion') was also a disciple of Hahnemann; in 1850 he wrote to John Epps, the homoeopathic doctor:[13]

> As a Protestant Dissenter I feel a natural sympathy for all those who hold opinions, whether theological or scientific, which are under the ban of legally-favoured professionals; and, however I might disavow such opinions, I should feel it my duty to assert for them the right to a fair hearing on their own merits.

For radicals and reformers the issues were clear enough. John Goodwyn Barmby, a Chartist and Owenite, writing in 1841, contrasted capitalist medicine (which, he argued, actually encouraged disease) with the superior health plan possible in a socialist community. Barmby argued that under the existing system doctors had an interest in not curing their patients too quickly because their fees depended on the length of treatment; whereas under communism preventive medicine would be pre-eminent.[14] It was also a complaint of the medical botanists that orthodox practitioners demanded full payment whether or not their patients were cured. In the case of *Harrison* v. *Toplis* (1853), for example, a Sheffield surgeon brought an action to recover his bill of £4 11s 6d., which the defendant, a working man, pleaded was excessive, he having been charged for twenty-one days' attendance in an unsuccessful treatment of diarrhoea. The defendant discharged the surgeon and brought in a botanic practitioner who cured him in twenty-three days and charged 22s. However, the defendant lost the case.[15]

But it was in cases where medical botanists were charged with manslaughter following the death of a patient that conflict with the orthodox medical profession was fiercest. Justice appeared to be denied when only regular practitioners could be called on to establish the cause of death at an inquest, and when the medical press provokingly refused to recognise medical botanists except by their previous occupations or trades, such as shoemaker or cotton spinner. The protest of the underdog against an oppressive establishment was well calculated to win the sympathy of radicals and dissenters — and was in fact perceived as part of the struggle for 'freedom' and liberal values. In 1867 Josiah Thomas, a botanical practitioner in Newcastle, was charged with manslaughter; Ernest Jones, a barrister and the most noted of the later leaders of Chartism, was retained for the defence. Before the trial John Skelton wrote to Jones reminding him of their earlier political comradeship and promising to let him have details of Thomas's case: 'You will have one of the best opportunities that could possibly arise for defending the right of free thought, and, if I mistake not, will take care to turn it to advantage.' Thomas was acquitted.[16]

Underlying the empiricism of anti-professionalism and self-help were deeper attitudes and convictions which were common to reformers and the medical fringe. Take for instance the concept of naturalism. Owen and his followers believed that existing society, with its inequalities, class divisions and competitive ethos, was artificial and unnecessary. The natural order of society was one which emphasised harmony and co-operation, not competition. Labouring people paid a high price in social and economic suffering for the 'progress' brought by the new industrial society, and until the middle of the nineteenth century hopes were nourished that the new order might not be permanent. The social evils of early Victorian England just could not be accepted by many thoughtful people, who looked for some alternative. Owenism offered them a critique of early industrial capitalism as an artificially imposed system, in contrast to the 'natural' society of the New Moral World. The Owenite labour theory of value was based in part on argument from natural right; and the religious beliefs of most Owenites (whether deists, freethinkers or members of some rationalist Protestant sect) contained a strong element of natural religion. Owenite views were diffused beyond the ranks of avowed Owenites, and Owenism was in any case largely a compound of popularly accepted Enlightenment and Utilitarian ideals and assumptions. The appeal to what was natural, in both a general and more specialist sense, was therefore likely to be quite widespread.

Certainly there was an answering echo among the medical botanists. In his 'epitome of botanic faith', Skelton declared: 'We believe that the true foundation of medical practice must be established agreeably with the economy of nature, for that only which agrees with the natural order of things can be found in practice to agree with the wants of men.'[17] But it was the vegetarian food reformers who most explicitly proclaimed the need for a return to natural ways.[18] Their symbol was the Garden of Eden, which represented the world as it was in its natural state and to which it might one day be returned. There is a long tradition which characterises Eden as vegetarian, and the Fall of Man marked (among other disjunctions) the introduction of meat-eating. The Owenite community was often represented in idyllic terms which had overtones of Eden.[19] Within Owenism there was a strong strain of pastoralism, derived largely from eighteenth-century sources. At the back of most Owenite plans for community was a utopian vision of a propertyless, egalitarian society; of men working together in the fields, taking from the common stock according to their needs, and engaging in intellectual pursuits in their ample leisure time. In such a society there was neither luxury nor want. Work was a source of satisfaction and independence; and feelings of anger, envy and all uncharitableness were dismissed as unworthy of a rational being. Harmony existed between man and man and between man and nature. Owenism was presented as community in a garden. It is not hard to see how the Edenic myth could be a bond of affinity between Owenite and vegetarian reformers.[20]

Thomas Low Nichols and his wife, Mary Gove Nichols, were enthusiastic American communitarian reformers of the 1840s (Yellow Springs Community, Ohio) who graduated via Fourierism, spiritualism, Grahamism and hydropathy, to Roman Catholicism. In 1861 they settled in England and campaigned for vegetarianism, sexual reform, women's rights and against compulsory vaccination.[21] In his *Esoteric Anthropology* (a handbook of popular sexual knowledge), Nichols argued that the natural taste of man was for vegetable food only: 'Man loves the vegetable world, and finds it full of beauty, and attraction, and gratification, because it is his. His nature is adapted to it; it is adapted to all his wants, and all his natural desires.'[22] Other movements of 'physical puritanism', especially hydropathy, homoeopathy and teetotalism, also emphasised their devotion to what was natural.[23] Purity and simplicity, as opposed to the corruptions of civilisation, were their watchwords. Hydropathy, despite its severely practical application of bath and blanket regimes, may have had some appeal as a reaction against the pollution of nineteenth-century industrial and urban life. The water cure, it has been suggested, was 'a lay return to nature, rather thinly if attractively disguised as the systematic medical use of pure cold water in natural surroundings, allied to a simple diet and frequent exercise'.[24] Water ('such a simple, pure, tasteless, scentless fluid') possessed curative powers because, claimed its advocates, 'it is in the most beautifully exact and harmonious accordance with the laws and operations of nature'.[25] To reformers it was axiomatic that what was natural was also good and just.

The devotion to nature, which reformers and the medical fringe alike perceived as attractive, was usually found in association with some form of holism. Owenites criticised competitive, industrial capitalism on the grounds that it was based on a fragmented, atomistic, partial view of what a society should be like. The social system, they claimed, should cater to the needs of all people and of the whole person. The central Chartist demand of universal suffrage was aimed at extending the political nation to the whole of the people, instead of just a section of them.

Among later socialists the significance of a holistic medical tradition was not lost. Edward Carpenter, the socialist guru of Edwardian England, remarked how the words health, whole and holy have the same etymology. He argued that the true conception of health should be positive ('a condition of the body in which it is an entirety, a unity') and, conversely, disease ('physical or mental, in society or in the individual') should be seen as a break-up of that unity.[26] This of course was not a new idea: 'They that be whole need not a physician,' says Jesus in St Matthew's gospel. But the logic of its practical application became one of the chief characteristics of fringe medicine.

Nowhere was this more so than in the case of homoeopathy. The followers of Samuel Hahnemann believed that 'disease . . . is life acting through a disordered organ: and the various symptoms are nothing but manifestations of that life struggling to recover health'.[27] They therefore rejected the principle of treating specific pathologies and instead emphasised the need to treat the whole person. The progress of a middle-class radical reformer to homoeopathy is well illustrated by the career of Dr John Epps.[28] As a young man he was a member of the Trial by Jury Society, which met annually to commemorate the trials of Horne Tooke, Thomas Hardy, John Thelwall and other democratic heroes of the 1790s. He described himself as 'a disciple of Major Cartwright', and took part in the Reform Bill agitation. Later he sympathised with Chartism (while condemning O'Connor and physical force), but was more enthusiastic for the Anti-Corn Law League. He attended the local phrenological society while still a medical student in Edinburgh in 1826, and subsequently achieved modest notoriety as 'the Christian phrenologist'. In about 1838 he became attracted to homoeopathy and rapidly published a series of little books on the subject, and so established himself as a leading advocate of the cause. He was interested in Swedenborgianism, and suffered distraint of his goods in 1844 for refusal to pay church rates. His autobiography reads like a catalogue of the liberal causes of the day, plus a roll call of the eminent radicals with whom he was acquainted. A similar career pattern — embracing Swedenborgianism, spiritualism, Fourierism, homoeopathy and much else — can be traced in the life of one of Epps's friends, James J. Garth Wilkinson.[29]

Holism was also a prominent part of the ideology of vegetarianism. Whole food meant food containing the whole grain or fruit. It was pure and natural. But quite apart from the nutritional aspect of the matter, words such as 'pure', 'natural' and 'whole', carried much wider implications. They created images which not only played a key role in vegetarian ideology, but which could also transfer meaning from one context to another.[30] Vegetarianism was concerned with more than diet reform (eating brown bread and raw vegetables, and avoiding meat); it carried with it certain attitudes towards life in general. Thus, whole food was associated in the vegetarian mind with ideas of psychic wholeness, the unity of body and mind and, ultimately, with the cosmic union of man and nature. Because vegetarianism, like other movements of physical puritanism, could be apprehended at different levels of experience, its followers were frequently associated with a variety of other movements and beliefs. From the communitarian reformers at Ham Common in the 1840s to Edward Carpenter's coterie of young socialists at Millthorpe in the 1880s and 1890s, the link with vegetarianism in both practice and ideology was close. There was a dreamlike, romantic quality in the 'higher' vegetarianism which Owenites of the 1840s and socialists of the 1880s could recognise sympathetically. Were not they too still looking for the perennial dawn, whether in the New Moral World or the New Age?

Like most thoughtful Victorians, members of the medical fringe sooner or later found themselves faced by questions involving religious belief. Many of them had had a strict Evangelical or Calvinist upbringing, and in some cases — like those of John Epps, Thomas Shorter and William Lovett — reacted against it. But few who abandoned their earlier beliefs remained untroubled by ethical questions, and the great imperative of Duty was always there to haunt them. The Victorian age was full of seekers looking for a creed — 'destitute of faith, yet terrified at scepticism', as Carlyle put it. The need and the search for a faith to live by are plain in the autobiographies of the people mentioned above. There was of course no single pattern. But common to them all was a dissatisfaction with orthodox and (usually) institutional religion, and a persistent desire to find answers to deep spiritual and intellectual problems of man and his place in society and the universe. Many of our herbalists and radicals were ordinary folk without any sophisticated education, and some may have had difficulty in expressing what they thought and felt. Yet there is no good reason to suppose that people who led apparently simple lives necessarily held simple beliefs. The ways of thinking of ordinary people are as complicated and difficult to unravel as are those of the more educated classes. But we are less familiar with the problems involved.

For those who could remain within the dissenting tradition the carry-over between religion, radicalism and fringe medicine presented no special difficulties. 'Medical botany is an eternal truth,' proclaimed

Skelton, and in his *Botanic Record and Family Herbal* he referred frequently to the 'botanic faith'.[31] Jesse Boot who as a young man carried on a medical botanist business with his mother in Nottingham came of parents and grandparents who were devoted Methodists. His father, John Boot, was a Wesleyan lay preacher with a strong sense of mission which he brought to his medical herbalism.[32] Salvation might be obtained through various channels. Given the emphasis on inner experience, on the rejection of outward forms, and the consequent elevation of individual at the expense of corporate or social effort, there was much in the nonconformist ethos that could be translated into the medical fringe.

For some Owenites and others who could not accept traditional dissent but who felt the need for some kind of religion, there was the possibility of spiritualism. Thomas Shorter was one who took this road. By trade a watchcase finisher in silver, he was a member of that small band of radical artisans who were leaders of London Chartism in the 1840s. He was friendly with Thomas Cooper, George Julian Harney and John Skelton, and in 1845 was secretary of the Finsbury Owenites. From 1849 he was drawn into the movement for co-operative working men's associations, and through this contact with the Christian Socialists became the first secretary of the Working Men's College, founded by F.D. Maurice and his friends in 1854. Shorter had at first denounced the Christian Socialists as deceivers of the people, and even after he was convinced of their sincerity, he remained a freethinker. But in about 1853-4 he investigated the 'phenomena' of spiritualism and accepted them as genuine. He published an account of his experiences, and from 1860 was joint-editor of the *Spiritual Magazine*. He originally turned to spiritualism at a time of sudden and painful bereavement, and may have been influenced by the example of Robert Owen, whom he admired. Later he came to value spiritualism as an antidote to secularism and as the expression of true religion. He was perplexed by problems of immortality, materialism, science, mind, the purpose of life. Shorter quoted with approval the testimony of Gerald Massey, another old Chartist who made the passage to spiritualism:[33]

> Spiritualism will make religion infinitely more real, and translate it from the domain of belief to that of life. It has been to me, in common with many others, such a lifting of the mental horizon and a letting in of the heavens . . . that I can only compare life without it to sailing on board ship with hatches battened down, and being kept a prisoner, cribbed, cabined, and confined, living by the light of a candle.

Beyond regular or orthodox nonconformity was what may be called the religion of nature, the belief that a walk in the woods was more beneficial than attendance at church. Doctrines of original sin and memories of repressive Evangelical childhoods were repudiated. Theology and creeds were not needed, only the determination to lead a simple, clean, 'good' life, and to 'Do unto others as you would be done by.' This type of ethical religion made its greatest impact in the later nineteenth and early twentieth centuries, when it was often allied with American transcendentalism and Indian theosophy. It then attracted socialists, vegetarians and progressive reformers of many kinds. This was perhaps the period of the greatest affinity between radicalism and the medical fringe. But in early Victorian England the same or similar connections were made. The concordium at Ham Common was transcendentalist, and Emersonianism was widespread among reformers. In Leeds, for instance, the *Truth Seeker* (1846-50) provided a focus for a small group of reformers interested in communitarianism, co-operation, associationism and transcendentalism. For James Hole (Owenite and associationist), F.R. Lees (temperance advocate) and January Searle (transcendentalist and adult educator), all reforms were part of their faith in 'Man the Reformer'.[34] Specific reforms and causes, whether in fringe medicine or social radicalism, were evidence of 'the great truth that every human being is morally bound, by a law of our Social condition, to leave the world somewhat better for his having lived in it'.[35] Or, as another Leeds reformer, Joseph Barker, promised when advertising his periodical, *The People*, it will be:[36]

> the Herald and Advocate of Reform in general. It pleads for Progress and Improvement in all things. It seeks to promote the free and full development of the whole human being and of the whole human family. Teetotalism, Phonography, and Phrenology, Reform in Theology, Dietetics, and the Healing Art, all share its aid. It is a wholesale and universal Reformer.

A central issue that troubled thoughtful reformers was materialism, or mind versus matter. For many of them, this appeared to go to the heart of such questions as the nature of man, his relation to the universe, and the origins of evil and suffering. Having rejected the orthodox Christian explanations of the churches, Owenites and Chartists were open to alternative answers to some of the great Victorian intellectual and spiritual conflicts. In two fringe movements — phrenology and mesmerism — partial answers at least were found. The days when these movements were regarded as little more than amusing Victorian parlour games or plausible pseudo-sciences are now over, and recent work has demonstrated their complex and sometimes contradictory social and cultural functions.[37] Phrenology had a peculiar fascination for Owenites, for its theory of brain could be interpreted as meaning that mind was material. It raised in acute form problems with which Owenites were already wrestling: materialism, free will and determinism:[38]

> As disseminated through [George Combe's] *Constitution of Man*, phrenology provided a rational religion or a type of intellectual deism for the masses. No other doctrine went quite so far or had quite as much effect in replacing supernaturalism with the Natural Laws of Man . . . . It was . . . a kind of secular Methodism legitimated by the existence of moral faculties.

Despite some philosophical inconsistencies, phrenology basically suited Owenites. It functioned to discredit traditional religion and so appealed to artisan radicals and middle-class sceptics; but it also sanctioned self-improvement of the individual and social harmony. Mesmerism, too, was characterised by similar complexities and ambiguities. It could be defended (as by Harriet Martineau) on rationalist grounds or by spiritualist arguments (as by Mary Gove Nichols). By Owenites it was welcomed as a reinforcement of the humanistic case against the religiously sanctioned social order. Phreno-magnetism, said a Sunderland Owenite, was[39]

> one of the most — if not *the most* — powerful agents in disseminating correct views of human nature, and indirectly, yet surely, destroying those old pernicious doctrines that have, in all ages, degraded humanity, and spread misery and suffering among the human race.

It has also been perceptively suggested that mesmerism put back (in a wholly secular way) into materialistic conceptions of natural reality certain elements of 'irrationality', like the passions and the emotions, which had previously been eliminated.[40] For Owenites, mesmerism thus afforded the means of making more complete and credible their comprehension of human personality and behaviour.

In their efforts to come to terms with the meanings of everyday life, to understand themselves, and to change things for the better, working people could find help in the philosophies of the medical fringe. As one reads their autobiographies or letters to the fringe journals, one recognises categories of thought which are familiar from other contexts. For the self-taught artisan with his thirst for improvement and the world of learning, there was the excitement of discovering esoteric knowledge through phrenology, mesmerism, or spiritualism. There was also the appeal to 'higher' things, and the rejection of 'animal propensities' which was strong in movements of physical puritanism. Meat-eating, for instance, was condemned by vegetarians as being animal-like; drunkenness to the teetotaller was bestial; and phrenology brought awareness of higher and lower faculties. The ethic of respectability put a high premium on such sentiments. As one Lancashire working man said in 1862:[41]

> The ignorant man had but few sources of elevated or refined joy, for he depended almost exclusively on the gratification of the mere animal faculties for his pleasure, and as those invariably flowed through one channel, the mind soon became completely satiated, and it was a question whether the pain did not counter-balance the momentary joys which he obtained . . . The intellectual man enjoyed a thousand sources of real pleasure, many of them being as pure and delightful, and as refined as could possibly be experienced.

At the same time the limitations of auto-didacticism are apparent: a certain narrowness of outlook, a weakness in the imaginative qualities, and an inclination to sectarian self-righteousness. After his initial enthusiasm, Skelton soon parted company with Coffin and accused him of slander. The phrenological world was similarly torn by the sectarian disputes of rival practitioners and their followers. An anti-intellectual element (and consequent populist appeal) was sometimes present. As part of their do-it-yourself appeal, and rejection of elite professionalism, fringe movements tended to disavow the need for any advanced learning. A preference for intuitive and instant forms of knowledge as part of a general anti-authoritarian stance may perhaps be detected here.[42]

The complexities, not to say ambiguities, of radical and medical fringe movements are well illustrated by their attitudes to sex. Because of his critique of the private family, his condemnation of the 'marriages of the priesthood', and the suspicion that he favoured artificial methods of birth control, Owen was attacked as an advocate of free love and sexual promiscuity. Owenites, and communitarians in general, favoured a liberal if not unorthodox approach to sexual relationships, and incurred much opprobrium for their alleged 'horrible abominations' — as did socialist followers of Edward Carpenter later.[43] But equally there were many Owenites who totally rejected such ideas and insisted on the need for moral respectability. Mesmerism carried sexual overtones because of the fear of one person dominating another, especially if the mesmerist was a man and the subject a young woman. Vegetarianism, particularly if practised in a community, could support ideas of sexual freedom and unorthodoxy; but more usually vegetarianism was associated with notions of purity and sexual abstinence. Movements of physical puritanism aimed at refining human nature and reducing the sensual appetites, especially sexual stimulation. Sexual eccentricity in reform and medical fringe movements could therefore take two forms: liberation in the free love tradition, or the purity and celibacy of an ascetic lifestyle. For those who had no taste for either of these extremes, there was the advice of sexual moderation dispensed in the popular health manuals of Frederick Hollick, T.L.Nichols and Sylvester Graham.

And so one could go on — documenting further the connections and associations between the medical fringe and radical social reformers. The two groups shared many common assumptions, attitudes and beliefs, and their personnel overlapped to some extent. Their functional role, too, seems to have been similar. In both groups we are dealing with people who were in some sense separate from, and indeed critical of, the society in which they found themselves. They were seeking self-knowledge; and some of them were also looking for ways to change the world. In so far as we can penetrate the mental world of these humbler Victorians, we have a way of seeing certain aspects of their society from a somewhat unusual angle — not exactly history from below, but from the corners and crevices.

Nevertheless, certain problems remain. First, there are difficulties of chronology. Although in some cases we can chart a progress from Owenism to spiritualism, or Chartism to botanic medicine, in others it is clear that the two sets of beliefs were held simultaneously. The problem is not only how or why a person should have moved from, say, Owenism to mesmerism, but how and why that person could be both an Owenite and a mesmerist at the same time. Again, this essay has dealt with the early and mid-Victorian period; but similar relationships between the medical fringe and various progressive causes can be found at the end of the century and into the 1900s. Second, it may be dangerous to generalise from the rather random selection of cases so far presented. Certain places seem to have been strongholds of the movements (Manchester, Leeds, Sheffield, Halifax, Keighley, Nottingham, Leicester and Bristol are frequently mentioned), and it may be that local or provincial studies would be the most profitable way of investigating further. Third, the concept of 'the fringe' may not be entirely satisfactory. It

212 Early Victorian Radicals

groups together a number of movements, some of which had little in common, or which had only an indirect concern with healing. Within each movement there were also differences of social class, ideological commitment, and geographical area which an omnibus label obscures. We have therefore to refine our methods before we can more fully locate the movements of fringe medicine in the social and intellectual context of early Victorian England.

Notes

It is not possible here to give full bibliographies of all the movements mentioned in this chapter, but the secondary authorities cited contain such information.

1. There is a very large literature on Chartism, and the fullest account of this is in J.F.C. Harrison and Dorothy Thompson, *Bibliography of the Chartist Movement, 1837-1976* (Sussex, Harvester Press, 1978). Recent studies which are relevant here are; James Epstein and Dorothy Thompson (eds), *The Chartist Experience* (London, Macmillan, 1982); and Dorothy Thompson, *The Chartists* (London, Temple Smith, 1984). On Owenism see J.F.C. Harrison, *Robert Owen and the Owenites in Britain and America* (London, Routledge & Kegan Paul 1969); Sidney Pollard and John Salt (eds), *Robert Owen: Prophet of the Poor* (London, Macmillan 1971); John Butt (ed.), *Robert Owen: Prince of Cotton Spinners* (Newton Abbot, David & Charles 1971); Barbara Taylor, *Eve and the New Jerusalem* (London, Virago 1983).

2. Logie Barrow, 'Socialism in Eternity: The Ideology of Plebeian Spiritualists, 1853-1913', *History Workshop*, 9 (1980) 37-69; *idem, Independent Spirits: Plebeian Spiritualists in Britain* (forthcoming). Also *idem,* 'Anti-Establishment Healing: Spiritualism in Britain', in W.J. Shiels (ed.), *The Church and Healing* (Oxford, Blackwell, 1982); and Janet Oppenheim, *The Other World Spiritualism and Psychical Research in England 1850-1914* (Cambridge, Cambridge University Press 1985).

3. *Two Worlds,* vol. 4 (1891), 65, quoted in Barrow, 'Socialism' (note 2), 55. Among the old Owenites and Chartists who became spiritualists were Joseph Gutteridge (a skilled Coventry silk-weaver, whose autobiography was published in 1893 as *Lights and Shadows in the Life of an Artisan,* and reprinted in Valerie E. Chancellor (ed.), *Master and Artisan in Victorian England* (London, Evelyn Adams & Mackay, 1969); Robert Dale Owen (one of his father's most enthusiastic young disciples and the author of two books on spiritualism); Alfred Russel Wallace (the Darwinist, who as a young man attended the Owenite Institute in John Street, and later defended phrenology and spiritualism); John Frost (Chartist, and a leader of the Newport Rising in 1839); John Culpan (a leading Halifax Chartist); William Stockton Cox (disciple and friend of Owen, who frequently stayed at his London hotel in Jermyn Street); Charles Jenneson (president of the Hoxton spiritualists and well-known Owenite); Gerald Massey (Chartist poet and later occultist).

For medical botany see particularly John V. Pickstone, 'Medical Botany (Self-help medicine in Victorian England)', *Memoirs of the Manchester Literary and Philosophical Society,* 119 (1976-7) 85-95; and *idem* 'Religious and Medical Belief-Systems', in Shiels (note 2). Also P.S. Brown, 'Herbalists and Medical Botanists in Mid-nineteenth-century Britain with Special Reference to Bristol', *Medical History,* 26 (1982) 405-420; Logie Barrow, 'Democratic Epistemology: Mid-19th Century Plebeian Medicine', *Society for the Social History of Medicine Bulletin,* 29 (1981) 25-9; E. Gaskell, 'The Coffinites', *Society for the Social History of Medicine Bulletin* 8 (1972) 12. There are also useful references in F.B.

Smith, *The People's Health, 1830-1910* (London, Croom Helm, 1979).

5. John Stevens, *Medical Reform or Physiology and Botanic Practice for the People*, 4th edn (London and Dudley, no publisher, 1849), x. The 1st edn was published in London in 1847, and a 2nd edn, London and Nottingham, 1848.

6. *Botanic Record* (1852), 4, 21.

7. Gaskell (note 4), 12.

8. See Brian E. Maidment, 'Magazines of Popular Progress and the Artisans', *Victorian Periodicals Review*, 17 (1984).

9. *Botanic Record* (1853), 229.

10. Stevens (note 5), xxi.

11. *Ibid.*, xi.

12. Cf. O. Phelps Brown, *The Complete Herbalist, or the People their own Physicians* (London, the author, 1870).

13. Letter from Miall to Epps, 11 March 1850, in Ellen Elliott Epps (ed.), *Diary of the late John Epps* (London, no publisher [1875]), 474.

14. John Goodwyn Barmby, 'Societarian Views on the Medical and Surgical Professions', *New Moral World*, 9 (1841), 187-8, 235-6, 395-7. There is an entry for Barmby in Joyce M. Bellamy and John Saville (eds), *Dictionary of Labour Biography* (London, Macmillan 1982), vol. 6.

15. *Botanic Record* (1853), 314.

16. Letter from Skelton to Jones, 7 February 1867, among Jones's papers in Seligman Collection, Columbia University, New York. I am indebted to Mrs Dorothy Thompson for a copy of this letter. There is also a reference to the case in W.E. Adams, *Memoirs of a Social Atom*, 2 vols (London, Hutchinson & Co, 1903), I, 231.

17. *Botanic Record* (1852), 35.

18. A thorough survey and analysis of vegetarianism, to which I am much indebted, is Julia Twigg, 'The Vegetarian Movement in England, 1847-1981: with Particular Reference to its Ideology' (unpublished PhD thesis, University of London, 1982). See also Stephen Willner Nissenbaum, 'Careful Love: Sylvester Graham and the Emergence of Victorian Sexual Theory in America, 1830-1840' (unpublished PhD thesis, University of Wisconsin, 1968). Among useful older works may be mentioned Charles W. Forward, *Fifty Years of Food Reform: A History of the Vegetarian Movement in England* (London and Manchester, no publisher, 1898).

19. Pictorial evidence of this is provided in the illustrations of Owenite communities. A particularly fine example was published in John Minter Morgan, *Hampden in the Nineteenth Century*, 2 vols (London, no publisher, 1834). The scene shows a classically moulded landscape, with gentle slopes, woods, rocks, and a river in the background. Buildings of stately proportions, somewhat like an Oxford or Cambridge college, occupy the left middle-distance, and sweeping lawns, dotted with a herd of deer, roll down towards the right of the picture. A building like a Greek temple is visible in the background. In the foreground groups of the happy colonists are amusing themselves in innocent diversions. A group of young females, dressed in simple flowing gowns, sits beneath the trees with their lyres; others converse on the grass or feed the deer. Children are picking flowers and looking at books, while a group of men dressed in short tunics rests upon their spades. Couples stroll beneath the huge trees in a parklike setting. No hint of industry or the machine mars the Arcadian bliss. The same illustration was later reproduced in George Fleming's journal, *The Union*, 1 (1842), 361, as an engraving of Harmony Hall. Other examples were printed in the *Co-operative Magazine*, 3 (1828) and in John Minter Morgan, *The Christian Commonwealth* (London, no publisher, 1845).

20. Nor can we be surprised that Henry Travis, one of the last of the old Owenites, should take the chair at a meeting of Sheffield medical botanists in 1854 to oppose the 'Medical Reform (Monopoly) Bill'. *Botanic Record* (1854), 368.

21. See Bernard Aspinwall, 'Social Catholicism and Health: Dr and Mrs Thomas Low Nichols in Britain', in Shiels (note 2), 249-270; Philip Gleason, 'From Free-love to

214   *Early Victorian Radicals*

Catholicism: Dr and Mrs Thomas L. Nichols at Yellow Springs', *Ohio Historical Quarterly*, 70 (October 1961), 283-307; Nissenbaum (note 18); and Thomas Low Nichols, *Forty Years of American Life, 1821-1861* (1864; reprinted New York, Stackpole & Sons, 1937).

22. T.L. Nichols, *Esoteric Anthropology (The Mysteries of Man)* (London, no publishers, 1873; revised edn, from American stereotype, London, nd), 157.

23. The phrase 'physical puritanism' is from a review article by Samuel Brown in the *Westminster Review*, April 1852, and reprinted in Samuel Brown, *Lectures on the Atomic Theory and Essays Scientific and Literary*, 2 vols (Edinburgh, T. Constable & Co., 1858), II. Very useful accounts of all aspects of physical puritanism in the 1860s are given in the periodical (edited by James Burns), *Human Nature: A Monthly Record of Zoistic Science and Intelligence*, 1-7 (1867-73).

24. Robin Price, 'Hydropathy in England, 1840-70', *Medical History*, 25 (1981), 270. Cf. Bulwer Lytton's recapture of the romantic vision of urban man regaining his health in natural surroundings in his *Confessions of a Water Patient*, 3rd edn (London, no publisher, 1847).

25. Joseph Constantine ['Practical Hydropathist, Manchester'], *A Handy Book of Hydropathy* (London, Whittaker & Co, 1860), 25. Cf. also Captain R.T. Claridge, *Every Man His Own Doctor. The Cold Water, Tepid Water, and Friction-cure, as Applicable to Every Disease to which the Human Frame is Subject* (London, J. Madden, 1849).

26. Edward Carpenter, *Civilisation: Its Cause and Cure* (1889; 13th edn, London, G. Allen & Unwin, 1914), 11, 12.

27. John Epps, *Homeopathy and its Principles Explained* (London, no publisher, 1850), 19.

28. Details from Epps (note 13).

29. For whom see Logie Barrow, 'An Imponderable Liberator: J.J. Garth Wilkinson', *Society for the Social History of Medicine Bulletin*, 36 (1985), 29-31; and his chapter in R. Cooter (ed.), *Alternatives: Essays in the Social History of Irregular Medicine* (forthcoming).

30. See Twigg (note 18), 18-19.

31. *Botanic Record* (1852), 35.

32. See Stanley Chapman, *Jesse Boot of Boots the Chemists: A Study in Business History* (London, Hodder & Stoughton, 1974), 32-7.

33. Thomas Brevior [Shorter], *Immortality in Harmony with Man's Nature and Experience: Confessions of Sceptics* (London, J. Burns, 1875), 19. Shorter's account of his experiences as a spiritualist is given in his *Confessions of a Truth Seeker: A Narrative of Personal Investigations into the Facts and Philosophy of Spirit Intercourse* (London, no publisher, 1859). See also Thomas Brevior [Shorter], *The Two Worlds, the Natural and the Spiritual* (London, F. Pitman, 1864); and *idem*, *Later Autumn Leaves: Thoughts in Verse* (London, Allan & Son, 1896), which contains a biographical sketch of the author. In the 1860s Shorter published several collections of poetry and prose, 'for school and home'. There are regular references to him throughout his life (1832-99) in the radical and spiritualist journals. See also J.F.C. Harrison, *A History of the Working Men's College, 1854-1954* (London, Routledge & Kegan Paul, 1954).

34. Cf. 'Man the Reformer', *Complete Works of Ralph Waldo Emerson* (New York, 1892), I. Details of the Leeds transcendentalists and Emersonians are given in J.F.C. Harrison, *Learning and Living, 1790-1960* (London, Routledge & Kegan Paul, 1961), ch. 3.

35. Horace Greeley, *Hints Towards Reforms* 2nd edn (New York, no publisher, 1853), 8.

36. *Cooper's Journal*, 17 January 1850, 48.

37. Most notably in Roger Cooter, *The Cultural Meaning of Popular Science: Phrenology and the Organization of Consent in Nineteenth-century Britain* (Cambridge, Cambridge University Press, 1984). There is an excellent review of the recent literature on phrenology by Cooter. 'Phrenology: The Provocation of Progress', *History of Science*, 14 (1976), 211-34. For Owenism and phrenology see also J.F.C. Harrison (note 1), 239-43; and David

de Giustino, *Conquest of Mind* (London, Croom Helm, 1975).

38. Cooter, 'Phrenology' (note 37), 216.

39. *New Moral World*, 20 May 1843, 377; and also quoted in Roger Cooter, 'The History of Mesmerism in Britain: Poverty and Promise', in Heinz Schott (ed.), *Franz Anton Mesmer und die Geschichte des Mesmerismus* (Stuttgart, Steiner, 1985), 152-62, to which I am indebted.

40. Cooter (note 39), 94.

41. *Ashton Reporter*, 12 April 1862, quoted in Neville Kirk, *The Growth of Working Class Reformism in Mid-Victorian England* (London, Croom Helm, 1985), 213-14.

42. Cf. Mary Douglas, *Natural Symbols; Explorations in Cosmology* (London, Barrie & Jenkins, 1973), 40.

43. See Raymond Lee Muncy, *Sex and Marriage in Utopian Communities: 19th Century America* (Bloomington, Indiana, Indiana University Press, 1973).

11 SOCIAL CONTEXT AND MEDICAL THEORY IN THE DEMARCATION OF NINETEENTH-CENTURY BOUNDARIES

P.S. Brown

By the mid-nineteenth century in Britain there were numerous groups on the fringe of medicine. Some were clearly separated from orthodoxy, while others represented medical heresies arising within the regular ranks. Established medicine was formalising its professional structure and needed urgently to define its boundaries. This paper examines the basis on which lines of demarcation were drawn between orthodoxy and three examples of the medical fringe — hydropathy, herbalism and the marketing of 'patent medicines'.

Proprietary Medicines

The supply of proprietary, or 'patent', medicines was in most cases clearly separated from orthodox medical practice: but before proceeding on this assumption it is best to discuss the areas in which the boundary between them was unclear. In the eighteenth century an established physician had patented a fever powder[1] and, in the first half of the nineteenth, patentees included five persons described as physicians, surgeons or apothecaries.[2] In the latter century, a licentiate of the Royal College of Physicians was suspended for becoming the proprietor of 'Water from the Pool of Bethesda' and a physician told a Select Committee that, 'in one or two instances', he still prescribed secret preparations. His evidence also implied involvement of regular practitioners in the retail market as he complained that young men intending ultimately to practise medicine, frequently financed their medical education by opening a shop to sell patent medicines and practise over the counter: it brought 'a class of men into the medical profession who ought not to be in it'. And another physician admitted that poverty compelled some medical men to 'sell quack medicines'.[3]

Some overlap between the domains of the patent medicine vendor and the medical profession therefore seems certain, but its significance should not be exaggerated. The proprietary market was very large and in the great majority of instances, patent medicines and regular medication were supplied in quite distinct and different contexts. Accepting this distinction, the question arises whether these two types of medicine showed equally distinct differences in the active substances they contained and the medical theories on which their composition was based. Studies of the patent medicines most often advertised in eighteenth-century newspapers have suggested that their composition closely resembled that of the official preparations used by the regular practitioners.[4] The similarity of proprietary and regular medicines was also suggested in a study of medicines advertised for treating the diseases of women in the eighteenth and nineteenth centuries,[5] and was supported by contemporary writers. Dr Henry Letheby of the London Hospital claimed in 1856 that analysis showed a large class of advertised medicines to be 'almost identical in their composition with the common Aperient Pills, which are dispensed at the public hospitals'. He defined other classes of proprietary medicines as containing orthodox medicaments, and referred to other medical authors supporting his views.[6] Regular and proprietary medicines seem therefore to have differed more in the context of their supply than in their composition.

The attitude of the patent medicine proprietors to the boundary between themselves and the medical profession was reflected in their advertisements. A systematic sample of advertisements for 100 medicines in seven Bristol newspapers published in 1851 and 1861, showed clearly that many advertisers wished to be identified with regular medicine. The title of 'doctor' was included in the names of twenty-eight medicines; the proprietor described himself by this title or as a surgeon in seventeen instances; use in regular practice was claimed for sixteen medicines; medical authorities were quoted in the text of eleven advertisements; and four printed testimonials, allegedly from medical men. Medical status was claimed for fifty preparations by at least one of the modes of association listed above. Possibly some claims had substance, but the two proprietors associated with Bristol who used medical titles were not what they implied. One could not be traced in any source except the advertisement, and the other described himself more prudently for the 1851 census as a patent medicine proprietor.

To the medical profession, the sale of proprietary medicines was objectionable on several counts. Their large-scale use meant that a substantial area of medical activity escaped control by the profession, and the great reputation of some patent medicines implied a body of therapeutic expertise, again outside the profession. And the competition could be seen in financial terms as proprietary medicines were probably used by all classes in the nineteenth century. George Crabbe, in *The*

Borough, claimed that they wasted no small portion of the poor man's pay, and Engels reported their extensive use by the working classes.[7] But the medical profession, more interested in their consumption by the wealthier, sometimes played down their purchase by the poor, who did not represent an important source of medical income. A practitioner from Bath claimed that 'It is not the lower classes of the community that buy and patronize the advertised nostrums, but the higher and educated.'[8]

The medical profession faced several difficulties in dealing with the problem of patent medicines. Professionals could only express their disapproval to individual patients or publish such articles as those 'On the Mischievous Effects of Quack Medicines' in the *Family Friend*,[9] in which Letheby wrote of 'the terrible mischief which results from the indiscriminate use of such medicines'. Some advertisements could be attacked on 'moral' grounds, to generate disapproval which would spread to the advertisements generally. A worthy target for attack were the alarm-provoking advertisements by the proprietors of pills for venereal disease, impotence and the results of 'secret vice'. There was talk of a 'Union for the Discouragement of Vicious Advertisements' and the *Lancet* editorial bubbled over with righteous indignation and prejudiced resentment.[10] But, in addressing the public, the regular profession could not compete with the bulk of advertising copy put out by the medicine vendors. The problem was illustrated by the discomfort of Sir Charles Locock, accoucheur to Queen Victoria, when his family name was being used to advertise medicines. Locock explained that publishing a disclaimer of any association with the medicine could not be effective unless it was printed at least as widely as the seemingly ubiquitous advertisements.[11]

Another major problem was the stamp duty on proprietary medicines, which seemed to give them official status and which provided a considerable item of government revenue. The tax offered some protection to unqualified practitioners, and when one was asked what he would do if the proposed Medical Act was passed, he replied, 'I shall then put a stamp on all the medicines I sell, and then the law cannot touch me.'[12] The importance of the revenue raised by the medicines was variously represented, estimates ranging from 'trifling' (in a report suggesting its abolition) to 'immense' (in the evidence to a Select Committee of a physician who had also taken into account the licence revenue and the associated advertisement duty). Withdrawal of the implied sanction of the medicine stamp was often urged but, presumably because of the opposition that the consequent loss of revenue might arouse, it was sometimes suggested that it was more important to deal with other aspects of 'quackery'.[13] It was even suggested that the suppression of quack medicines should not be discussed at public meetings on medical reform because the threatened loss of revenue might frighten off political support for more important measures.[14]

By the middle of the nineteenth century, then, the marketing of proprietary medicines was largely separated from orthodox medical practice with a small equivocal area of overlap. The boundary was based on different modes of supplying proprietary and orthodox medicines, rather than on any radical difference in their pharmacological composition. Most of the medicine vendors were anxious to gain by implied association with medical orthodoxy, while the medical profession was not able to suppress their activities. Already the proprietors had developed notable financial muscle and it was reported that a meeting of the owners of medicines in 1864 quickly contributed nearly £3,000 for a committee to resist legislation.[15] Not surprisingly, the trade in proprietary medicines went from strength to strength in the later decades of the century.[16]

In stressing the desire of the medicine vendors to fit comfortably beside regular practice, an important exception has been ignored. This was James Morison, who has been studied in detail by Helfand.[17] Morison was frankly and aggressively anti-medical, the title page of one of his publications declaring that 'The old medical science is completely wrong,' a theme developed in the text with the observation that the medical profession, 'having called in the aid of minerals and chemistry . . . there has been no end of their fruitless tortures, trials, and experiments on the human body'.[18] Rejecting orthodox medicine, Morison developed his own system which postulated a common cause for all diseases and a universal vegetable pill to cure them; and the consequent confrontation with the medical establishment resulted in battles, often fought in coroners' courts and the columns of the *Lancet*. Morison challenged the medical profession socially and in terms of medical theory: in these attitudes and their consequences, he resembled the next group of fringe practitioners to be considered.

Herbalists

Medical botanists of the Thomsonian school were clearly distinct from the regular practitioners and they entered the field with a blatant social challenge to the medical profession. Albert Isaiah Coffin had arrived in Britain in 1838, bringing the botanic system from America where

Samuel Thomson, its originator, had been involved in legal confrontation with regular medicine.[19] Coffin continued the fight and by his lectures and publications was able 'to carry on the war of aggression with the old allopathic system'.[20] One aim of his *Botanical Journal and Medical Reformer* was 'to expose . . . and to reform the abuses of the profession', this being necessary because the influence of the medical profession had been 'accumulating for centuries, until they vainly imagined themselves to be the only rightful oracles of the science'.[21] The medical world had acquired 'the prescriptive right of killing or curing at pleasure', but now it was time for Coffin's followers to 'throw off the yoke of medical despotism'.[22]

John Skelton, another leader of the Thomsonian movement in Britain, believed that 'the so-called science of medicine, as now taught in the schools, imposed upon society, and supported by law, is one huge deception alike injurious to all'. It was the monopoly of the privileged allopathic doctor who has[23]

> a brass plate upon his door, and a coloured lamp over it, and besides this he rides in his own vehicle: he has a brother a minister, another a lawyer, his father practiced before him; his son too is studying for the profession, his reputation is as extensive as his practice, and therefore being so respectable and respectably connected, he cannot possibly be wrong.

But thousands among the poor can scarcely find bread for their children and are in no condition to pay doctors' bills: for them Skelton is determined 'to brave all prejudice and opposition so that he can assist to rescue the poor and needy from medical bondage'.[24] Similar themes were pursued by John Stevens, another Thomsonian, whose book *Medical Reform* (1847) celebrated the social and political reforms already achieved but saw reform in the practice of medicine as the most needed one of all, the regular practitioners being 'licensed to kill'.[25]

The medical botanists sought to 'demystify' and 'deprofessionalise' medicine. In Coffin's view,[26]

> That which has been falsely termed science in medicine, is no more than a tissue of incongruities, interwoven with the obsolete and unmeaning language of the schools of antiquity, invented for no end, save the final prostration of the human intellect at the shrine of monopoly, in order to dignify and confer wealth on a few individuals, and to support institutions which have thus grown upon us. The

learned have combined together for the purpose of throwing dust into the eyes of the people, in support of which fallacy they have invented a language peculiar to themselves.

By contrast, the system of medical botany was 'so easy to be understood, that every member of society may learn it if disposed'. To aid understanding, Coffin's *Botanic Guide* has been 'freed . . . from all technicalities', and understanding could be translated into practice so that 'every father can now discharge the duties of physician to his own household'.[27] These sentiments were echoed by John Stevens, who wrote that 'however lofty Medical Science has appeared when clothed in mystery, or flaunting in the false airs of pedantic learning, it is not, if stripped of that mystery, higher than the reach of the ordinary mind, or beyond the attainment of common sense'.[28]

Debunking established medicine and setting up a new medicine for the people required new standards — and who should set those standards but 'the people'? This idea was most clearly linked with the demystification of medicine by Skelton. He did not believe that medical practice was 'a difficult, abstruse, mysterious science', but that it only seemed so because 'of its being a sealed profession, from which the public mind is excluded'.[29] He believed that medicine should be simplified and popularised, and that the only way of doing so was 'to proselytize the people'.[30] The public had the right to judge its medicine as much as it had the right to judge its food, and 'The only "established" criterion or standard by which the practice of medicine should be determined, is the will of the public.'[31] And in accordance with their aim of involving the people, Thomsonian herbalists encouraged the establishment of local botanic societies for medical self-help.

The medical botanists and the orthodox profession were thus sharply divided by socially defined barriers: they served different social groups and they viewed society from totally different perspectives. The uncompromisingly aggressive views of the botanists provoked an equally vigorous condemnation from the regular profession. But demarcation of their territories was not only in social terms, there being clear conflict of medical theory to support them. Indeed, it would be artificial to separate the theoretical from the social considerations as they represented two aspects of the same situation which were mutually reinforcing. The medical profession represented the institutionalised expression of the therapeutic ideas which the herbalists abhorred.

The medical botanists saw orthodox treatment as a lethal combination of depletion and poisoning. In typical style, Coffin wrote that 'The seeds of disease and death, are sown in the vitals of society, by the use of poisonous medicines.'[32] By contrast, they claimed, the medicines of the botanists were 'natural' and innocuous. Not surprisingly the medical profession did not agree, and took pains to establish the toxicity of the herbalists' favourite medicine, *Lobelia inflata*. This conflict of opinion has been discussed elsewhere,[33] but the botanists' ideas on 'natural' remedies are worth considering further because they involve attitudes towards the healing power of nature which have been increasingly important in characterising the 'fringe' since the nineteenth century.

Trust in the healing power of nature, particularly in contrast to reliance on the use of toxic medicines, was regaining ground in orthodox medicine in the first half of the nineteenth century,[34] and has been considered in the British context by Price when discussing hydropathy.[35] It became a common theme in the teaching of many sections of alternative medicine, culminating in its purest form in Britain as the local brand of naturopathy or nature cure. Traces of this optimistic philosophy can be detected in the writings of the Thomsonian herbalists in this country.

The naturopathic emphasis on the idea that disease was due to the violation of nature's laws can be seen, for instance, in Stevens's explanation that 'man, by the abuse of his privilege of free will, is constantly living and pursuing habits in opposition to all the laws of health and life, and consequently suffering disease, debility, and degeneration'.[36] Fox and Nadin warned that 'The result of a violation of the physical laws of our nature, is to produce misery and disease; in proportion to the extent of those violations.'[37] Skelton also wrote that disease was due to such a violation, but concluded that disease was natural to man. This view would not have been shared by the later naturopaths, and was challenged by the herbalist W. Dale, both in Skelton's own journal and in a fuller defence of the proposition that disease was not a necessary consequence of life.[38]

Coffin also considered that most diseases were 'in our power entirely to prevent' and, in common with medical systems which relied upon nature, saw acute disease not as a foreign entity to be attacked and vanquished, but as a manifestation of the salutary efforts of the body to eliminate impurities from the system. Accordingly, Coffin wrote that 'we always regard fever as a friend, or the result of an exertion of nature to throw off the obstruction, and which only wants assistance instead of opposition'.[39] And similar views were expressed by other Thomsonian botanists.[40]

Although these themes can be detected in the writings of the early Thomsonians in Britain, they were frequently mixed with almost contradictory ideas. Reliance on powerful herbal medicaments — stimulants, astringents, tonics, diuretics, cathartics — was itself a contradiction of naturopathic ideas, though Fox and Nadin pointed out that the stimulants used by the botanists did not 'increase the pulsation beyond its natural standard'.[41] Later in the century the herbalists drew strength and support from naturopathy,[42] and it was even claimed by a herbalist that Coffin had been the pioneer of 'nature cure *principles*' in Britain.[43] But common antipathy to the medical profession, and some shared belief in what they considered to be natural remedies, did not line up the medical botanists close beside any of the other groups of unorthodox practitioners in the mid-nineteenth century. Coffin attacked homoeopathy and hydropathy in the same breath as he condemned allopathy.[44] The hydropaths, who are to be considered next, resembled the herbalists in their condemnation of orthodox medicine, but they did not replace one *materia medica* with another and their particular universal remedy of water had a far better claim to be called 'natural'.

Hydropathy

Price has discussed hydropathy during its first three decades in England, concentrating on the resulting struggle within the medical profession.[45] Most of those involved in the water cure at this time were medically qualified and their beliefs can be seen as heresies within medicine, while orthodox practitioners could claim that any successes of hydropathy merely reflected the virtue of bathing already well known to the profession.[46] There were, however, important hydropathic practitioners outside the profession and the present discussion will concentrate on their activities and relationship with the medically qualified.

British interest in hydropathy was stimulated by Richard T. Claridge, a contractor in asphalt, who wrote and lectured enthusiastically on the water cure of Priessnitz.[47] An early unqualified practitioner in England was James Ellis, a lace merchant and temperance worker, who had gained medical experience but apparently no formal qualification on the continent. While practising at Sudbrook Park in the 1840s, he arranged special accommodation for patients unable to pay the usual fees, and later started a free hydropathic sanatorium for working people in London.[48] At the start of the next century, Ellis was hailed by the British Nature Cure Association as 'the first really great apostle of Naturopathy as we now practise it'.[49] He wrote under the title of 'Dr Ellis', and did not appear anxious to distance himself from the regularly qualified.[50]

The best known of the non-medical practitioners was John Smedley, who became interested in the system when he paused after a hard but highly successful struggle to modernise and develop his father's hosiery-manufacturing business.[51] A long illness impressed him with the inefficiency of regular medicine, but finally his ailment yielded to the efficient yet harsh water cure at Ben Rhydding in Yorkshire. Smedley was converted to hydropathy and at the same time replaced his formal self-satisfied worship in the established church with 'the unbounded joy and confidence' of a new religious fervour.[52] Highly critical of the established clergy, he built and maintained chapels for the Methodists and preached or lectured regularly in a marquee, but apparently was unable to commit himself fully to any religious sect.[53] He started to practise hydropathy by providing free facilities for his workmen at Lea Mills in 1851; then, at the rapidly expanding Matlock Bank Hydropathic Establishment, Smedley developed a mild version of the water cure. His wife supervised the female patients and published a *Ladies' Manual* for their use.[54] The success of hydropathy in Matlock attracted other non-medical practitioners to the area and several of Smedley's bathmen and their wives were encouraged to set up satellite establishments.[55]

A pioneer Scottish hydropath was Archibald Hunter, a cabinet-maker with a degree from the Hydropathic Institute of New York. He entered practice in 1855 and eventually built up a hydropathic establishment at Bridge of Allen.[56] His idealistic and benevolent attitudes are expressed in his specifications for the ideal physician.[57] Other unqualified hydropaths are mentioned by Metcalfe,[58] but one of particular interest was Spencer T. Hall, who practised briefly but apparently not successfully in Matlock around 1862 before moving eventually to Windermere.[59] Hall, the son of a Quaker cobbler, became known chiefly for his literary work and his association with mesmerism and phrenology. He used the title of 'Doctor' by virtue of a PhD (Tübingen), but his clinical practice did not save him from eventual poverty.[60] Finally, Samuel Kenworthy, though not born until 1838, should be mentioned as an important editor and writer on hydropathy. Metcalfe describes him as deeply and sincerely interest in 'hydrotherapeutics, sanitation, Christianity, total abstinence, and the general moral and spiritual well-being of the people'.[61]

The gulf between the lay hydropaths and the regular practitioners was clear enough. The unqualified could find no virtue in orthodox medical doctrine. Claridge wrote of the faculty's errors and prejudices and of their pernicious drugs which might destroy the whole species if unchecked.[62] Smedley thought that the patient always came off the loser from the doctors' drugs and other inventions to force nature's hand; and that death and misery resulted from the medical profession's fundamental error of seeing disease as something to be subdued and driven out.[63] But, perhaps as a result of his social background as a successful factory-owner, Smedley allowed that regular practitioners were usually of high principles, intelligent and philanthropic — it was only the evil effects of allopathic practice that he deplored.[64]

No violent reactions to Smedley's pronouncements seem to have figured in the medical journals and he does not appear to have been subjected to attack in the law courts. Smedley's success and his non-profit-making practice[65] might well have aggravated any reaction of the regular practitioners to his attacks on their theory and practice, and they could have dismissed his benevolence as humbug. But Smedley probably did not provide the medical profession with ammunition for attack: even if they had found suitable inquests, it would have been difficult for the doctors to maintain that his mild water cure was the cause of death as they did the herbalists' lobelia or Morison's pills. James Ellis had been less fortunate in 1846 when hydropathy was being actively debated and when a death at his hydropathic establishment had elicited a charge of manslaughter, though not a conviction.[66] But the medical journals generally concentrated their attack on the medically qualified hydropaths, orthodoxy being less concerned about activity well outside the profession than about the breach in its own defences.

One might have expected demarcation between the unqualified and the medically qualified hydropaths to be less clear. But it was clear enough because, not surprisingly, the regularly qualified hydropaths were extremely anxious to retain and defend their position within the profession. Also, years of medical training made it difficult for them to reject all drugs. Although James Wilson declared physic and the water cure to be as incompatible as fire and water, Dr Gully admitted that some medicines could never be dispensed with in rational therapy.[67] Thomas J. Graham, the writer on domestic medicine who ran a hydropathic establishment at Stansteadbury, advocated drugs in preparation for courses of hygienic treatment; while Robert Hay Graham was critical of Priessnitz but thought that a combination of water treatment with medication might be more effective.[68] And Abraham Courtney, the naval surgeon, used medicines if his patients wanted them, but believed he had a more powerful remedy in the water cure.[69]

Edward Johnson, also medically qualified, did not reject drugs entirely, and his views illustrate the attitude of the medical hydropaths to the unqualified. Johnson implied that it was the 'unlettered and unprofessional practitioner' who wished to abolish drugs completely:

he knew nothing of their actions and sought to 'bring down the science of healing diseases to the level of his own knowledge and acquirements'.[70] Similarly, James Wilson considered the study of anatomy, physiology and pathology to be indispensable to the understanding and safe practice of the water cures;[71] and John Goodman thought it strange that, because the old system of medicinal dosing had sometimes proved injurious, the whole accumulated wisdom of medicine should be swept away and that the unlearned and medically uneducated should be considered competent to treat the sick.[72]

The lay practitioners, in their turn, criticised the medically qualified hydropaths. Smedley, humble about his lack of medical education but believing that his work led him in the path that God had designed for him, claimed that some took to the water cure because they had not succeeded in regular practice. Excellent physicians, however, might make poor hydropaths because their professional attitudes prevented them from condescending to 'the unprofessional and common employment of seeing personally to the important minutiae of their patients' treatment.[73] But Smedley finally handed over his practice to William Bell Hunter (MD Glasgow),[74] while Ellis was followed at Sudbrook Park by Edward R. Lane (MD Edin) and Samuel Kenworthy was succeeded by his medically qualified son.[75] Despite these takeovers by regular practitioners, there was also a continuing tradition of lay practice. The doctor chosen by Smedley was the son of Archibald Hunter, and the latter's medically unqualified widow, Mrs A.S. Hunter, remained active in hygienic medicine and was later described as the 'Mother of the [nature cure] movement' in Britain.[76] And hydropathy remained an important element in naturopathic medicine in the early twentieth century.[77]

Hydropathy represented one of several forms of reaction to the unsatisfactory state of orthodox therapeutics. To the medically qualified it offered a road to the reform of medicine and, to the lay practitioners, a means of extending their humanitarian activities. Examination of the other beliefs and systems adopted by the hydropaths helps to explain their motivation and suggests that hydropathy was attractive to those already in a reforming state of mind. Some, for instance, came to the water cure through the temperance movement, hydropathy preaching a temperance in all things. Teetotallers naturally approved of medical treatment based only on water and the *Bristol Temperance Herald* noted 'the intimate connexion between Hydropathy and Total Abstinence'.[78] Edward Johnson, Ralph Grindrod and Abraham Courtney all wrote in the temperance cause before hydropathy had reached Britain.[79] They were already reformers before the water cure offered them a means of reforming medicine.

Homoeopathy was a heretical system greatly favoured by hydropaths and McMenemy has pointed out its prevalence among the water doctors of Malvern.[80] Interest in the two systems was not confined to Malvern practitioners, another notable example being William Macleod, the physician of Ben Rhydding. He wrote of homoeopathy and hydropathy that 'these two systems must go hand in hand' and that they 'harmoniously work together'.[81] As editor of the *Water Cure Journal* he published a letter on homoeopathic treatment by William Forbes Laurie, who ran a hydropathic establishment at Dunstable: Laurie also wrote in the *Journal of Health* that he practised both systems.[82] Among the non-medical hydropaths, Smedley was not in favour but Spencer Hall summed up his enthusiasms with the statement that 'were there no Hydropathy, I would be a Homoeopathist; or, were there no Homoeopathy, I would be a Hydropathist'.[83]

Why then should homoeopathy and hydropathy be adopted by the same practitioners? The two systems shared some common ground in medical theory. Hydropaths believed that the manifestations of disease were the body's salutary reactions to undesirable agents and that these reactions should be encouraged rather than suppressed; the homoeopaths might be seen as encouraging such reactions by using medicines which provoked similar symptoms. But the infinitesimal doses of homoeopathy raised particular problems of acceptance. So the similarity of the two systems was somewhat tenuous and probably the adoption of both hydropathy and homoeopathy represented a general reaction to medical authority — both to unsatisfactory allopathic therapeutics and to the allopathic establishment. This view is supported by the interest shown in other unorthodox medical ideas by the hydropaths. They were exposed to the American Health Reform movement through the writings of William Alcott and Sylvester Graham printed in the *Journal of Health*, published in Britain under the editorship of Grindrod during 1851. And the same journal published a long phrenological analysis of Priessnitz.[84] Forbes Laurie wrote of his treatment of epilepsy by electro-biology, using zinc and copper discs, and among the non-medical practitioners, Spencer Hall held a very full hand being a homoeopath and a hydropath who was also prominent in mesmerism and phrenology.[85]

Conclusion

It has been argued that the business of supplying proprietary medicines differed from orthodox medical practice primarily because of differences in their social and commercial contexts. The medical profession could not deal with the type of competition involved and, as the nineteenth century progressed, the section of the medicine-producing industry responsible for 'patent medicines' continued to flourish. With the rise of 'scientific medicine' in the present century, another section of the medicine-producing industry has engineered a great proliferation both of pharmaceuticals and of profits. Sometimes continuity between the different phases of the industry's activity can be traced across the centuries, as for instance from the humble origins of Beecham's Pills to the scientific 'breakthrough' of Beecham's semi-synthetic penicillins.[86] And the concept of proprietary medicines has shifted ground but gained in importance, so that for several decades the drug-manufacturers have been able to manipulate a large section of medical practitioners to think of official medicines by their proprietary rather than their generic names. The pharmaceutical companies which supply the items of the complex modern *pharmacopoeia*, under generic or proprietary names, as well as their proprietary preparations sold over the counter, cannot now be seen in any way as on the medical fringe. They have established themselves as a powerful element inextricably involved in modern established medicine.

Some differences based in medical theory were probably needed for practitioners to be recognisable as forming a 'fringe' group. But some groups could exist and be separated from the medical profession by social and administrative barriers alone. There were, for example, unregistered practitioners after the Medical Act and chemists who practised over the counter.[87] Both groups were accused of ignorance and lack of skill, but they were not usually accused of subscribing to a different medical theory. Presumably they based their practice on that of regular medicine and were seen as second-rate doctors offering a second-rate service to the poor, rather than as a fringe group supplying an alternative type of therapy.

Identification of differences in medical theories held by fringe groups and the medical profession is not always straightforward, if only because the collection of beliefs which characterise orthodoxy is constantly changing. Ideas may first be harboured and then rejected by orthodoxy, while other beliefs by a reverse process may become newly acceptable. Astrology, once an integral part of medicine, was later rejected:[88] it found a lodging with herbalism but eventually was rejected in turn by the herbalists.[89] On the other hand, mesmerism — which was once a desperate heresy — later became acceptable to medicine on a more empirical basis and under the guise of hypnotism.[90] And at any one time established medicine might contain a wide spectrum of beliefs. Attitudes and emphases differ in different schools of medicine and disparity between the outlooks of physicians and general practitioners was recognised in the nineteenth century as relevant in the discussion of medical heresy.[91]

It was not a single idea or belief held in isolation that characterised a medical cult or fringe group. Herbalists did not believe only in treatment by herbs; and, in any case, herbal medicines were prominent in the orthodox *pharmacopoeia*. Hydropaths did not believe only in treatment by water; and again, the regular profession admitted some value in such treatment. By the time that a fringe group could be identified, its members had developed a complex assemblage of interrelated ideas: some of those ideas might be found also in the assemblage characteristic of orthodoxy but, as assemblages, the two were distinct. Herbalists, for example, used herbal medicines, preferably in a simple form and not as refined chemical extracts; they used no mineral medicines, which they considered unnatural, and no preparations which they considered to be poisonous in any dose, be they mineral or vegetable; they considered their remedies to be 'natural' and emphasised temperance in food, drink and action; they considered the regular doctors' treatment to be lethal, and their disapproval of such therapy extended to the practitioners who used it and to the practices such as vaccination and vivisection which they saw as characteristic of allopathic medicine.[92]

An individual might formulate such a package of ideas, but if he were an isolated regular practitioner who developed a distinctive and unusual set of beliefs, he would probably have been dismissed as no more than eccentric. He would hardly be seen as a challenge to orthodoxy until he had formed a group of similarly minded individuals or projected his views in some organised setting such as public lectures or a commercial enterprise. It was the 'public exhibitions' of mesmerism to which the Medical Committee of University College Hospital took particular exception in the censure of John Elliotson, resulting in the resignation of his professorship.[93] And hydropathy became a challenge to orthodoxy when it could be seen as the inspiration of a group of practitioners who developed their characteristic hydropathic establishments and publicised their dogma in books and journals. The idea that there can be a characteristic set of beliefs and practices presupposes a number of individuals sharing them, so that a fringe activity can only be identified and characterised when such a group of practitioners has been formed. The group must have some social organisation and this social, organisational aspect is as important in the demarcation of the group from

230 Social Context and Medical Theory

orthodoxy as the medical theories it holds. And a socially definable group will also tend to share attitudes and outlooks in relation to problems outside medicine. Demarcation of the 'fringe' is therefore a matter both of medical theory and of social boundaries. As the developing medical profession was deeply concerned with its organisation and social cohesion, so increasingly were the fringe groups. From the second half of the nineteenth century, the herbalists can be seen moving away from their network of local botanic societies for self-help, and attempting to formalise their group organisation with the appearance of national societies, journals, training programmes, examinations for diplomas and agitation for legal recognition.[94] The herbalists' efforts at survival had only limited success and, with the passage of time, the hydropathic movement also lost vigour and enthusiasm.[95] A less aggressive hydrotherapy became absorbed into accepted physical medicine and the reforming zeal of the early hydropaths shifted to other manifestations of alternative medicine.

Notes

1. P.S. Brown, 'Medicines Advertised in Eighteenth-century Bath Newspapers', *Medical History*, 20 (1976), 152-68.
2. *Patents for Inventions. Abridgments of Specifications Relating to Medicine, Surgery and Dentistry, 1620-1866* (London, Patent Office, 1872).
3. *Report from the Select Committee on Medical Registration* (1847), evidence of J.A. Paris, Q. 50; *Report from the Select Committee on Pharmacy Bill* (1852), evidence of J.R. Cormack, Qs 2402 and 2407; and in *ibid.*, E. Crisp, Q. 2314.
4. Brown (note 1); idem, 'Some treatments of Skin Disease in Eighteenth Century Bath', *International Journal of Dermatology*, 21 (1982), 555-9
5. P.S. Brown, 'Female Pills and the Reputation of Iron as an Abortifacient', *Medical History*, 21 (1977), 291-304.
6. Henry Letheby, 'On the Mischievous Effects of Quack Medicines', *Family Friend*, 3rd series, 11 (1856), 7-9, 31-2, 91-5, 121-3.
7. Frederick Engels, *The Condition of the Working-class in England in 1844*, trans. F.K. Wischnewetzky (London, George Allen & Unwin, 1892), 104-5.
8. George King, 'Sale of Quack Medicines', *Provincial Medical & Surgical Journal* (1844), 596-7.
9. Letheby (note 6).
10. Editorial, *Lancet*, 1 (1851), 72-3.
11. Charles Locock, letter, *Lancet*, 1 (1846), 311.
12. 'The Medical Reform Bill and Quackery', *Lancet*, 1 (1854), 218.
13. 'Quackery and Illegal Practice', *Lancet*, 1 (1841-2), 138-9; *Select Committee Pharmacy Bill*, evidence of E. Crisp, Q. 2313 (note 3).
14. King, (note 8).
15. 'The Medical Act', *Lancet*, 1 (1864), 26.
16. Stanley Chapman, *Jesse Boot of Boots the Chemist* (London, Hodder & Stoughton, 1974), 203-5.

17. William H. Helfand, 'James Morison and his Pills', *Transactions of the British Society of the History of Pharmacy*, 1 (1974), 101-35.
18. James Morison, *Morisoniana* (London, British College of Health, 1868), title page and v.
19. Alex Berman, 'The Thomsonian Movement and its Relation to American Pharmacy and Medicine', *Bulletin of the History of Medicine*, 25 (1951), 405-28.
20. John Skelton, 'A Brief Record of the Botanic Progress in England', *Dr Skelton's Botanic Record and Family Herbal* (subsequently *Skelton's Record*), 1 (1852), 3-4.
21. *Coffin's Botanical Journal and Medical Reformer* (subsequently *Coffin's Journal*), 1 (1847), 1-3.
22. A.I. Coffin, *A Botanic Guide to Health*, 5th edn (Manchester, The Author, 1846), ii, ix.
23. John Skelton, *Skelton's Record*, 1 (1852), 7, 97-100.
24. John Skelton, *The Epitome of the Botanic Practice of Medicine* (Leeds, Samuel Moxon, 1855), v.
25. John Stevens, *Medical Reform*, 3rd edn (London, Whittaker, 1848), xii-xxv.
26. A.I. Coffin, *Botanic Guide to Health*, 31st edn (London, The Author, 1859), 69-70.
27. *Ibid.*, xv.
28. Stevens (note 25), x.
29. John Skelton, *A Plea for the Botanic Practice of Medicine* (London, Watson, 1853), 20.
30. John Skelton, *Skelton's Record*, (1855), 1-2.
31. Skelton (note 29), 242-8.
32. Coffin (note 22), 70.
33. P.S. Brown, 'Herbalists and Medical Botanists in Mid-nineteenth Century Britain, with Special Reference to Bristol', *Medical History*, 26 (1982), 405-20.
34. J.H. Warner, ' "The Nature-trusting Heresy": American Physicians and the Concept of the Healing Power of Nature in the 1850s and 1860s', *Perspectives in American History*, 11 (1977-8), 291-324.
35. R. Price, 'Hydropathy in England 840-70', *Medical History*, 25 (1981), 269-80.
36. Stevens (note 25), 116-17.
37. William Fox and Joseph Nadin, *The Working Man's Family Botanic Guide* (Sheffield, Dawson, 1852), 84.
38. *Skelton's Record*, 1 (1852), 20, 54-5; W. Dale, *The Principles and Practice of the Botanic System of Medicine* (Glasgow, Murray, 1855), 20.
39. 'Causes of Disease', *Coffin's Journal*, 1 (1847), 5-6; Coffin (note 26), 345-6.
40. Skelton (note 24), 69-70. Fox and Nadin (note 37), iv.
41. Fox and Nadin (note 37), 39.
42. P.S. Brown, 'The Vicissitudes of Herbalism in Late Nineteenth- and Early Twentieth-century Britain', *Medical History*, 29 (1985), 71-92.
43. *Herb Doctor and Home Physician*, 25 (1928), 36.
44. Coffin (note 26), xxii.
45. Price (note 35).
46. For example, J.A. Symonds, 'Some Truths in Medicine that may be Heresies', *Lancet*, 1 (1842-3), 244-5.
47. R.T. Claridge, *Hydropathy; Or the Cold Water Cure*, 3rd edn (London, J. Madden, 1842).
48. Richard Metcalfe, *The Rise and Progress of Hydropathy in England and Scotland* (London, Simpkin, Marshall, Hamilton & Kent, 1906), 50-7.
49. *Nature Cure Annual* (London, Macgregor Reid & Shaw, 1907-8), 81.
50. Dr Ellis, *Pain: Its Alleviation, Suspension and Cure* (London, W. Tweedie, 1871).
51. Joseph Buckley, *Matlock Bank, (Derbyshire), As It Was, and Is* (London, J. Caudwell, nd), 47-52.
52. John Smedley, *Practical Hydropathy*, 4th edn (London, S.W. Partridge,

1861), ix-xiv.
53. Henry Steer, *The Smedleys of Matlock Bank* (London, E. Stock, 1897), 15-22.
54. Caroline Anne Smedley, *Ladies' Manual of Practical Hydropathy*, 12th edn (London, W. Kent, 1870).
55. Buckley (note 51), 7, 37-41.
56. Metcalfe (note 48), 164-71.
57. Archibald Hunter, *Hydropathy*, 3rd edn (Edinburgh, J. Menzies, 1887), 38-40.
58. Metcalfe (note 48), 84, 86.
59. Buckley (note 51), 41.
60. 'Hall, Spencer Timothy', *Dictionary of National Biography*.
61. Metcalfe (note 48), 115-16.
62. Claridge (note 47), 35, 87.
63. Smedley (note 52), iii-v; and *idem*, 14th edn (London, J. Blackwood, 1872), p. 4.
64. Smedley, (note 52), v.
65. Smedley, (note 63), 350.
66. *Lancet*, (1846), 666-7, 707-8; *The Times*, 22 June 1846, 7d.
67. James Wilson, *The Water Cure. Stomach Complaints and Drug Disease* (London, Churchill, 1843), 123; J.M. Gully, letter, *British Medical Journal*, 2 (1861), 543-4.
68. Thomas J. Graham, *The Best Methods of Improving Health and Invigorating Life*, 6th edn (London, Simpkin, Marshall, 1851), 368-95; Robert Hay Graham, *Graefenberg* (London, Longman, Brown, Green & Longmans, 1844), 90.
69. A. Courtney, *The Water Cure* (London, Gilpin, 1843), 25.
70. Edward Johnson, *The Domestic Practice of Hydropathy* (London, Simpkin, Marshall, 1851), viii, x-xi.
71. James Wilson, *The Water Cure. A Practical Treatise*, 2nd edn (London, Churchill, 1842), 17-18.
72. John Goodman, *Hydropathy or the Philosophy of Bathing* (London, Horsel, 1859), 149-53. See also *Water Cure Journal*, 30 (1850), 411-15, 446-52, 482-4.
73. Smedley, (note 52), 67-71.
74. Smedley, (note 63), 4.
75. Metcalfe (note 48), 57, 115-16.
76. *Nature Cure Annual* (1907-8), legend to photograph of Mrs A.S. Hunter.
77. See, for example, V. Stanley Davidson, *Nature Cure* (London, Thorsons, 1936), 27-42.
78. *Bristol Temperance Herald*, 7 (March 1843), 23.
79. E. Johnson, *The Philosophy of Temperance* (Oxford, 1837); Ralph Barnes Grindrod, *Bacchus* (London, J. Pasco, 1839); A. Courtney, *The Moderate Use of Intoxicating Drinks* (London, New British & Foreign Temperance Soc., 1840). See also N. Longmate, *The Waterdrinkers* (London, Hamish Hamilton, 1968), 61-2.
80. W.H. McMenemey, 'The Water Doctors of Malvern', *Proceedings of the Royal Society of Medicine*, 46 (1952), 5-12.
81. William Macleod, *The Treatment of Small Pox . . . by the Water Cure and Homoeopathy* (Manchester, W. Irwin, 1848), 1-2.
82. *Water Cure Journal*, 1 (1847-8), 211-12; W. Forbes Laurie, letter, *Journal of Health*, new series, 2 (1852), 210-11.
83. Smedley, (note 63), 7-8; Spencer T. Hall, *Homoeopathy and Hydropathy* (London, Leath & Ross, 1865), 1-6.
84. *Journal of Health*, 2 (1851), 1-6, 21-6, 41-2.
85. 'Hall', *Dictionary of National Biography*; W. Forbes Laurie, 'Electro-biology as a Curative Agent', *Journal of Health*, new series, 2 (1852), 251-6.
86. Anne Francis, *A Guinea a Box* (London, Hale, 1968); H.G. Lazell, *From Pills to Penicillin* (London, Heinemann, 1975).
87. P.S. Brown, 'Defining the Medical Profession in Mid-nineteenth Century Bristol', *Bristol Medico-Chirurgical Journal*, 96 (1981), 4-7.

88. Peter W.G. Wright, 'A Study in the legitimisation of Knowledge: The "Success" of Medicine and the "Failure" of Astrology', *Sociological Review*, monograph 27 (1979), 85-101.
89. Brown, 'The Vicissitudes of Herbalism' (note 42).
90. Terry M. Parssinen, 'Professional Deviants and the History of Medicine: Medical Mesmerists in Victorian Britain', *Sociological Review*, monograph 27 (1979), 103-20.
91. 'Doctors and Quacks', *Saturday Review*, 6 (1858), 30.
92. Brown, (note 42)
93. 'University College and Hospital,' *Lancet*, vol 1 (1839), 561-2.
94. Brown, (note 42).
95. Metcalfe (note 48), Preface.

12 MEDICAL SECTARIANISM, THERAPEUTIC CONFLICT, AND THE SHAPING OF ORTHODOX PROFESSIONAL IDENTITY IN ANTEBELLUM AMERICAN MEDICINE

John Harley Warner

In the historiography of orthodox-fringe conflict in American medicine, no proposition is more firmly entrenched than the notion that between about 1820 and the outbreak of the Civil War in 1861, the sectarian assault upon orthodox practices was among the principal propellants of the decline of heroic therapeutics. According to this model, Thomsonians, homoeopaths, eclectics, hydropaths and other sundry irregular healers denounced violent regular or orthodox therapies and offered alternative sources of medical care to the public. As the sectarian attack led to a popular outcry against heroic drugging, orthodox physicians made their therapies increasingly milder to render them less vulnerable to sectarian ridicule and more palatable to paying patients. At the same time, the apparent success of mild homoeopathic and hydropathic treatment convinced many orthodox physicians that perhaps their own patients' cures owed more to the healing power of nature than to medical art, seconding the move away from traditional heroic remedies. The sectarian challenge thereby encouraged regular practitioners to shed their more aggressive therapeutic ways.[1]

The actual influence of medical sectarianism on regular therapeutics, I want to suggest, was at once more complex and less unidirectional in its action. Regular therapies were not just instruments of medical practice; they were also concrete expressions of the physician's professional creed. Sectarianism did indeed encourage regular physicians to distance themselves from the more energetic excesses of past therapeutics. But simultaneously it gave rise to the conflicting impulse among regular practitioners to hold on all the tighter to the therapies that represented their own professional tradition. While sectarianism fostered therapeutic change, it also engendered a dogmatic adherence to tradition that made change difficult and at times professionally suspect.

The conservative influence of medical sectarianism that the case of therapeutics illustrates was, I propose in this paper, the leading force in the creation of medical orthodoxy in the United States. Only with the rise of sectarian strength from the 1820s did a self-conscious group awareness of being orthodox emerge among regular physicians. The divisions between regular and sectarian practitioners often remained blurred. Yet this ambiguity in the boundary lines delineating the fringe, which troubled regular physicians because of the very real threat posed to them by sectarian competition and criticism, made the self-perception of being orthodox important to physicians anxious to clarify their own professional place. Sectarians set up a socio-economic and intellectual environment that forced regular physicians to turn inwards to established tradition to find a stable core of professional definition and distinctiveness.

It is more than simply the clarity with which it displays the conservative influence of sectarianism that makes therapeutics an apt context in which to examine the process by which medical sectarianism formed orthodox professional identity. The imagery of medical therapy was central to this process. For both regular physicians and their sectarian competitors, therapy provided the most conspicuous hallmark of their own professional creed and stigmata of the misdirection of other medical belief systems. Accordingly, medical therapeutics was the pivot upon which orthodox-sectarian conflict in America turned. Vigorous sectarian assaults on such traditional therapies as bloodletting and calomel transformed them into potent symbols that regular physicians upheld as badges of their orthodoxy, and avowed allegiance to these symbols became the touchstone by which professional regularity was tested. In the United States, where legal distinctions among various species of medical practitioner were virtually abolished during the antebellum period, these therapeutic symbols were the chief device used to define orthodoxy, and institutional discriminations between regular and irregular practitioners all coalesced around them. The extent to which medical sectarianism moulded orthodox professional identity that this reveals, though not the pattern itself, may represent a peculiarly American relationship between medical orthodoxy and the medical fringe.

The Sectarian Challenge and the Definition of Orthodox Symbols

Before the early nineteenth century, medical sects did not exist in the United States, and not until the 1820s did sectarianism become an important factor in American medicine. To be sure, many healers practised at the fringes of the dominant medical tradition: root and herb doctors, Indian healers, bone-setters, nostrum-mongers, cancer doctors and spiritual curers offered the sick public a variety of alternatives to regular medical care. Yet these individual healers did not belong to sects which possessed some formal organisational structure and shared creed. Only in 1806, when Samuel Thomson began to market 'family rights' to his botanical system of domestic practice (patented in 1813), were some Americans recruited to a true medical sect. During the 1820s and 1830s Thomsonianism's following and strength grew markedly. Eclecticism — a parallel system of botanical healing in which professional medical practitioners supplanted the self-help care of the early Thomsonian plan — began to flourish in the 1840s and 1850s.[2] During the same two decades homoeopathy, first introduced to America in the mid-1820s, became the country's most prominent medical sect.[3] Hydropathy, or the water cure, the other major sect to emerge during the antebellum period, became well entrenched from the late 1840s.[4]

Medical sectarianism was far from monolithic. In social origin, education, distribution, economic standing and constituency, there was vast diversity among different categories of sectarian practitioners. Especially during homoeopathy's early decades in America, many of its practitioners held MD degrees from regular medical schools, and before their conversion some had ranked among the regular medical elite. In some locales, homoeopaths occupied a higher socio-economic position and served a more affluent clientele than their regular counterparts.[5] By and large, homoeopaths were most common in the urban centres of the northeast. In contrast, Thomsonians and later botanical sectarians infrequently held regular medical degrees, were prevalent chiefly in the more rural south and west, and served a less affluent patient population. Further, the beliefs and practices of various sectarian groups were widely divergent, and members of different sects often assailed each other's systems. Botanics commonly ridiculed the homoeopathic theory of infinitesimals, while hydropaths roundly condemned the bold use of potent plant drugs by eclectics.[6] Therefore, sectarians cannot be typified as a group on the basis of either their medical theories or socio-economic characteristics.

Nor can they be characterised by any shared posture towards professionalism. True, assaults upon medical monopoly were common in the rhetoric of all sects. These were most vehement in Thomsonian writings, where they were sustained by the populist political ideology of the Jacksonian era and the impulse to democratise all knowledge and institutions. Early Thomsonians urged the abolition of the authority of doctor, lawyer and clergyman alike. But most sectarians were not driven by any animus against professionalism and directed anti-monopolistic rhetoric only against regular power and privilege. Indeed, eclectic and homoeopathic practitioners never doubted that they were members of 'the medical profession' (though regulars denied it), and claimed only the added distinction of having moved beyond regular bondage to tradition.[7]

What all sectarians did share was the proclaimed objective of overturning medical orthodoxy. It was their common goal of destroying the established medical order that gave them definition as a group. William Henry Holcombe, for example, a prominent homoeopathic practitioner and editor, was typical in his repeated calls for the rupture of medical orthodoxy, which homoeopaths also called allopathy. In his mind, his dual commitment to homoeopathy and Swedenborgianism forged the link between his opposition to medical and religious orthodoxy. The structures that sustained these orthodoxies, he maintained, had to be torn down before the new order could be erected: 'As it is impossible for the old bottles to contain our *new wine*, I strongly recommend the immediate demolition of all Orthodox Theological Schools and all apothecary Shops,' he wrote in his diary.[8] The changes Holcombe desired could not come about within existing orthodox frameworks. 'I felt how useless it is to argue with any body whose whole life has been given to the contemplation and defense of certain dogmas,' he complained one day in 1855 after reading a regular medical journal. 'The present race of Old Church theologians and of Allopathic doctors has to *die out* before the good seed can spring up on the place of those weeds in the garden of the world.'[9]

The desire of physicians like Holcombe to overthrow orthodoxy — their inbuilt urge to dissent — was unambiguous, but what delineated orthodoxy in their minds was not so clear. Defining medical orthodoxy was not always a simple task for sectarians who wished to assail it. In England, as elsewhere in Europe, regular physicians were distinguishable by their legislated status, by licensing and legal sanctions that granted them special privileges and set them apart as a readily defined group. But in the United States, especially after the collapse of licensing laws starting in the 1830s, no legal distinction discriminated between the orthodox physician and the sectarian. Medical practice was open equally to all comers, and the individual practitioner's identification as regular or sectarian was largely a matter of personal choice. Professional identity derived above all from practice, not official decree, and therefore any intuitively persuasive criterion for judging orthodoxy had to derive in the first instance from medical practice itself.[10]

It was in the context of this situation that in sectarian rhetoric, certain therapies identified with regular practice became the most powerful, widely recognised signs of the orthodox medical profession. Regular therapeutic practice in the early nineteenth century was characterised by its heroic use of depletive treatments. Physicians believed that in most diseased conditions the body was morbidly over-stimulated; therapy, therefore, sought to lower the patient's system down to a healthy balance by draining off excessive vital energy. Commonly, this was accomplished by bloodletting (leeching, wet cupping, or using a lancet to venesect) and by administering purgatives, the most drastic of which included mineral drugs such as the mercurial cathartic calomel and the antimony-containing tartar emetic. Orthodox physicians extensively used these therapies, but by no means employed them by rote. Nevertheless, bloodletting and purgative mineral drugs became the distinctive emblems of regular practice.[11]

Sectarian iconography of the orthodox physician centred upon aggressive drugging, and especially the use of these key therapies. Typically, a Virginia planter who had become a convert to Thomsonianism used the term 'old time MD' interchangeably with 'Calomel Doctor' in his diary, clearly reflecting the identification of regular physicians with their drugs.[12] This imagery was pervasive in sectarian medical journals, where regular practitioners were portrayed as 'Mineral Doctors', 'Mineralites', 'the poison depletive quacks', 'Mercury dosers', 'drug doctors', and 'the knights of calomel and the lancet'. Orthodox medicine, in turn, was styled 'the drugging system', 'the calomel and blue pill school of medicine', 'the Bleeding, Mineral, Reducing System', and 'the mineral, humbuggery practice'.[13] Visual representations of orthodox physicians depicted them brandishing oversized lancets in bellicose poses, pressing poisonous pills on an innocent public, or mindlessly preparing drugs.

The use of heroic therapies as symbols by which to identify orthodox medicine aided the sectarian campaign against the regular profession. Sectarian practitioners targeted regular therapy as the system's worst evil, and identified orthodox physicians with their therapies only in order to denounce them both. Professors in sectarian schools routinely illustrated their lectures by cases 'treated by the murderous systems' of orthodox medicine,[14] while sectarian editors gave over a large proportion of the space in their journals to displaying the dire consequences of regular drugging.[15] A term such as 'calomel doctor' not only identified the orthodox physician, but also derided his practice as dangerous to the people's health. Sectarians were free to assail regular practice as murderous without in any way indicting their own treatments. 'The essential difference,' one homoeopath noted, 'between the old and new school, consists in an entire rejection by the latter, of the materia medica, and therapeutics of the former.'[16] Bloodletting and large doses of mineral drugs had been virtually banished from sectarian practice: botanics substituted sometimes equally aggressive plant remedies; homoeopaths employed only very minute doses of any drug; and hydropaths replaced all such treatments with the creative use of water.

The sectarian attack upon regular therapy was given real force by the socio-economic realities of medical practice in antebellum America. A surplus of practitioners meant that for many physicians it was enormously difficult to earn a living practising medicine.[17] A young physician who in 1831 had just put up a sign for his new office in New Orleans wrote to his brother than 'one of the old Doctors died off [and] 14 new ones arrived to divide the spoils, and those of the most ravenous kinds, but I will try to keep my spirits up and do my best'. He consoled himself with the prospect that 'the John Fever [a corruption of *jaune*, or yellow, fever] must kill or frighten some of them'.[18] Within the year he had given up on New Orleans, but continued to complain about the overabundance of physicians in Maryland, where he again attempted to set up practice. 'If the town should increase [in population],' he wrote, 'they will be as thick here as hail. The country around is swarming with them.'[19] Even a busy practice was no guarantee of earning a living. A physician in search of a place to settle wrote home that the citizens of one prospective location 'told me in May that if I went there I could get as much practice as I wanted, but they told me at the same time that I would have to wait for my pay for at least one or two years'.[20]

Competition from sectarian practitioners compounded the problem, for orthodox physicians routinely expected the arrival of a new species of sectarian healer in their neighbourhood to diminish their own practices. 'The competition now prevailing in medicine,' an Ohio physician explained in 1851, 'has been brought to a very [high] pitch . . . [It] is certain that even the longest established and most estimable physicians have yielded large and lucrative portions of their practice to homoeopathy &c.'[21] A recent medical school graduate who was trying to establish practice in Mississippi wrote home to his wife that 'the steam doctors [that is, Thomsonians] . . . will likely interfere with me. One has located within a mile and will get a part of the practice, as it is a new thing here and some are in favor of the system.' He noted with satisfaction, however, that the recent execution by hanging of men plotting a slave uprising had somewhat reduced the competition. 'Five or six white men and about twenty negroes have been executed,' he wrote. 'Among these were two celebrated steam doctors, whose medicines were found to avail nothing against hemp.'[22]

This intense competition for patients made regular practitioners acutely sensitive to public opinion. The explicit objective of widely publicised sectarian charges that physicians poisoned their patients with heroic doses of such drugs as mercury was to undermine public confidence in the orthodox profession. 'We shall . . . exert ourselves, to the extent of our ability, to destroy the confidence of the community in their detestable practice,' the editors of the *Boston True Thomsonian* pledged in 1841;[23] echoing this statement a decade later, the editor of the *American Journal of Homoeopathy* explained that 'the public good demands, that we should . . . exhibit to the public the evil of a system of medicine which is destroying the health of our citizens, and filling thousands of graves prematurely'.[24] 'Popular prejudice' in the realm of treatment became a common euphemism for the threat of sectarian competition. A patient dissatisfied with the treatment his physician offered could turn to another regular physician, to one of a variety of sectarian healers, or to any number of self-help medical systems. Sectarian charges that bleeding and mineral drugs ruined patients not only struck at orthodox physicians' tradition but also threatened their very livelihoods.

The Institutionalization of Orthodox Identity

Medical orthodoxy in the United States was created with the rise of sectarianism. Prior to the emergence of medical sects, a broad spectrum of practitioners — diverse in social background and intellectual attainment — shared the self-perception of being legitimate, regularly educated practitioners. They seldom questioned each other's regularity. Physicians educated in one of the handful of American medical schools, or trained in European centres such as Edinburgh, acknowledged that the worst apprenticeship-trained practitioner might still be a physician, regular — however regrettable. Certainly, many practitioners disparaged signs of inadequate knowledge or idiosyncratic ways among their fellows. And some physicians established organisations such as the Massachusetts Medical Society to distinguish themselves as members of a well-educated elite. But those groups of physicians who sought to separate themselves from other practitioners did so by and large because they saw the latter as ignorant, not heterodox or heretical. Orthodoxy was not the issue.[25]

As sectarian attacks upon regular medicine mounted after the 1820s, however, those physicians who continued to identify with the dominant medical ways were compelled to reflect upon their relationship to those who were assailing them. The rise of medical sectarianism heightened regular practitioners' awareness of their group identity and its rooting in allegiance to a shared tradition. At the same time, those who chose to bind themselves to established tradition self-consciously began to consider who among their brethren shared their beliefs and who dissented from them, a distinction that could not be reduced to education or skill alone. For the first time in American medicine, heresy — not just ignorance — became a crucial professional issue. With the strengthening concept of orthodoxy, regular physicians looked for ways of setting themselves apart from heterodox healers and purifying their own ranks.

It seemed increasingly unlikely that orthodox physicians could draw upon any legal distinction to separate themselves from other medical practitioners. Repeal of medical licensing laws by the individual state legislatures, from the 1830s onwards, exaggerated the openness of American practice and exemplified growing sectarian power. Licensing had never been more than honorific, granting minor legal privileges such as the right to sue for fees in court, and did not prevent anyone who wished from practising medicine. But it had provided one institutional distinction by which medical societies, which ordinarily held licensing power, could distinguish between the quack and the trained practitioner. Thomsonian assaults upon this invidious legal favouritism for the regular medical belief system precipitated the downfall of medical licensing and the abolition of legal distinctions among practitioners.[26]

Growing awareness of orthodox identity after the 1820s was expressed most visibly by the proliferation of explicitly orthodox medical institutions. Local and state medical societies multiplied and in 1847 the national American Medical Association was formed, in part to distance regulars from sectarians. The number of regular medical schools trebled between 1820 and 1850, and the socialisation students received in these institutions forcefully impressed upon them their participation in orthodox tradition. Orthodox medical journals, which rapidly multiplied, also served as a forum for denouncing sectarian ways and consolidating orthodox identity.[27]

By the 1840s and 1850s such institutions in principle rigidly upheld orthodoxy by enforcing an official policy of discrimination against irregular practitioners. Sectarians were barred from regular medical societies and thereby denied access to one source of professional distinction, knowledge and business. Further, the code of ethics to which society members pledged themselves forbade regulars from consulting with sectarian practitioners, and some members who violated this stipulation were charged with unethical conduct and expelled.[28] The medical practices employed by the individual physician, not his training or knowledge, constituted the most common criterion by which regular societies assessed his orthodox or sectarian status.

Similarly, to ostracise sectarians, regular medical schools closed their doors to unorthodox practitioners who sought an MD degree; revoked the diplomas of alumni who took up sectarian ways; expelled students who associated with sectarians or themselves practised sectarian medicine between terms; and refused to allow students who had been apprenticed with sectarian practitioners to attend lectures or become degree candidates. In 1845, for example, a Dr Carter, who had graduated from the orthodox Medical College of Ohio, returned to that school to refresh his knowledge by attending lectures. But the faculty discovered that since his graduation Carter had advertised himself as an eclectic or botanic physician. When confronted, Carter confessed 'that he put [up] a sign as "Botanical Doctor" to be enabled to get those who preferred that kind of practice & he confessed that he was a Botanical physician'. The faculty resolved that Carter had 'deserted the profession and renounced his Diploma', barred him from the school, and returned his matriculation fee.[29] In a like fashion, the faculty of the Medical College of the State of South Carolina refused to consider one student as a candidate for graduation when they learned that his father, with whom he had apprenticed, had converted to homoeopathy. The fact that the student had attended lectures, and that the father held an MD degree from that same orthodox school, did not alter their decision.[30]

In their day-to-day management of affairs, however, regular and unorthodox practitioners were much less rigidly partitioned. Sectarians often accused orthodox physicians of using irregular therapies without giving them credit: 'many of them', one botanic complained in 1842, 'compelled by public opinion, are pursuing a mixed practice, half regular and half Thomsonian'.[31] Orthodox practitioners, for their part, routinely charged that some sectarians prescribed regular remedies; 'the clever rogues among the homeopathists take good care to give active doses of medicine, under cover of their infinitesimal humbug'.[32] Moreover, some regulars did not rigorously denounce sectarian remedies, and at times even endorsed them. A regularly trained South Carolina physician studying in Paris wrote to his father than in his mother's illness, 'the employment of the *homeopathist* is a very good idea; and one which will be the most likely to succeed'.[33]

More troubling still to the upholders of orthodoxy was the suspicion that homoeopaths sometimes presented themselves as orthodox practitioners, and that many regular physicians were complacent about this subterfuge. James Otis Moore, for example, a Maine homoeopath practising in the Union Army during the Civil War, represented himself as a regular physician in order to secure the post of surgeon. When a regular medical colleague learned of Moore's homoeopathic background from a mutual acquaintance from Maine, he did not report the deception and merely told Moore, 'I care nothing about it of course, as long as you do your duty as well as you have done it.'[34] Belying any implied rapport between the two medical orientations, however, Moore's letters to his wife expressed his growing horror at the harm done by orthodox treatment.

Many orthodox physicians were more tolerant of social and professional interaction with sectarians than the official policy of discrimination dictated. The young John Leonard Riddell was by no means unique in having both orthodox and sectarian medical friends, though his tactic of playing the prejudices of each group against the other — criticising either the regulars or the eclectics, depending upon with which group he was communicating — may have been more unusual.[35] Social intercourse between regulars and irregulars was not the rule, but neither was it rare. Even some unimpeachably regular physicians occasionally had professional associations with homoeopaths. When James Jackson, Sr, was asked to consult with a Salem homoeopath in 1857, for example, he did not balk at the idea of consulting with an irregular practitioner but only wanted to be sure that the homoeopath was an honourable gentleman. In a letter boldly marked '*Private*', Jackson, a Harvard medical professor and the acknowledged elder of the medical profession in New England, asked a Salem friend for more information. 'I know Dr. G[ersdoff] to be a Homoeopath, or Semi-Homoeopath. I wish to know whether there is any objection to his character', Jackson wrote. 'My rule', he explained, 'has always been to meet Homoeopaths, as I have other M.D.'s whose practice I disapproved, provided they would adopt my plans.'[36]

The Ideology of Orthodoxy

The expression of orthodoxy in the profession's cognitive structures was even more thoroughgoing, though less obvious, than in its social structures. It was precisely because the institutional and behavioral boundaries distinguishing between regular medicine and the fringe in America remained blurred that clearly objectifying the concept of orthodoxy in regular medical thought became so important. Key symbols standing for the orthodox faith became rigidly established among regular physicians, and the idea of orthodoxy that a proclaimed commitment to these symbols represented became far sharper than the reality of distinctions among medical practitioners ever was. The sectarian onslaught tended to make those who saw themselves as defenders of regular medicine think in terms of an absolute dichotomy between heterodoxy and its opposite, and demand that other practitioners declare their allegiance to one side or the other. Sectarianism unmistakably shaped regular physicians' thought and practice in ways that defined and fortified the concept of orthodoxy.[37]

Nevertheless, most historical attention to the relationship between medical orthodoxy and the medical fringe in America has stressed how sectarianism compelled regular physicians to shed traditional ways and bring their practice into line with the sectarian example. This has been argued hardest in explaining the transformation of therapeutics. During the past two decades, historians have become dissatisfied with earlier explanations for therapeutic change that focused narrowly on progress in medical science. Instead, they have sought sources of change outside of the regular medical profession and identified the power of alternative healers and the public as crucial. According to this newer explanation, the example of sectarian success in practice showed regular practitioners that cure could often be effected with very mild therapeutic intervention. More important, the sectarian assault upon orthodox therapy incited patient resistance to heroic therapeutics, and in a competitive market this compelled regular physicians to renounce their traditional mainstays. What limits this perspective is that it tends to see sectarianism (as an earlier view saw science) as the revealer of a therapeutic truth that inevitably discredited regular therapies and ordained their rejection. Deterministic models of therapeutic change, whether centred upon high-culture knowledge or marketplace forces, are simplistic.

There can be no doubt that sectarianism led regular physicians as a group to diminish their use of aggressive depletive therapies. Homoeopathy's example in particular generated one forceful impulse to regular therapeutic change. Many regular physicians acknowledged that the recovery of patients under homoeopathic care was impressive, although this did not indicate to them that homoeopathy ever actively cured patients. In their view, prescribing the infinitesimal doses of homoeopathy was physiologically tantamount to doing nothing. 'Homeopathy, is another beautiful system of refined nonsense . . . But from it we may be taught several important lessons,' one regular physician urged in the early 1850s. Homoeopathy 'teaches us the important truth, that the great majority of the complaints of mankind, do not necessarily endanger life and may get well under almost any plan of treatment, or if you will, without any course of treatment at all'.[38] Thus, homoeopathic successes urged regular physicians to recognise the tendency of most cases to satisfactory resolution without heroic intervention, and encouraged therapeutic moderation. 'There is good in everything', an orthodox practitioner asserted, 'and if Homeopathy with all of its fallacies has opened the eyes of all or at least of many to the evils of drugging patients, it has been of service.'[39]

Public resistance to heroic drugging and demand for milder treatment, which sectarian polemics informed, was clearly also one engine of regular therapeutic change. 'Not only have the regulars lost most of their practice', one botanic practitioner gloated in 1839 about the influence of his sect on patients' opinions, 'but the few patients they have retained, are so much aroused to a sense of danger of regular quackery, that their first salutation to the old family doctor is, "Doctor, you must not bleed me, I can't take calomel, opium is a poison, I won't have a blister on me, I don't believe they do any good," &c. &c. Poor Doctor, what can he do?'[40] This botanic practitioner was overly sanguine about public opposition to orthodox remedies; yet regular physicians noted it as well. Typically an Alabama physician observed that regular practitioners had begun to look at such remedies as mercury 'through glasses, adapted to the *focus* of popular prejudice'.[41] After recording the case history of a patient who had just died, an Ohio physician complained in his diary in 1836, 'This patient was strongly opposed to the use of the lancet & calomel', and therefore 'the former was not used at all & the latter in too small quantities to do good or hurt'.[42]

Yet patient-generated demand is more problematic as a factor in regular therapeutic change than is suggested by a simple model that identifies it as the vehicle for sectarian influence. Certainly, extreme competition for paying patients did make regular physicians malleable to the therapeutic inclinations of those whom they treated. However, sectarian success in changing the American public's assessment of traditional heroic therapies should not be over-estimated. Regular physicians frequently complained that public insistence on traditional treatments was a leading impediment to therapeutic change. In the case record books of American hospitals from the antebellum decades, instances of patients' requests for heroic therapies far outnumbered instances of resistance to them.[43] 'The people love strong measures in the management of the sick,' one practitioner put it simply.[44] Physicians argued that their efforts to move away from massive doses of cathartics and emetics, for example, often were blocked by 'this "morbid public taste, this voracious appetite for medicine" '.[45] 'How often', one physician asked, was the young practitioner 'forced by patients and their friends to give medicine when it is not plainly indicated, when he would gladly watch and await the efforts of nature? This privilege is denied him; he must cure *quickly*, or *give place to a rival*.'[46] A physician practising with his father recorded in his diary that, one Sunday in 1842, they were summoned in haste to attend a young boy who had been thrown from a horse. 'The parents', he wrote, 'were very desirous that he should be bled — The coldness of the skin — the feebleness of the pulse & respiration &c all contraindicated the use of the lancet but in order to satisfy the minds of the parents the median cephalic vein was opened & blood to a very small quantity was permitted to flow — But this little amount seemed too much — for he seemed to sink.'[47] Patients' demands, in other words, may have hampered a move from heroic therapeutics as much as it encouraged it.

The reigning historiographic emphasis on how sectarianism forced regular practitioners away from therapeutic tradition does more than just over-simplify a complex relationship. It also ignores the extent to which medical sectarianism operated as a powerfully conservative force on regular medicine. Sectarianism set up a socio-economic context for medical practice that urged regular physicians firmly and persistently to reaffirm their regularity. It drove them hard back to medical tradition in search of the enduring features of their practice that could help them understand and define orthodoxy and for a secure platform from which they could proclaim their own identity. Medical sectarianism thus fostered not only regular stability, but also reaction — and was the critical element in transforming regular physicians' confidence in their heritage into a rigid ideology of orthodoxy. Put simply, sectarianism made the regular profession think and behave like a sect.

The principal symbols of orthodox tradition to which regular physicians turned were heroic depletive therapies, especially bloodletting and calomel. The identification of these treatments with regular physicians, and their function as emblems of the profession, were by no means new; but between the 1820s and the 1850s their standing as symbols of orthodox medicine became stronger and more rigid. Regular physicians praised their worth with unprecedented vigour, and avowed belief in their value became the central touchstone of orthodoxy. Reaffirming allegiance to traditional therapies offered regular physicians a vehicle for dramatising their distinctiveness from sectarians that did not depend on such unsure methods as pointing to educational differences, seeking legal sanctions, and preserving institutional purity. It was these therapeutic symbols, more than any other nucleus, about which the concept of orthodoxy crystallised.

The stridency with which regular physicians defended these therapies in spite of their sharply declining use in actual practice during the antebellum period underscores the symbolic role they had assumed. At the same time that regular physicians employed bloodletting and calomel more and more infrequently at the bedside, the symbolic importance of these practices was elevated. Indeed, the profession of faith in these therapies became loudest at mid-century when the eclipse of heroic depletive therapy from regular practice appeared a real possibility. The members of the St Louis Medical Society concurred in a discussion of bloodletting in 1859 that the lancet was only very rarely used; yet the secretary could record that 'we find none opposing blood-letting, and ... we must conclude, that the lancet holds the same place as a remedial measure, among well educated medical men, that it ever did'.[48] It was to the value of these therapies in *principle*, not so much in *practice*, that orthodox physicians pledged their faith.[49]

In selecting badges of orthodoxy, it is ironic that regular physicians elected to take up the same symbols sectarians had fixed upon to identify old-school medicine. In one sense it was of course an obvious choice, as all of the competing groups of medical practitioners in nineteenth-century America used their therapies as the most lucid sign of their professional distinctiveness. Further, by asserting that bloodletting and calomel were valuable treatments, regular physicians were defending their goods against the slanders of their competitors in a buyer's market. But more than this, the very fact that non-believers so violently assailed these signs of orthodox faith gave the avowals of belief in them made by regular physicians added meaning. Sectarian assaults upon bloodletting and calomel sharpened and empowered their utility to regulars as symbols. With the ascendancy of sectarianism, a statement endorsing these therapies could no longer be professionally neutral. It bespoke a commitment to orthodox ways and confirmed orthodox identity.

As a professional credo, the assertion of the value of bloodletting or calomel was also reassuring to regular practitioners. From the 1820s through mid-century, regular physicians shared with members of all professions in the United States a perception of decline in power and position. 'Our own profession, what with its ignorance, its heresies, and its moral sense, has lost the respect of the community and sunk to the level of a trade less honest & less useful than that of the rudest mechanic,' one prominent Philadelphia physician lamented in 1857, in a letter to a Boston colleague. 'Alas! it should be so when every year is adding to the learning & science, & skill of our leading men & those around them.'[50] As mounting sectarian assaults aggravated the sense of professional instability, there was comfort in a ritual affirmation of belief in the mainstays of traditional therapeutics, which pointed to the sturdy links binding the regular practitioner to two millennia of medical thought and practice. Clinging tightly to these symbols of orthodoxy was one means of preserving confidence and order at a time of severe professional dislocation.

The Spectre of Heresy and the Conservative Influence of Sectarianism

The conservative influence exerted by sectarianism pervaded regular medical thought. But because therapies assumed such a powerful role as symbols of orthodoxy, this influence can be seen with exceptional clarity in regular therapeutic discussion. Expressions of therapeutic doubt were often checked by the fear that they would be interpreted as lapses in orthodox belief. After all, when the accusation of heresy was brought against a physician, it was almost always grounded upon a charge of therapeutic unorthodoxy. Openly questioning the worth of established therapies invited attack from other members of a profession very much on the lookout for signs of heterodoxy within its ranks.[51]

Regular physicians were preoccupied with maintaining an appearance of therapeutic unity. Dissension, they feared, would be exploited by sectarians in pillorying orthodox practice before the public. To avoid this, medical societies stipulated in their codes of ethics that therapeutic disagreements arising in consultation, for example, were to be discussed and resolved without allowing the public to become aware of professional disharmony. 'Neither the subject matter of such differences nor the adjudications of the arbitrators should be made public as publicity in a case of this nature may be personally injurious to the individuals concerned and can hardly fail to bring discredit on the faculty,' the Committee on Ethics of one medical society insisted.[52] An underlying fear was that confrontation between regular physicians in consultation could drive patients to sectarians. 'If censure is cast upon a former attendant, the conclusion on the part of the patient is, that he had been shamefully maltreated', a Cincinnati physician observed, 'and, perhaps, instead of acquiring confidence in the kind censor, he too becomes a subject of distrust, and the *finale* is, that an unblushing empiric, who loudly condemns all physicians, supercedes the regular practitioner.'[53]

Yet it was not just in the public forum that sectarianism made regulars reluctant to voice therapeutic criticism. It is easy to see — though difficult to show — that the atmosphere sectarianism created forcefully suppressed therapeutic self-criticism within regular professional circles as well. This can be clearly displayed, however, by the reaction of regular physicians to those among them who did point out the shortcomings of orthodox practice.

The most distinguishable group of regular physicians who questioned the therapeutic power of the orthodox armamentarium during the antebellum period was made up of those who emphasised the healing power of nature. Especially from the 1830s, some practitioners began to argue that often nature more than medical art was responsible for curing the sick. Encouraged by contemporary movements in French medical philosophy, the nature-trusters were also reacting against the excessive bleeding and purging of early-nineteenth-century heroic practice. Physicians' power actively to break up disease by therapeutic intervention was considerably less than the profession generally believed, they proposed, for nature deserved much of the credit conventionally ascribed to art. These physicians did not reject traditional therapies in principle or practice; but they did suggest that perhaps these treatments did more harm and less good than was usually assumed.[54]

Debate over the relative merits of art and nature in dispelling disease was hardly new in the nineteenth century. Critics of nature's American devotees during the antebellum period were merely repeating longstanding objections when they charged that the physician's excessive faith in nature endangered the patient. A reliance on nature 'blinds the physician to the true action of therapeutical agents, and destroys his patient', one South Carolina practitioner argued in 1851.[55] The physician who carried his doubts about the power of medical art with him into the sickroom would be poorly prepared for the prompt and bold action required of the successful therapeutist. 'Salutory and rational effort may be paralyzed by medical scepticism', another physician warned, and the practical utility of medical art would thereby be diminished.[56] It was imperative that the practitioner at least make an effort to interrupt the course of a disease. As an Ohio physician asserted, 'I do not believe it is our duty to stand by and do nothing: we ought to study every disease, and interfere.'[57]

But from the early 1830s onwards, as sectarian power became increasingly menacing, the concerns voiced by those critical of a dependence upon nature expanded. Added to the objection that nature-trusting enfeebled the physician's ability to cure was the much more vehement charge that it could represent betrayal of the orthodox profession.

Practitioners who emphasised nature's power were derisively termed therapeutic sceptics to highlight their lapse of confidence in not only orthodox therapy, but also in the orthodox profession. Sceptics were branded with 'infidelity to the healing art'.[58] Excessive faith in nature, critics charged, was tantamount to a loss of faith in art, which violated the physician's profession of his ability to heal, 'which', in the assessment of one practitioner, 'virtually proclaims the existing medical profession worse than useless'.[59] Further, it indicted the practices of physicians who retained their confidence in drugs and used them aggressively. Nature-trusting, according to one critic, held that all medicine was 'absurd in itself and dangerous to the patient', and 'convicts all those upon whom this marvelous revelation has not fallen, of stultification and criminality at every step of their professional career'.[60]

In the eyes of his assailants, the sceptic's loss of confidence would in turn dissipate that of the public. 'Skepticism and distrust', a Boston physician argued, '[are] inconsistent with proper activity and perseverence in the use of means of cure. Surely faith and confidence are essential to the successful prosecution of our art, and we cannot inspire our patients with what we have not ourselves.'[61] A New York physician who wrote in 1859 to vindicate 'the character and honor of the profession', expressed the opinion of many physicians when he charged that the notion 'that all the physician does is to amuse the patient whilst nature cures the disease' was 'a labored effort to destroy public confidence in the medical profession'.[62] The physician who doubted his own effectiveness could not expect to instil the confidence in his patients that was required for the cure of disease.

The most insidious implication of the belief that nature healed, in the perception of critics, was that the physician became superfluous; his professional role was annulled. If the profession were to take up the faith of nature, one physician asserted, then 'it is time to abandon the practice of medicine to homoeopaths and old women'.[63] A Philadelphia medical professor commented on the idea that the course of disease could not be curtailed by art, 'Could I believe this opinion to be correct, I would at once without hesitation strike the flag of my profession, and cease to pilfer a generous public of their money by such a fraud and impostance.'[64] By implication, those practitioners who did persist in seeing patients while at the same time extolling nature were behaving unethically.

Many critics maintained that the rising emphasis on nature's role in healing was an injudicious response to sectarian therapeutics, and especially to homoeopathic infinitesimals. One version of this argument held that some physicians were capitulating to sectarian rhetoric that denounced regular drugging to the public. Such physicians were guilty of giving in to ill-informed public demand in order to make themselves more competitive, and thereby of responding to an illegitimate source of therapeutic change. Another version began with the premiss — widely shared among regular physicians — that homoeopathic treatment was physiologically equivalent to therapeutic abstinence, and therefore to relying entirely on nature. Some physicians, this argument continued, believed that clinical statistics purportedly showing homoeopathic successes both illustrated nature's power and suggested that regulars had been attributing to art much that was in fact due to nature. Critics scoffed at the reliability of homoeopathic statistics and denounced regular physicians who pointed to homoeopathic recoveries, even if they gave nature rather than Samuel Hahnemann (homoeopathy's founder) credit for the cure. 'Absurdity and heresy can go no farther', one Cincinnati practitioner declared.[65]

The link between sectarianism and an allegiance to nature had another, more threatening, dimension. Whether or not the emphasis some regular physicians placed on the healing power of nature was actually caused by the homoeopathic example and propaganda, many practitioners believed that it would inevitably be taken by sectarians as an endorsement of their systems. And indeed, the use sectarians made of statements by regular practitioners extolling nature fully justified this concern.[66] Sceptics, one orthodox Nashville physician typically commented, were 'of considerable value in exercising some check upon the "overdosing" we are too apt to fall into; but again deplorable in their too often giving a handle to quackery, and supplying hydropaths, homoeopaths, and others with theories and facts, which they do not fail to turn to their own advantage'.[67] Regarded in this way, scepticism directly harmed the regular profession by endorsing its enemies.

It is significant that religious metaphor was among the most common vehicles for criticism of *scepticism*. Nineteenth-century American physicians were well aware of that term's theological resonance, and exploited it in their rhetoric. Sceptics were guilty of the sin of disbelief in the efficacy of medical art and of proclaiming their new faith in nature. 'The worshippers of this faith look upon drugs as meddlesome, if not profane interferences, downright polypharmacy and "damnable heresy",' one practitioner charged.[68] Although it was the 'sceptic' Oliver Wendell Holmes, an eminent regular physician, who coined the phrase 'nature-trusting heresy' to describe the therapeutic movement in which he was participating, the term *heresy* used without his jocularity was frequently employed to stigmatise the position he defended.[69] The nature-truster's apostasy threatened to corrupt not only his individual standing, but also that of the professional community. By renouncing his profession of faith in the redemptive power of medical art, the sceptic weakened the collective faith and confidence of orthodox physicians.

Those regular American physicians who were committed to the healing power of nature and who expressed their scepticism about the extent to which traditional therapies healed the sick, typically shared several characteristics — above all, security. These physicians tended to belong to both medical and social elites. They were among the best-educated practitioners in the country, and often had experience in the hospitals of Europe. They occupied leading positions in regular medical institutions as professors at medical schools, physicians to hospitals, and officers in societies. And often they were known for their medical publications. They possessed, in other words, all of the outward signs of professional grace that were available in American society. Further, they tended to reside in older cities where patterns of deference were long established. Their own esteem often came from family and community ties as much as from their role as physicians. Even though they tended to see themselves as among the leadership of the regular medical profession, individually they were less vulnerable than the vast majority of their brethren to sectarian attacks and competition, and were thus less preoccupied with the maintenance of orthodox purity.[70]

No one among regular physicians doubted that the most vocal nature-trusters had all the trappings of professional eminence. Yet to some of their colleagues, they were doubtfully orthodox. What was in question was the firmness of their allegiance to the therapies that had become the symbols of orthodoxy, and thereby their orthodox standing. The vehement criticism brought against sceptics for their putative lapse of faith illustrates the measure of pressure weighing upon all practitioners who had chosen to identify with orthodoxy to conform to tradition and curb any doubts about it they might have. If prominent, secure physicians could withstand such attacks, ordinary practitioners — more marginal economically and socially — could ill-afford to arouse their colleagues' ire. Sectarianism set up fidelity to the symbols of regular tradition as the cardinal test of orthodoxy, and the link thus forged between intellectual conservatism and professional respectability hobbled the minds and utterances of regular American physicians.

American Fringe and American Orthodoxy

There was nothing peculiarly American about the fact that medical sectarianism exerted a conservative — not just change-inducing — effect on the regular profession. Sectarian-orthodox interactions were intrinsically polarising, and encouraged those who saw themselves as orthodox to celebrate their own tradition all the more fervently. In large measure, heterodox sects and orthodoxy were defined in terms of their opposites, and therefore mounting sectarian power heightened regular physicians' self-consciousness of their orthodoxy and what it meant. To this extent, the considerable strength medical sects attained in early- and mid-nineteenth-century America may simply have generated, in exaggerated form, a polarisation at work whenever established and alternative groups both claim the possession of incommensurate truths.

Medical sectarianism may have had a special relationship to the shaping of orthodox professional identity in the American context, however. In contrast to England, for example, in America the available institutional, social and legal structures failed to provide a framework capable of defining and supporting medical professional identity. Instead, professional identity derived chiefly from practice. The *qualified* practitioner in England was a man duly examined and licensed by one of several legally chartered bodies. In America, on the other hand, the physician established himself as *qualified* in an open market only by winning the confidence of patients and his fellows in his practice. For regular and irregular physicians alike, professional identity and esteem ultimately rested not upon sanctions given by formal education, licensing, or society membership, but upon practice.

This singular dependency of American physicians on practice for their professional definition was the chief reason why the sectarian attack on regular practice — made more troubling by the severe competition for patients — was so strong a force in moulding orthodox professional identity. Sectarianism encouraged regular physicians to think in terms of orthodoxy; set up symbols by which faith in orthodoxy could be proved; and largely contributed to the instability in regular practice and image that made orthodox solidarity matter. In the absence of legal distinctions to define orthodoxy, the use of therapies as symbolic ones may also have been especially compelling in America. Certainly, treatments like bloodletting and calomel became symbols of the orthodox profession and were actively exploited in the rhetoric of medical politics elsewhere as well. But in a society committed to egalitarianism, in which artificial, legislated discriminations among practitioners were regarded as dubiously legitimate (indeed, unAmerican), the symbols of medical orthodoxy derived from practice were particularly powerful and useful. The values and realities of an egalitarian society sharpened the significance of symbols that were recognisable to practitioners and the public alike, but not at odds with an aggressively democratic ethos. In the process of defending their practices and the tradition in which they were rooted against sectarian assaults, regular physicians also articulated an ideology of orthodox professional identity.

Notes

This essay was supported in part by National Institutes of Health Grant LM 03910, from the National Library of Medicine; a research award from an Arthur Vining Davis Foundation grant to the Department of Social Medicine and Health Policy, Harvard Medical School; a NATO Postdoctoral Fellowship from the National Science Foundation; and a research fellowship from the Wellcome Trust. I am grateful to Ronald L. Numbers and Roy Porter for their suggestions on an earlier draft of the paper.

1. The most lucid expression of this view is William G. Rothstein, *American Physicians in the Nineteenth Century: From Sects to Science* (Baltimore and London, Johns Hopkins University Press, 1972).
2. There is still no book-length study of Thomsonianism in the United States. On antebellum botanic sects, see Alex Berman, 'The Impact of the Nineteenth Century Botanico-Medical Movement on American Pharmacy and Medicine' (unpublished PhD thesis, University of Wisconsin-Madison, 1954); idem, 'Neo-Thomsonianism in the United States', *Journal of the History of Medicine and Allied Sciences*, 11 (1956), 133-55; idem, 'The Thomsonian Movement and Its Relation to American Pharmacy and Medicine', *Bulletin of the History of Medicine*, 25 (1951), 405-28 and 519-38; idem, 'Wooster Beach and the Early Eclectics', *University of Michigan Medical Bulletin*, 24 (1958), 277-86; Jonathan Forman, 'The Worthington School and Thomsonianism', *Bulletin of the History of Medicine*, 21 (1947), 772-87; Barbara Griggs, *Green Pharmacy: A History of Herbal Medicine* (London, Jill Norman & Hobhouse, 1981); Philip D. Jordan, 'The Secret Six: An Inquiry into the Basic Materia Medica of the Thomsonian System of Botanic Medicine', *Ohio Archaeological and Historical Quarterly*, 52 (1943), 347-55; Joseph F. Kett, *The Formation of the American Medical Profession; The Role of Institutions, 1780-1860* (New Haven and London, Yale University Press, 1968), 97-131; Ronald L. Numbers, 'The Making of an Eclectic Physician: Joseph M. McElhinney and the Eclectic Medical College of Cincinnati', *Bulletin of the History of Medicine*, 47 (1973), 155-66; and Frederick C. Waite, 'Thomsonianism in Ohio', *Ohio State Archaeological and Historical Quarterly*, 49 (1940), 322-31.
3. Of a large literature on homoeopathy in America, the most useful studies include Harris L. Coulter, *Divided Legacy: A History of the Schism in Medical Thought*, 3 vols (Washington, D.C, McGrath, 1973), vol. 3: *Science and Ethics in American Medicine, 1800-1914*; idem, *Homoeopathic Influences in Nineteenth-century Allopathic Therapeutics: A Historical and Philosophical Study* (St Louis, Formur, 1973); Martin Kaufman, *Homeopathy in America: The Rise and Fall of a Medical Heresy* (Baltimore and London, Johns Hopkins Press, 1971); and Kett (note 2), 132-64. Synthetic treatments of sectarianism include Elizabeth Barnaby Keeney, Susan Eyrich Lederer and Edmond P. Minihan, 'Sectarians and Scientists: Alternatives to Orthodox Medicine', in Ronald L. Numbers and Judith Walzer Leavitt (eds), *Wisconsin Medicine: Historical Perspectives* (Madison,

University of Wisconsin Press, 1981), 47-74; Ronald L. Numbers, 'Do-it-yourself the Sectarian Way', in Guenter B. Risse, Ronald L. Numbers and Judith Walzer Leavitt (eds), *Medicine without Doctors: Home Health Care in American History* (New York, Science History Publications, 1977), 49-72; Paul Starr, *The Social Transformation of American Medicine* (New York, Basic Books, 1982), 47-59; and Frederick C. Waite, 'American Sectarian Medical Colleges before the Civil War', *Bulletin of the History of Medicine*, 19 (1946), 148-66.

4. On hydropathy, see Marshall Scott Legan, 'Hydropathy in America: A Nineteenth Century Panacea', *Bulletin of the History of Medicine*, 45 (1971), 267-80, and Harry B. Weiss and Howard R. Kemble, *The Great American Water-cure Craze: A History of Hydropathy in the United States* (Trenton, New Jersey, Past Times Press, 1967). On the broader health reform movement to which hydropathy was linked, see Stephen Nissenbaum, *Sex, Diet, and Debility in Jacksonian America: Sylvester Graham and Health Reform* (Westport, Conn., Greenwood Press, 1980); Ronald L. Numbers, *Prophetess of Health: A Study of Ellen G. White* (New York, Harper & Row, 1976); and James C. Whorton, *Crusaders for Fitness: The History of American Health Reformers* (Princeton, Princeton University Press, 1982).

5. Michael Philip Duffy, 'A Progression of Sectarianism: Homeopathy in Massachusetts from 1855 to 1875' (unpublished AB thesis, Harvard University, 1982).

6. Typical instances are Joseph R. Buchanan, 'Sixth Annual Address of the Faculty of the Eclectic Medical Institute, to the Members of the Medical Profession', *Eclectic Medical Journal*, 2 (1850), 391; J.G. Peterson, 'Incorrigibility of Drug Doctors', *Water-cure Journal, and Herald of Reform*, 17 (1854), 52-3; and 'On the Present Condition of Medicine in the United States', *Western Medical Reformer*, 2 (1837), 276-7.

7. This is clear, for example, in [Joseph R.] B[uchanan], 'Medical Reform', *Eclectic Medical Journal*, (1849), 178-83; 'Educational Requirements of the Homoeopathic Physicians', *Homoeopathic Examiner*, 1 (1840), 17-22; 'Introduction', *American Journal of Homoeopathy*, 1 (1846), 1; and 'The Ohio Medical Convention', *Botanico-Medical Recorder*, 6 (1838), 124-5.

8. William Henry Holcombe, 'Diary and Notes, 1855-7' (Southern Historical Collection, University of North Carolina, Chapel Hill), entry for 4 April 1855. 'Alas! for poor Allopathic practice!' Holcombe wrote in his diary, adding five days later, 'Alas! for poor tottering Old Church Orthodoxy!' Some months later he recorded, 'To-day when speaking rather bitterly of Roman Catholic mummeries, my mind following a familiar undercurrent of thought, I misnamed it *Allopathic* mummeries. The differences between Old and New Church are very similar to those between Old and New medicine. Indeed I am a Homeopath simply in a primary view because I was previously a new Churchman' (entries for 22 February, 27 February, and 4 April 1855).

9. *Ibid.*, entry for 3 March 1855.

10. On professional identity in nineteenth-century American medicine, see Marti S. Pernick, *A Calculus of Suffering: Pain, Professionalism, and Anesthesia in Nineteenth-Century America* (New York, Columbia University Press, 1985); Barbara Gutmann Rosenkrantz, 'The Search for Professional Order in 19th-Century American Medicine', in Judith Walzer Leavitt and Ronald L. Numbers (eds), *Sickness and Health in America: Readings in the History of Medicine and Public Health*, 2nd edn (Madison and London, University of Wisconsin Press, 1985) 219-32; and John Harley Warner, *The Therapeutic Perspective: Medical Practice, Knowledge, and Identity in America, 1820-1885* (Cambridge, Mass. and London, Harvard University Press, 1986).

11. Alex Berman's 'The Heroic Approach in 19th-Century Therapeutics', *Bulletin of the American Society of Hospital Pharmacists*, 11 (1954), 320-7, remains the only study explicitly on heroic therapeutics in America. On antebellum therapeutics, see Charles E. Rosenberg, 'The Therapeutic Revolution: Medicine, Meaning, and Social Change in Nineteenth-century America', *Perspectives in Biology and Medicine*, 20 (1977), 485-506; John Harley Warner, 'From Specificity to Universalism in Medical Therapeutics:

Transformation in the Nineteenth-century United States', in Yosio Kawakita (ed), *The History of Therapy* (Tokyo, Taniguchi Foundation, in press); and Warner (note 10).

12. John Walker, 'Diary, King and Queen County, Virginia, 1826-49', 3 vols (Southern Historical Collection, University of North Carolina, Chapel Hill), vol. 3, entries for 12 August 1834 and 28 March 1835.

13. The terms are from 'Botanico-Medical Convention', *Botanico-Medical Recorder*, 8 (1840), 267; 'Drugging System', *American Journal of Homoeopathy*, 2 (1847), 161; 'Mineral Doctors', *Botanico-Medical Recorder*, 6 (1838), 292; 'Preface', *Botanico-Medical Recorder*, 8 (1840), 3; 'Retrospect', *Western Medical Reformer*, 6 (1846), 25-8; and 'Spread of Hydropathy in the United States', *Water-cure Journal*, new series, 1 (1845), 107.

14. George Washington Bowen, 'Notes Taken on Lectures Given by Chas. D. Williams on the Institutes and Practice of Homoeopathy, Cleveland Institute of Homoeopathy, 1851-2' (Western Reserve Historical Society, Cleveland, Ohio).

15. Examples abound in virtually all mid-nineteenth-century sectarian medical journals. Typical articles are 'Deleterious Influences of Calomel', *Western Medical Reformer* 4 (1844), 2-5; 'Horrors of Calomel', *Boston True Thomsonian*, 3 (1843), 349-50; 'Mercury — No. 1', *Botanico-Medical Recorder*, 6 (1838), 12-14; and 'The Use of Poisons, Calomel, and Depletions', *Water-cure Journal*, 3 (1847), 271-2.

16. 'Some Things Explained', *American Journal of Homoeopathy*, 1 (1846), 13-14.

17. A useful study of overcrowding is William Barlow and David O. Powell, 'To Find a Stand: New England Physicians on the Western and Southern Frontier, 1790-1840', *Bulletin of the History of Medicine*, 54 (1980), 386-401. The proliferation of proprietary medical schools was one source of this problem. 'Heaven only knows what is to become of all the Doctors ground, or rather bolted, out of the unnumerable mills from Maine to Texas. They should be sent as pioneers to Oregon', one eminent physician observed (Alfred Stillé to [George Cheyne] Shattuck, Philadelphia, 26 March 1844 (Massachusetts Historical Society, Boston, Shattuck Papers)).

18. Burdon Randall to Alexander Randall, New Orleans, 6 February 1831 (Manuscripts Department, Alderman Library, University of Virginia, Charlottesville, Randall Family Papers).

19. Burdon Randall to Alexander Randall, Williams Port, Maryland, 7 September 1831 (Randall Family Papers).

20. William D. Somers to 'My Dear Wife', Memphis, 9 July 1867 (Manuscript Collection, William R. Perkins Library, Duke University, Durham, North Carolina, William D. Somers Papers).

21. C.G. Comegys to Diathea [M. Tiffin], Cincinnati, 13 January 1851 (Western Reserve Historical Society, Matthew Scott Cook Papers).

22. William H. Thomson to 'My Dear Wife', Hines County, Mississippi, 12 July 1835 (Southern Historical Collection, Ruffin Thomson Papers). 'This country is overrun with half educated physicians', Alfred Stillé complained in a letter to George Cheyne Shattuck, 'besides whole brigades of quacks, and the chances of earning one's meat & drink are just about in proportion to one's disregard of truth, honor, and modesty' (Philadelphia, 3 June 1844 (Shattuck Papers)).

23. 'Preface', *Boston True Thomsonian*, 1 (1841), viii.

24. 'The Allopathic School', *American Journal of Homoeopathy*, 6 (1851), 2.

25. Some of the considerations at issue in judging a medical practitioner's legitimacy during the colonial period are examined in Margaret Humphreys Warner, 'Vindicating the Minister's Medical Role: Cotton Mather's Concept of the *Nishmath-Chajim* and the Spiritualization of Medicine', *Journal of the History of Medicine and Allied Sciences*, 36 (1981), 278-98. And see Whitfield J. Bell, Jr, 'A Portrait of the Colonial Physician', *Bulletin of the History of Medicine*, 44 (1970), 497-517; Walter L. Burrage, *A History of the Massachusetts Medical Society, with Brief Biographies of the Founders and Chief Officers, 1781-1922* (Norwood, Mass. Plimpton Press, 1923); and the essays in Philip Cash, Eric H. Christianson, and J. Worth Estes (eds), *Medicine in Colonial Massachusetts 1620-1820* (Boston, Colonial Society of Massachusetts, 1980).

26. On the decline of licensing, see Kett (note 2), 1-96; Rothstein (note 1), 63-100; and Richard Harrison Shryock, *Medical Licensing in America, 1650-1965* (Baltimore, Johns Hopkins University Press, 1967). For a comparison of professional regulation in the United States with Europe, See Matthew Ramsey 'The Politics of Professional Monopoly in Nineteenth-century Medicine: The French Model and its Rivals', in Gerald L. Geison (ed.), *Professions and the French State, 1700-1900* (Philadelphia, University of Pennsylvania Press, 1984), 225-305.

27. On medical schools, see Martin Kaufman, *American Medical Education: The Formative Years, 1765-1910* (Westport, Conn., and London, Greenwood Press, 1976), and William Frederick Norwood, *Medical Education in the United States before the Civil War* (Philadelphia, University of Pennsylvania Press, 1944). On societies, see James G. Burrow, *AMA: Voice of American Medicine* (Baltimore, Johns Hopkins Press, 1963); Ronald L. Numbers, 'Public Protection and Self-interest: Medical Societies in Wisconsin', in Numbers and Leavitt (note 3), 75-104; and Rothstein (note 1), 63-121.

28. For typical charges, see the accusations brought against an orthodox society member for consulting with steamers and practising homoeopathy in 'Minutes of the Miami Medical Association', in William C. Langdon, Record Book, 1853-1900' (Manuscripts Collection, Cincinnati Historical Society, Cincinnati, Ohio), entry for 4 July 1854.

29. 'Medical College of Ohio, Faculty Minutes, 1831-52' (Special Collections Department, University Library, University of Cincinnati, Cincinnati, Ohio), entries for 17 and 27 December 1845.

30. 'Minutes of the Faculty of the Medical College of the State of South Carolina, 1873-83' (Waring Historical Library, Medical University of South Carolina, Charleston), entry for 30 October 1874; and see 'Miami Medical College, Faculty Minutes, 1852-81' (Special Collections Department, University of Cincinnati), entry for 2 February 1867.

31. 'Preface', *Boston True Thomsonian*, 2 (1842), iii.

32. 'Death Caused by Homoeopathic Pills', *Western Lancet*, 1 (1842-3), 93; and see 'Morality in Medicine', *Western Lancet*, 2 (1843-4), 339-40.

33. Edward E. Jenkins to 'Dear Father', Paris, 6 June 1854 (Manuscripts Division, South Carolina Library, University of South Carolina, Columbia, John Jenkins Papers). And see Theosur Blatchford to John W. Francis, Troy, 27 July 1842 (Manuscripts Division, Astor, Lenox, and Tilden Foundations, The New York Public Library, New York, John W. Francis Papers), and C.W. Short to J.C. Short, Mayfield, Kentucky, 21 September 1855 (Manuscripts Collection, Cincinnati Historical Society, Short Family Papers).

34. James Otis Moore to Lizzie Moore, Williamsburg, [Virginia?], 12 April 1864 (Manuscript Collection, Perkins Library, Duke University, James Otis Moore Papers); and see letters from various camps dated 10 July 1864, 18 June 1864, 2 July 1864, and 17 March 1865. On a similar circumstance, see S.G. Jarrard to George Washburn, Camp Seward, Virginia, 1 November 1862 (Department of Archives and Manuscripts, Library, Louisiana State University, Baton Rouge, Simon G. Jerrard Papers).

35. See letters copied into John Leonard Riddell, 'Notebooks', 21 vols, especially vol. 5, 10 August 1832-7 September 1832, Worthington, Ohio, and vol. 9, 25 July 1833-17 December 1833, Worthinton, Ohio (Special Collections Division, Howard-Tilton Memorial Library, Tulane University, New Orleans, Louisiana, John Leonard Riddell Manuscript Volumes); and J.L. Riddell to S.P. Hildreth, Worthington, Ohio, 15 January 1833 (Archives, Dawes Memorial Library, Marietta College, Marietta, Ohio, Samuel P. Hildreth Papers).

36. James Jackson to Edward B. Peirson, Boston, 4 August 1857 (Oliver Wendell Holmes Hall, Francis A. Countway Library of Medicine, Harvard Medical School, Boston, Massachusetts).

37. For other instances in which regular physicians' therapeutic thinking was fundamentally shaped by the socio-economic context of practice in antebellum America, see John Harley Warner, 'The Idea of Southern Medical Distinctiveness: Medical Knowledge and Practice in the Old South', in Leavitt and Numbers (eds), *Sickness and Health in America* (note 10), 53-70; and idem, 'The Selective Transport of Medical Knowledge: Antebellum

American Physicians and Parisian Medical Therapeutics', *Bulletin of the History of Medicine*, 59 (1985), 213-31.
   38. W. Taylor, 'Changeability of Disease', *Proceedings of the Medical Association of the State of Alabama, at Its Sixth Annual Meeting, Begun and Held in the City of Selma Dec. 13-15, 1852, with an Appendix and List of Members* (Mobile, Dade, Thompson, & Co, 1853), 77 and 78.
   39. 'The Relation of Drugs to Treatment [Review of Edward H.Clark, An Introductory Lecture before the Medical Class of 1856-1857, of Harvard University]', *Cincinnati Medical Observer*, 2 (1857), 43.
   40. 'Preface', *Botanico-Medical Recorder*, 7 (1839), vii-viii.
   41. 'Letters from Saml.D. Holt, M.D., upon Some Points of General Pathology. Letter No. 15', *Southern Medical and Surgical Journal*, new series, 12 (1856), 594.
   42. Job Clark, 'Medical Diary and Notes of Cases, November 1836-November 1837, [Ravenna, Ohio]' (Manuscripts and Archives, Sterling Memorial Library, Yale University, New Haven, Connecticut), entry for 23 November 1836.
   43. This is based on a study of the male medical ward case history books of the Massachusetts General Hospital in Boston (384 vols, 1823-85, Holmes Hall, Countway Library) and of the Commercial Hospital in Cincinnati (51 vols, 1837-81, History of the Health Sciences Library and Museum, University of Cincinnati, Cincinnati, Ohio); see Warner (note 10), 133-5.
   44. John P. Harrison, 'On the Evacuant Indication of Treatment', *Western Lancet*, 1 (1842-3), 49.
   45. R.E.H., Review of '*Nature and Art in the Cure of Disease*. By Sir John Forbes', *Nashville Medical and Surgical Journal*, 14 (1858), 57.
   46. [E.D.], 'Review of Homoeopathy, Allopathy, and "Young Physic," by John Forbes, . . . (Phila., 1846)', *New Orleans Medical and Surgical Journal*, 2 (1845-6), 761.
   47. R.P. Little, 'Diary', nd but commenced 28 November 1842 (Duke University Medical Center Library, Durham, North Carolina, Trent Collection, P. Washington Little Papers).
   48. Thomas Kennard, 'Proceedings of the St Louis Medical Society', *St Louis Medical and Surgical Journal*, 17 (1859), 311-12.
   49. This point is developed in Warner (note 10), 4-7, 162-84, 207-32. When the sectarian challenge to orthodoxy became especially severe, precipitating an awareness of professional crisis, regular physicians may have returned to traditional heroic remedies in practice, not just principle; see John Harley Warner, 'Professional Power, Sectarian Conflict, and Orthodox Identity in Mid-Nineteenth-Century American Medicine: Therapeutic Change at the Commercial Hospital of Cincinnati', *Journal of American History*, forthcoming.
   50. Alfred Stillé to [George Cheyne] Shattuck, Philadelphia, 5 October 1857 (Shattuck Papers). The perception of professional decline is explicated in Daniel H.Calhoun, *Professional Lives in America: Structure and Aspiration, 1750-1850* (Cambridge, Mass. Harvard University Press, 1965), 178-97, and Ronald L. Numbers, 'The Fall and Rise of the American Medical Profession', in Leavitt & Numbers (eds), *Sickness and Health in America* (note 10), 185-96.
   51. On conflict in American therapeutics, see (in addition to sources cited in notes 2, 3, 4 and 11), Gert H. Brieger, 'Therapeutic Conflicts and the American Medical Profession in the 1860s', *Bulletin of the History of Medicine*, 41 (1967), 215-22; John S. Haller, Jr, *American Medicine in Transition, 1840-1910* (Urbana, Chicago, and London, University of Illinois Press, 1981); and Guenter B. Risse, 'Historical Vignette: Calomel and the American Medical Sects during the Nineteenth Century', *Mayo Clinic Proceedings*, 48 (1973), 57-64.
   52. 'Report of the Committee on Ethics, Minutes of the Miami Medical Association', in Langdon, Record Book, entry for Madisonville, [Ohio'[, 29 March 1853.
   53. 'Patronage of Quackery', *Western Lancet*, 1 (1842-3), 190.
   54. This movement in therapeutic thought is analysed in John Harley Warner, ' "The Nature-trusting Heresy": American Physicians and the Concept of the Healing Power of

Nature in the 1850's and 1860's', *Perspectives in American History*, 11 (1977-8), 291-324.

55. W.J. Summer, 'On the Vis Medicatrix Naturae', *Southern Medical and Surgical Journal*, new series 7 (1851), 203. The best general histories of the concept of nature's healing power remain Max Neuburger's 'An Historical Study of the Concept of Nature from a Medical Viewpoint', *Isis*, 35 (1944), 16-28, and his *The Doctrine of the Healing Power of Nature throughout the Course of Time*, trans. Linn J. Boyd (New York, New York Homeopathic Medical College, 1933; first pub. 1926).

56. Jas. W. Hughes, 'A Few Thoughts Suggested by the Present Phase of Medical Skepticism', *Cincinnati Lancet and Observer*, 19 (1858), 655.

57. Remarks of John P. Harrison at meeting of 1 March 1849, Hamilton County [Ohio] Medical Club, Minutes of Meetings, 21 May 1842-4 April 1850 (History of Medicine Division, National Library of Medicine, Bethesda, Maryland).

58. Alex. McBride, 'A Chemico-Pathological Classification of Fevers, and Hints at Treatment Based Thereon', *Cincinnati Lancet and Observer*, 25 (1864), 23. This tacit condemnation of medical tradition, another physician commented, was 'well calculated to derogate from the honor and utility of medicine' ('Nature and the Physician in the Cure of Disease', *Boston Medical and Surgical Journal*, 33 (1845-6), 461).

59. Bennet Dowler, 'Speculative and Practical Researches on the Supposed Duality, Unity, and Antagonism of Nature and Art in the Cure of Diseases', *New Orleans Medical and Surgical Journal*, 15 (1858), 789.

60. Review of 'Brief Expositions of Rational Medicine . . . by Jacob Bigelow', *Medical Journal of North Carolina*, 2 (1859), 359.

61. George C. Shattuck, 'The Medical Profession and Society', *Medical Communications of the Massachusetts Medical Society*, 10 (1866), 421.

62. C.B. Coventry, *Nature and Art in the Cure of Disease, Read before the Medical Society of the County of Oneida, July 1859* (Utica, New York, Roberts, 1859), quotations on pp. 4, 7, and 3.

63. Warren Stone, 'On Inflammation', *New Orleans Medical and Surgical Journal*, 16 (1859), 765.

64. Samuel Murphey, 'Notes Taken on Lectures Given by [Nathaniel] Chapman, 1830', 2 vols, vol. 1 (University Archives, University of Pennsylvania, Philadelphia).

65. Review of 'John Forbes, *Homoeopathy, Allopathy, and "Young Physic"* (1846)', *Western Lancet*, 5 (1846-7), 198. And see J.R. Black, 'Thoughts on the Prevalence of Quackery', *Cincinnati Lancet and Observer*, 22 (1861), 599, and B. Dowler, Review of '*Brief Exposition of Rational Medicine:* By Jacob Bigelow', *New Orleans Medical and Surgical Journal*, 16 (1859), 902-3. For many regular American physicians, the link between clinical statistics and sectarian therapeutics was sufficient to discredit this method of inquiry. That many American physicians virtually rejected the validity of the numerical method as a way to gain therapeutic knowledge in part because of its homoeopathic associations is a clear instance of the social context of medical practice influencing physicians' epistemological commitments. James H. Cassedy also discusses the relationship between antebellum sects and statistics in *American Medicine and Statistical Thinking, 1800-1860* (Cambridge, Mass. Harvard University Press, 1984).

66. See, for example, Neidhard, 'Preface', *Miscellanies on Homoeopathy*, 1 (1839), 1-2; 'Progress of Homoeopathy and the Abandonment of Allopathy', *American Journal of Homoeopathy*, 7 (1852), 110; and the articles in *Indian Arcana; Devoted to Illustrations of Indian Life, Indian Medicine, Science, Art, Literature, and General Intelligence*, 5, no. 7 (1860).

67. Review of '*Brief Expositions of Rational Medicine* . . . By Jacob Bigelow', *Nashville Journal of Medicine and Surgery*, 16 (1859), 57.

68. Bennet Dowler, 'Critical and Speculative Researches on the Fundamental Principles of Subjective Science in Connection with Medical and Experimental Investigations, with Remarks on the Present State of Medicine', *New Orleans Medical and Surgical Journal*, 15 (1858), 46.

69. Oliver Wendell Holmes, *Currents and Counter Currents in Medical Science, an Address Delivered before the Massachusetts Medical Society, at the Annual Meeting, May 30, 1860* (Boston, Ticknor & Fields, 1860), 16. One critic tellingly denounced Holmes for his 'free thinking' in therapeutics ('Dr. Holmes *vs.* the Medical Profession', *Medical Journal of North Carolina*, 3 (1860), 619). On the charge of heresy, see for example review of '*Science and Success: A Valedictory Address Delivered to the Medical Graduates of Harvard University, at the College in Boston. Wednesday, March 9, 1859.* By Henry Jacob Bigelow', *Nashville Journal of Medicine and Surgery*, 17 (1859), 252, and 'The Water Cure or Hydropathy', *Western Lancet*, 5 (1846-7), 393.

70. See Warner (note 10) 31-6.

INDEX

Abernethian Creed 183
Abernethian Society, bone-setting sessions 172 (note)
Abernethy, John (1764-1831) 183
  Surgical Observations on the Constitutional Treatment of Local Diseases 183
Académie Royale de Médicine 100
advertising in 18th century
  handbills 36
  newspaper advertisements 36-7
Alcott, William 227
Allen, Hanbury & Barry 149
Allen, William FRS (1770-1843) 184-9
Allen & Howard 148
allopathy 237
Alsop, Robert (1803-1876) 151
America, toppling of state medical registration laws 190
American Health Reform movement 227
American Journal of Homeopathy, quoted 240
American medicine, ante-Civil War 234-60
  American fringe/American orthodoxy 253-4
  bloodletting 246, 247
  competition from sectarian practitioners 239-40
  conservative influence of sectarianism 248-52
  definition of orthodox symbols 235-40
  discrimination against irregular practitioners 241-2
  heresy 241, 248-52
  homeopathy 236, 242-3, 244-5
  ideology of orthodoxy 243-8
  institutionalization of orthodox identity 240-3
  lack of legal distinction, orthodox physician/sectarian 237
  medical journals 241
  medical schools 241, 242
  medical secretaries 241, 242; codes of ethics 241
  National Medical Association 241
  nature trustees 249-52
  physicians' characteristics 252
  physicians identified with their drugs 238
  physicians' qualifications 253
  proprietary medical schools 256 (note)
  repeal of licensing laws by state legislatures 241
  sectarian challenge 235-40
  surplus of doctors 239-40
  therapeutics 244-8
  therapeutic unity 248
'Amicus', letter to *Gazetteer* 69-70
Ancell, Henry (1803-1863) 146, 156 (note)
ancien régime of medicine 175
Andree, John
  mercury for syphilis 16
  source of venereal disease in body 13
Answer to a Pamphlet written by Dr. Lettson . . . 63
antimony, for syphilis 17
anti-professionalism 201
apothecaries 42-3
  antagonism of physicians 108
  attacks on wealth/practice 45
  prosperity in 18th. century 108
Apothecaries Act 1815 106, 119
  current views on 123
  dispensing druggist named as guilty party 45
  licensing of 'general practitioners' 2
  repeal mooted 128
apothecaries shop, bottles/jars in 31
'aquillea millefeuilles' 90
Archer, Lord, patient of Myersbach 5
Aristotle's Masterpiece 13, 27 (note)
Armstrong, John (1709-1779), publication on venereal disease 11
Association of Apothecaries and Surgeon-Apothecaries 119

Index

Association of General Medical and Surgical Practitioners, opposition to repeal of Apothecaries Act 128 (note)
astrology 228
Astruc, Jean (1684-1766) 23
Attfield, John (director of Pharmaceutical Society's laboratory) 145

Bacher, Alexandre-André-Philippe-Fréderic 86
Bacher, George-Fréderic 86
Bacon, Francis (1561-1626), experimental programme 176
Balm of Soriacum 113
balneology 176, 179-80
 Presbyterianism associated 180
Barailon, Jean-Francois 88
barber-surgeons
 apprentices 42
 fate after 1745 41-2
 free treatment for poor 33
 Old Parsley (Bristol) 42
 regalia 31
 regulation of fees 33
 shop 31
 split with surgeons 31
Barclay, Captain 185
Barker, Sir Herbert (1869-1950) 166, 168, 172 (note)
Barker, Joseph (reformer), quoted 208
Barmby, John Goodwin 202
Barron, Charles (pharmacist) 150
Barry, John Thomas (1789-1864) 148, 149
Bateman, Dr. 126
Bateman's Pectoral Drops 43, 112
Bath 44
bath 189
 public 190
bathing cures 31
Battley, Richard (1770-1856) 151-2
Battley & Watts 152
Beddoes, Thomas (1760-1808) 45, 48-51, 186
 A Letter to Joseph Banks 49
 Edinburgh Royal Infirmary denounced by 49
 hostility to apothecaries 51
 medicalisation of social life 50
 opinion of John Brown 49
 publication on venereal disease 11
 quackery denounced by 49-50
 quoted on quackery 40
Beecham's pills 228
Bell, Jacob (pharmacist) 129, 130, 135-7 *passim*
 assistants, competent, difficulty in obtaining 138
 Historical Sketch of the Progress of Pharmacy in Great Britain, 129, 140
 monthly scientific meetings 138-9
 on raising qualifications of chemists 139-40
 'pharmaceutical tea party' 133
 pharmacy as a profession 140-2
Bell, John (pharmacist) 149
Belloste, Jean-Baptiste 97, 99
Belloste, Michel-Antoine 97, 99
Belloste's pills 97
Benvenuti, Dr. Georgslanger 30, 34
Bennett, G. Matthew (bone-setter) 167
Ben Rhydding
 homeopathy at 227
 hydropathy at 224
Berkshire, regulars/irregulars in 125
Bew, J. *The New Method of Curing Diseases by Inspecting the Urine Examined* 65
Bichat, Xavier 187
bill to regulate the practice of pharmacy (1830) 130-1
Bird, Dr. Golding 146
Birkbeck Laboratory, University College, London 139
Blake, John *Letter to a Surgeon on Inoculation* 44
bleeding *see* bloodletting
'Bleeding, Mineral, Reducing System' 238
bloodletting (bleeding)
 American 235, 239, 246, 247
 barber's shop 42
Boerhaave, Hermann, (1668-1738) 181
bone-setter 117
 Employers 'Liability Acts' effect on numbers 162
 families 170 (note)
 female 170 (note)
 'hereditary' ('natural') 160
 itinerant 160
 manslaughter case against (Ffestiniog) 162
 orthopaedists' complaint 165
 rural situation 160
bone-setting 158-73

Index 263

as sideline 160
  learning of 160
  Rosen's views 158-9
  sixteenth-seventeenth centuries
    159-60
booksellers, sellers of patent medicines
  112
Boot, Jesse (medical botanist) 207
Boot, John (Weslyan lay preacher)
  207
Boston True Thomsonian, quoted 240
Boswell, James (1740-1795)
  attacks of venereal disease 12
  treated for gonorrhoea 11-12
Brest, Vincent (surgeon and
  cupper) 14
Bridge of Allen hydropathic
  establishment 224
Bristol, 18th century
  apothecaries 42-3
  barber-surgeons 41-2
    apprentices 42
  dispensary for eye diseases 46
  honorary hospital posts 33
  Hotwells 31, 32;
    Smollett's Ferdinand Fathom
      at 34
  infirmary 33;
    annual march of practitioners/
      subscribers 36
  medicine in 29-39
  number of medical practitioners/
    apothecaries 43
  patent medicines 43
  population 43
  St. Peter's Hospital 33
  waters 33-4
Bristol, 19th, century
  Bedminster 46
  Bristol General Hospital 47
  Clifton 46
  Clifton Dispensary 47
  directory-cited regulars 45
  geographical distribution and class
    organization 46
  medical grouping 48
  medical institutions 47
  Old Market 46
  Port Street 46
  quack medicines 48
  religious segmentation 47
  St. Paul's 46
  St. Peter's Hospital 47
  Thomsonians arrive 46

British Drug Houses Ltd, 150
Broderip, Billy (Bristol apothecary) 110
Brodum, Dr. William 75
Brodum's Nervous Cordial 75
Broussais, François Joseph Victor
  (1771-1838) 183
Brown, John (1735-1788) 48
Brown, Samuel (literary critic) on
  'physical puritanism' 174
brucine 143
Brunonian medicine 48
Buchan, Alexander, guaiac's co-
  operation with mercury 17
Buchan, William (author) 182, 191
  Domestic Medicine 13, 155, 179
  *Observations Concerning the
    Prevention and Cure of the
    Venereal Disease* 14
  recommends mercury 15
Burrows, George Man (President of
  Association of Apothecaries and
  Surgeon-Apothecaries) 121, 126
  (note)

Cabarus, Georges *Du Degré de
  certitude de la médicine* 82
Cadogan, William *Essays on Nursing* 32
caffeine 143
Calés, Jean-Marie 88
Callot, Jean-Gabriel 87
calomel (mercurous chloride) 183, 235
'calomel and blue pill school of
  medicine' 238
'calomel doctor' 238
Cambridgeshire, regulars/irregulars in
  123
Campbell, R. *London Tradesmen* 8-9
Camplin, Reverend Mr., patient of D.
  Smith 44
cancer cures 114
Carlisle, Sir Anthony (surgeon) 190
Carlyle, Thomas (1795-1881), quoted
  206
Carpenter, Edward (1844-1929) 205
  followers 206; attacks on 210
Carter, Dr. (American botanic
  physician) 242
'Cassius', pseudonym of J.C. Lettsom
  71
Chadwickian emergency sanitary
  measures 190
Challice, Dr. (of Bermondsey) 186
Chambers, William (1800-1883) 164,
  166

264　Index

Chartism 198-9
  strongholds 211
Chassier, François (professor of anatomy, Paris) 93
chemistry
  development in 19th. century 146
  Paracelsian 176
chemists
  criticisms of 153
  nineteenth century development 149
Chemists and Druggists of the Metropolis, The 130
Chesterfield, Lord (Philip Stanhope) (1694-1773) 178
Cheyne, George (1671-1743) 178
  Essay of Health and Long Life 178
childbirth, in public 31
cholera 187
'chymical' doctor 176
cinchonine 143
Cincinatti physician, quoted 248
Claridge, Richard T. (hydropath) 223, 224
Clark, Dr. (physician and oculist) 30, 34
  'lamp of light' 30
cleanliness
  physical necessity 175
  social history 174
  social virtue 175
Clegg, James (minister-physician) 107
Clias, Peter H. 185
Clinical Society of London, bone-setting sessions 172
Clowes, William (1540?-1604) 9
Cocchi, Antonio *The Pythagorean Diet* 178
Cockle's Compound Anti-bilious Pills 113
codeine 143
cod liver oil 149
Coffin, Albert Isiah (botanic physician) 200, 201, 219-23
  attack on homeopathy and hydropathy 223
  fever as friend 222
  pioneer of nature cure principles 223
  poisonous medicines condemned 221-2
  prevention of disease 222
  quoted on science in medicine 220-1
Coffins's Botanical Journal and Medical Reformer 200, 220, 221

Colas's elixir of long life 88
colchicine 143
coldness, as guarantor of godly life 176-7
cold water
  fasting associated 180
  health/beauty associated 180
  'Spare Diet' associated 180
cold-water nurse 180
Coleridge, Samuel Taylor (1772-1834) 51, 178-9
'College and Hall' qualification 45
College of Pharmacy 88
  regulation of secret remedies 88
Coltheart, P.C., definition of quack 107
Combe, Andrew (author) 182, 187-8, 190
  The Art of Preserving Health 187
Combe, George 187
Comfort, Alex *The Anxiety Makers* 5
Comité de Salubrité 87
  secret remedies discussed 87
Committee of Chemists and Druggists (1814-15) 131
Committee on public education (France) 103 (note)
Conolly, John *Working Mans' Companion* 186
consilia 175
Contagious Diseases Act, 'syphilis' not mentioned in debate 6
Cooper, Thomas 201
Corbyn & Co 147
Cordial Balm of Gilead 112, 115, 126 (note)
Cornaro 186
Council of Five Hundred (France), report to 88
Courtney, Abraham (naval surgeon) 225, 226
Coutelet (Paris parasol dealer) 91
Cox, William Stockton (Chartist) 212 (note)
Cox's Companion to the Family Medicine Chest and Compendium of Domestic Medicine 155
Crabbe, George (1754-1832), on proprietary medicines 217
creosote 150
Crown and Anchor tavern, public meeting at 129, 133
Crowthers (bone-setter) 170 (note)
Cullen, William (1710-1790) 178, 186

Cullenite medicine 48
Culpan, John (Chartist) 212 (note)
'curers by imagination' 117
Curil (Curle), Edmund 27 (note)
Curtis, J. Harrison 186, 188

Dagge, Abel (Bristol surgeon) 35
Dale, W. (herbalist) 222
dames' schools 201
Deacon, H. 25 (note)
  A Compendious Treatise on the Venereal Disease, Gleets, etc. 25 (note)
deafness
  disappearance of specialists in 43
  treated by quacks 114
Declaration of Rights of Man (France) 81, 85
democratic polemic 175-7
Devonshire, regulars/irregulars in 125
di Dominiceti, Bartholomew 30, 31, 34-5
  certificate of integrity/judgement 34
  Short and Calm Apology 44
'digestibility' scale 184
Dinneford, Charles (pharmacist) 149
disease as violation of nature's laws 222
doctor's surgery, dispensing in 154
Dolman, John (surgeon) 48
domestic medicine chest 155
Dorsetshire, regulars/irregulars in 124
Douglas, Alexander, treats Boswell for gonorrhoea 11, 12
Dover, Thomas (1664-1742) 33
Dr. Anderson's (Scotch) Pill 112
Dr. Bateman's Pectoral Drops 3, 112
Dr. Boerhaave's Red Pill 112
Dr. Borthwick's 'vegetable remedies' 113
Dr. Norris's Fever Drops 113
Dr. Radcliffe's Elixir 112
'drug doctors' 238
'drugging system' 238
druggist, dispensing 108-11
  as quack 111
  collusion with physicians 110
  criticisms 153
  described by J. Power 125 (note)
  source of prosperity in 19th century 154
  South-west England, 18th-early 19th centuries 109 (table)
Druggists' Association 131

Druggists' Provident Association 130
'drug-grinders' 150
drugs
  pure, preparation of 143-4
  supposed properties 83
drug-taking self-helper as quack 53
Dubois, Louis-Nicolas-Pierre 90
Duckett, Mr. (specialist in poor hearing) 43
Durham, regulars/irregulars in 124

eclecticism 236
Edenic myth 203-4
Edinburgh Royal Infirmary, denounced by Beddoes 49
Elcocks, Dr., urine-casting by 115
electro-biology, treatment of epilepsy by 227
electro-therapy 163
Elliotson, John 229
Ellis, James (hydropath) 223, 225
emetine 143
empiricism 64
  prolix 83
Employers' Liability Acts (1880 and after), effect on number of bone-setters 162
English, Mr. ('practitioner in physic') 113
epilepsy, treatment by electro-biology 227
Epps, Dr. John 205, 206
Essay on the Inspection of the Urine . . . An, by a physician 62
Essence of Coltsfoot 48
Essex, regulars/irregulars in 125
Estlin, John Bishop (1785-1855) 46, 51
ether inhaler, first 151
Evans Medical Ltd 149-50
Evans & Lescher 149
Evelyn, John (1620-1706) 178
eye disease, quack activity in (1820-30) 45-6

Fairclough (oculist) 34
Family Oracle of Health, gibes against vegetarianism 184
farriers, as midwives 127 (note)
Fergusson, Sir William (surgeon) 164
Floyer, John (balneologist) 179
Fluid Magnesia 149
folk medicine 155
Forbes, Duncan, treats Boswell for gonorrhoea 11

266 Index

Forsyth, J.S. 184
Fothergill, Dr. John (1712-1780),
  letter to *Gazetteer* 74
Foulger, Samuel (pharmacist) 150
freedom of trade and enterprise
  (France) 81
Fresenius, C.R. (pupil of Liebig) 145
Friendly United Medico-Botanic Sick
  and Burial Society 201
Frochet, Nicolas-Thérèse Benoît,
  (prefect of police) 88
Frost, John 212 (note)
Fuller, Francis *Medicina Gymnastica*
  185

Gachet, Louis-Etienne
  elixir against gout 85
  Le Manuel des goutteux 85-6
  Problème médico-politique: pour ou contre les arcanes, ou remèdes secrets 85
'Galen', poem by, in *Public Ledger*
  72-3
galvanic therapy 163
Gammage, R.G. (Chartist) 198
Gentleman's Magazine, list of
  nostrums/patent medicines (1748)
  11
Gardner, Dr. (itinerant irregular) 115
Garrick, David (1717-1779)
  patient of Myersbach 57
  quoted 57
Gazette de santé, rejects
  advertisements for secret remedies
  84
Gazetteer
  Amicus's letter to 69-70
  John Fothergill's letter 74
  John Willan's letter to 68-9
  J.S.'s letter to 70-1
  'London spy's' letter to 70
General Association of Chemists and
  Druggists of Great Britain, The
  129-30
General Pharmaceutical Association of
  Great Britain 110
general practitioner
  dispensing of drugs by 121-2
  despise druggists 121
  higher standards of
    education/knowledge 120
  licensing 2
  LSA (Licence of Society of
    Apothecaries) 121

MRCS (Membership of the Royal
  College of Surgeons) 121
Germinal law on secret remedies
  (France) 89-92
Giessen University, Liebig's laboratory
  at 144
gleet 13, 15
Globe Tavern, meeting of chemists
  and druggists at 130
Gloucester, attendance at druggists 118
gluttony 184
'Golden Age of Physic' 108
Goldsmith, Oliver (1728-1774) 178
Goldwyn, Thomas (surgeon) 48
gonorrhoea, surgical prerogative 9
Goodman, John 226
Grace, James (surgeon-apothecary,
  Bristol) 39 (note)
Graham, James 30, 45
  as cracked in the head 56
  'Great Empire' 54
  view of vegetable-eating 79
Graham, Sir James 122
Graham, Robert 225
Graham, Sylvester 211, 227
Graham, Thomas J. 185, 185-6, 225
Granville, A.B. *Catechism of Health*
  186
Greenland doctors 117, 124
Greenough, Mr. (chemist), Society of
  Apothecaries case against 135
Gregory, John, treats Boswell for
  gonorrhoea 12
Grimaldi, Joseph (surgeon/dentist) 30
Grindrod, Ralph (temperance reformer)
  226
guaiac 9, 17, 18
Guillotin, Joseph-Ignace 87
gullibility of English people 65
Gully, Dr. 225
Guthne 122
Guybon, Francis, definition of quack
  106-7

Hahnemann, Samuel, followers of 205
Halin's jelly 90
Hall, Spencer T. (hydropath) 224, 227
Ham Common concordium 208
Hamilton, Gustavus 185
Hanbury, Daniel (pharmacist) 148
Hancocke, John (d. 1728) 179, 180
Hands (surgeon/man midwife) 34
Hardy, Antoine-François 88-9

Index 267

Harrington, Lady, patient of Myersbach 59
Harrison, Dr. Edward (Horncastle) 118
  investigation by 111-12, 118 123-5
Harrison v Toplis 202
Hartley, David (1705-1757) 178
Harvey, Gideon (1640?-1700?) 9
Harvey & Barron 150
Haussman (Myersbach's apothecary's assistant) 64, 71
Hawes, Benjamin 130
Hawke, Lord, patient of Myersbach 58-9
Hayward, Thomas (Bristol apothecary) 38
health 'genre' 182
Heath, D.W. 200
Herapath, William (1796-1868) 46
herbal(s) 175
herbalists 219-23, 229
herbal medicaments, reliance on 223
hernia, topical remedy 96
heroic therapy 48
Herring Brothers 150
Herring, Thomas (1785-1864) 150
Herring, Thrower Buckle (pharmacist) 150
Herring's vegetable powders 150
High German Dr. Symon 114
Hill, Thomas Hyde (pharmacist) 149
Hillman, Dr. (counsellor to court of King of Prussia) 34
Hill's medicine for mad dog bite 43
'Hippocrates', poem by, in *Morning Chronicle* 73
Holcombe, William Henry (homeopath) 237, 255 (note)
Hole, James (Owenite) 208
Holism 205
Hollick, Frederick 198, 211
Holmes, Oliver Wendell (1809-1894) 251, 260 (note)
home medicine chest 155
homeopathy 174, 227
  American 236, 242-3, 244-5
Homer & Sons 147
Hood, Wharton (surgeon) 164
  A Treatise on Bone-setting 164, 168
Horner, Edward (pharmacist) 147
'Hortator' 184
Hospital for the Ruptured and Crippled (New York) 171 (note)

hot-cold polarity 176
hot water, suspicions of 180
Howard, John (1726?-1790) 178, 180
Howard, Luke FRS (1772-1864) 148
Howard's Quinine, Borax and Tartaric Acid Works 148-9
Hudson, W.B. (druggist) 130
Hufeland, C.W. (German hygienist) 187
Hull irregulars c. 1780-1830 112-16
Hunter, Archibald (hydropath) 224
Hunter, A.S., Mrs (hydropath) 226
Hunter, John (1728-1793) *Treatise on the Venereal Disease* (1786) 11, 12
Hunter, William Bell (medical hydropath) 226
Hutton, Richard (1801-1871) 162-3
Huttons (bone-setters) 170 (note)
hydropathy 174, 223-7, 229
  America 236
hydro-therapy 163
hygiene
  core beliefs 174
  specialist periodicals, first 191
  specialist study in academic curriculum 191

Imposter Detected or the Physician the Greater Cheat. . . . The 63, 66, 67
incunabula (1450-1500) 175
Innes, Mr. (surgeon?) 116
inoculation, effect on pregnant women 44
inoculators 44
insensible perspiration 189
irregulars, pre-Victorian
  attempted suppression 118-23
  classification into groups 117
  continuation in practice after Apothecaries Act 120
  druggists 117; *see also* druggist, dispensing
  Hull, c. 1780-1830 112-16
  individuality 116-17
  itinerant 114-15, 117
  local (stationary) 117
  medical reform and 116-17
  midwives 117
  noble patronage 113
  pamphleteering 112-16
  part-time healers 117
  salesmanship 116-17
  variety 116-17

268 Index

Jackson (Bristol druggist) 109
Jackson, James Snr. 243
James's Fever Powders 43
Jenkins, Edward E. 257 (note)
Jenneson, Charles (Owenite) 212 (note)
Johnson, Dr. (Hull) 114
Johnson, Edward (medical hydropath) 225-6, 226
John Webb's cordial 48
Jones, Ernest (barrister) 202
Jones, Sir Robert (1857-1933) 159, 165, 168
Jordan, L. 113
Jordan, R. 113
J.S., letter to *Gazetteer* 70-1
juniper 17
jurys médicaux 90

Keating, Thomas (pharmacist) 149 †
Keating's Powder 149
Kennedy, Gilbert, MD. (c. 1680-1780) 12
Kennedy's Lisbon Diet Drink, taken by Boswell 12
Kenworthy, Samuel (hydropath) 224
Kilgour, A. *Lectures on the Ordinary Agents of Life* 190
'knights of calomel and lancet' 238

Laffecteur's vegetable 'rob' 92
Lambert, Dr. (itinerant irregular) 114
Lancashire working man, quoted 210
Lane, Edward R. (medical hydropath) 226
Laurie, William Forbes (hydropath) 227
Law, William (1686-1761) 178
Leake, John (1729-1792) 27
  Dissertation on the Properties and Efficacy of the Lisbon Diet-drink and its Extract 27 (note)
Leake's Diet Drink 27 (note)
Leake's pill 27 (note)
Lechat, Armande-Geneviève-Elisabeth Lechat (widow Belloste) 97-9
Lees, F.R. (temperance advocate) 208
Lescher, J.S. (pharmacist) 149, 150
Letheby, Dr. Henry 217
  'On the Mischievous Effects of Quack Medicines' 218
Lettsom, John Coakley (1744-1815) 57
  anti-quack exposés in *Medical and Physical Journal* 74-5
  attack on William Brodum 75
  confrontation with T. von Myersbach 57, 62-75
  investigates Myersbach's drugs 62
  medical position 63-4
  Observations Preparatory to the Use of Dr. Myersbach's Medicines. . . . 62
  pseudonym 71
  support for 62-3
  see also Myersbach, Theodor von
Liebig, Justus (1803-1873) 144-5
  address to British Association for the Advancement of Science 146-7
  as business man 147
  fermentation explained by 145-6
  law of contagious molecular action 146
  physicians' reactions to his ideas 146.
  visits Morson's 'Science Sunday Evening' 150
  visits Pharmaceutical Society's laboratory 145
Liebig's Extract of Meat 147
Lincoln, attendance at druggists 118
Lincolnshire Medical Benevolent Society 111
Linstead, H.N. *Jacob Bell and Some Others* 129
lithotomy, in public 31
Lobelia inlata 222
Locke, John (1632-1704) *Some Thoughts Concerning Education* 179
lock hospitals
  existence in London 7
  new, foundation in 1747 7
Locock, Sir Charles 218
'London spy', letter to *Gazetteer* 70
Long, St. John (irregular) 128 (note)
Lovett, William 198, 206

Macleod, William (homeopath) 227
mad dog bite, Hill's medicine for 43
Magendie, François (1783-1855) 143
  Formularie pour la préparation et l'emploi de plusiers nouveaux médicaments 143
Mainduc, de, lecturer on animal magnetism 53 (note)
male midwives 97
Maltbys (bone-setters) 170 (note)
Malvern, homeopathy in 227

Index 269

Mapp, Sarah, ('Crazy Sally') 163, 170 (note)
Marat, Jean-Paul (1743-1793) 85
Marsh, Howard (surgeon) 166-7
  'On Manipulation . . . as a means of Surgical Treatment' 164
Marten, John *Treatise. . . . of the Venereal Disease in both Sexes* 14, 14-15
Mary Barton (E. Gaskell), Alice Wilson in 154
Martineau, Harriet (1802-1876) 258
Maryland, abundance of physicians in 239
Masons (bone-setters) 170 (note)
Massachusetts Medical Society 240
massage 163
Messey, Gerald (Chartist) 207, 212 (note)
materialism (mind versus matter) 208
Matlock Bank Hydropath Establishment 224
Matthews (bone-setter) 170 (note)
Maurice, F.D. 207
mechano-therapy 163
Medical Act (1856), *Medical Register* established 2
Medical Adviser, gibes against vegetarianism 184
Medical and Physical Journal, letters from Lettsom to 74-5
medical botanists 203, 221-2
medical botany, as eternal truth 206
medical gymnastics 163
medical empiricism 64
medical registration (1858) 106
medical police 187
Medical Reform Bill (1841) 130
  committee meetings opposing 132
Medicine Act (1802), modification 129
Medicine Stamp Acts, penalties under 129
Merck, Sharp & Dohme Ltd 150
mercurous chloride (calomel) 183
mercury
  complications of treatment with 16
  fifteenth-century use 9
  metallic breath due to 16
  recommended by Buchan 15
  salivation due to 16
  syphilis treated with 6, 9, 15-17
'mercury dosers' 238
mesmerism 174, 208-9, 228
  public exhibitions 229

sexual overtones 211
Meyrick, William *New Family Herbal* 17
mezereon 17, 18
Mezger, Johnn (Dutch doctor) 171 (note)
Miall, Edward 201-2
midwives 117
  farriers as 127 (note)
  male 7
  unqualified women 201
mind versus matter (materialism) 208
'mineral doctors' 238
'mineral, humbuggery practice' 238
'mineralites' 238
Minister of Interior (France) 89-90
Mississippi doctor 239
Montrose, regulars/irregulars in 125
Moore, James Otis (Maine homeopath) 243
More, Henry (1614-1687) 177
Morgan, John Minter *Hampden in the Nineteenth Century* 213 (note)
Morison, James ('The Hygeist') 184, 219
Morning Chronicle, poem by 'Hippocrates' in 73
morphine 143, 150
Morson, Thomas Newborn Robert (1799-1874) 150
Mortimer, Jabez (bone-setter in Young's *Dr. Bradley Remembers*) 165
Mountjoys, Thomas (father and son) 35
Mr. Lignum's Royal Anti-scorbutic Drops 112-13
Myersbach, Theodor von 3, 57
  as abortionist 77 (note)
  confrontation with J.C. Lettsom 57
  charges 59
  diagnostic technique 61
  drugs provided by 61-2
  early career 57-8
  exposé 60-1
  lack of medical training, degrees, membership of learned societies 65
  replies to critics 63
  return to Germany, followed by return to England 74
  servants' gathering of information about patients 60
  urine examination 59-60

270 Index

vindicators 67-71 *passim*
   see also Lettsom, John Coakley
mystic neo-Platonic phases 178

Napier, Richard 125 (note)
narceine 143
Nashville physician quoted 251
'national debility' in urban populations 187
National Constituent Assembly (France) 87
National Medical Association (USA) 241
Natras, Dr. (Hull) 114
nature's healing power 222
nature-trusters, American 249-52
'nature-trusters, American 249-52
'nature-trusting heresy' (O.W. Holmes) 251
naturopathy 223
Newberry, Francis (proprietor of Dr. James' Powder) 44
New Method of Curing Diseases by Inspecting the Urine Explained . . . The 62, 65, 77 (note)
New Moral World 200
New Orleans physician 239
New System of Vegetable Cookery, A 184
Newton, Isaac, (1642-1727) 178
Newton, J.F. (vegetarian writer) 178
New York physician quoted 250
Nichols, Mary Gove 204, 209
Nichols, Thomas Low 204, 211
nitrous oxide, for syphilis 24
Norman James (Bristol surgeon) 35
Northumberland, regulars/irregulars in 124
'nosographies' of symptoms of disease 82
Nottingham, regulars/irregulars in 124
Nottingham Medico-Botanic Society, report from 200
Nottinghamshire District, regulars/irregulars in 124

obstetrics, develoment of 7
oculists, quack, operations in public 31
Ohio physicians quoted 239, 247
Old Parsley (Bristol barber-surgeon) 42
ophthalmology, origin as marginal specialism 6
orthopaedics, progress of, due to Lister, not to bone-setters, claim 167
Oswald, John (vegetarian writer) 178
Owen, Robert (1771-1858) 198
   attacks on 210
Owen, Robert Dale 212 (note)
Owenism (Owenites) 198-204 *passim*, 207
   mesmerism suited to 209
   phrenology suited to 209
   strongholds 211

Paget's disease of bone 166
Paget, Sir James (1814-1899) 166
   On the Cases that Bone-setters Cure' 159, 163, 163-4
Paley, William (1743-1805) 178
Palmer, Samuel 20
pamphleteering by irregulars/regulars 112-16
paper qualifications in medicine 66
Paracelsian chemistry 176
Paracelsianism 193 (note)
Paris Faculty of Medicine (formerly Paris School of Medicine) 91, 93
   assessment of new remedies 100
Parisian medicine, respect for 48
Paris School of Medicine 90
patent medicines, English 79
Paulin, Mr. (patient of D. Smith) 44
Payne, Charles James (vice-president of Pharmaceutical Society) 145
Pearson, John (1758-1826) 24, 28 (note)
   nitrous oxide for syphilis 24
   Observations on the . . . Lues Venerea 24
Pelletier, Pierre-Joseph (1788-1842) 143
Penn, John (specialist in poor hearing) 43
Pereira, Dr. Jonathan 147-8
Péroutet (petitioner to Minister of Interior) 94
Pharmaceutical Journal 145
   'Illustrations of the Present State of Pharmacy in England' 152
Pharmaceutical Society of Great Britain
   centenary celebration 129
   establishment 132-4
   examinations 139-40
   laboratory 139, 145; visited by Liebig 145

library 139
museum 139
professional education of members 138
Royal Charter of Incorporation 134
School of Pharmacy 139
scientific committee for the promotion of pharmacological knowledge 147
scientific meetings 139
transfer of money to 133
pharmacological companies 228
pharmacopoeia syphilitica 17
Philadelphia physician, quoted 247-8
Philadelphia professor, quoted 250
Phillips, Richard (editor, translator) 145
phrenology 174, 187, 208-9, 210
physical exercise 185
physical puritanism 174-212, 214 (note)
  1820s 182-6
  1830s 186-91
  physically cool 177
physicians, proprietary medicines sold by 216
Pigeon, Richard Hotham (1789-1851) 150-1
Pinel, Philippe (1745-1826)
Nosographie philosophique 82
Pinel woman, wife of Le Boulanger, falsely calling herself midwife 104 (note)
Pinney, Joel (temperance author) 184, 186, 190
Pneumatic Institute 49
'poison depletive quacks' 238
pollution fears 175
Ponsonby, Hon. Spencer, treated by R. Hutton 162
poor hearing *see* deafness
Poor Man's Friend, The 115-16
Pope, Alexander (1688-1744) 178
popular physiology 174, 186
Pott, Percival (1713-1788) treats Boswell for gonorrhoea 11
Power, D.J. (Bosworth), description of druggists 125 (note)
practica 175
pregnant women, inoculation effect on 44
priapism, herbal treatment for 95
Prichard, James Cowles (1768-1848) 47, 54 (note)

Priessnitz, phrenological analysis of 227
Priessnitz water cure 223, 225
Pringle, Sir John (1707-1782), treats Boswell for gonorrhoea 12
Profily, John MD 21-2
  An Essay and Exact Method of Curing the Venereal Disease 21
prolapse of uterus, recipe for plaster 95
prolix empiricism 83
proprietary medicines 216-19
  Bristol advertisements 217
  sold by physicians 216
  stamp duty on 218-19
  use by all classes 217-18
psychiatry, development of 7
Public Ledger, poem by 'Galen' in 72-3
publishing, early English 175
purification 176
Pustule, Peter de 30
Pythagoreans 177

quacks (quackery)
  advertisements 29-30
  definition 29, 106-7; Coltheart's 107; Guybon's 106-7
  drug-taking self helper 53
  female 37 (note)
  humble 30
  itinerant life 31
  lack of concern about 35
  local examples of cures 35
  nineteenth century scare 46
  ruptures treated by 114
  venereal disease treated by 114
  warnings against 30
  see also irregulars
'qualified medical practitioner', term with no precise limits 106
quinine 143, 150
quinquina 81

Radcliffe, Dr. John (1650-1714) views on urine-casting 58
rationality, in therapeutics 82
Redwood, Theophilus 147
Rees, George 7, 14
Reform Act (1832) 181
regimens 175
regular practitioners, patients/diseases treated by 118
Reily, Jane (patient of Dr.

Index

Myersbach) 64
religion of nature 208
religious faith of Victorian medical fringe 206-8
Report as to the practice of Medicine and Surgery by Unqualified Persons in the United Kingdom (1910) 162
revolutionary assemblies, (France) medical deregulation by 81
Richerand, Anthelme-Balthasar 90
Richmond, Duke and Duchess of (patients of Myersbach) 5
Riddell, John Leonard 243
right of property (France) 81
Ritson, Joseph (vegetarian writer) 178
Roberton, John 190, 191
Robinson, Nicholas (1697-1775) publication on venereal disease 11
Rocquemonty, Carouge de (proprietor of elixir of long life) 91
Rosen, George, on bone-setting 158-9
Royal College of Physicians, London Harrison's plan defeated by 118
  v. Rose 110
Royal Southern Hospital (Liverpool) 171 (note)
Rumsey, H.W. (Gloucester surgeon) 118
ruptures, treated by quacks 114

Saffory, Henry, publication on venereal disease 11
St. Louis Medical Society, bloodletting discussed by 247
Saint Peter's Hospital (Bristol) 33
Saint Sauveur, tailor's remedy for scrofula 90
Salmon-Maugé (remedy proprietor) 95
Salzman, C.G. 185
Samuel Foulger & Son 150
sanitarianism 191
sarsparilla 17, 18
sassafras 17, 18
Savory, John (druggist) 130
Scabby skin eruptions 114
Scorbutic symptoms 114
Scotch (Dr. Anderson's) Pill 112
Scrofula, infallible remedy for 90
scurvy 114
Searle, January (adult educator) 208
secret remedies in France (1789-1815) 79-105
  Commisson on secret remedies 93-100; remedies submitted to 94-8
  cure for specific disease 81
  Decree of 1810 92-3
  during Revolution 81, 85-9
  Germinal law 89-92
  pharmacist forbidden to sell 89
  see also Société Royale de Médicine
Seine, health council (France) 90
self-help, collective/mutual 201
self-medication 154-5
semiologist, clinician as 82
Shelley, Percy Bysshe (1792-1822) 179
Sherborne, regulars/irregulars in 124
Shorter, Thomas (Chartist) 206, 207, 214 (note)
shower 189
'simples', complexity of 83
Sinclair, Sir John (1754-1835) 178, 185
Skelton, John (Chartist) 199-200, 201, 207, 210
  Botanic Record and Family Herbal 200, 207
  demystification of medicine 221
  letter to E. Jones 202-3
  medical monopoly attacked 220
  Plea for the Botanic Practice of Medicine 200
skin, sense impressions of 187
Smedley, John (hydropath) 224, 224-5
Smedley, Mrs. John 224
Smiles, Samuel (1812-1904) 164, 166
Smith, Daniel, M.D. 35-6
  An Apology to the Public for Commencing the Practice of Physic 36, 44
Smith, John (cold water enthusiast) 180
Smith, Richard (Bristol surgeon) 53 (note), 108
  Bristol druggists 109
  Memoirs 41, 42, 53 (note)
  secret entrance for venereal patients 53 (note)
Smollett, Tobias George (1721-1771)
  The Adventures of Ferdinand, Count Fathom 34
Smyth, J.M.D. 22
  A New Treatise on the Venereal Disease 22-3
Société Royale de Médicine 80
  abolished 88

attack on 87
remedies approved by 80, 83, 84
Society of Apothecaries 119
actions by 120
first case against chemist 135
Solomon, Dr. (Gilead House, nr. Liverpool) 112, 126 (note)
Sourget, remedy for intermittent fevers 95
Southampton, attendance at druggists 118
South Carolina physicians, quoted 242, 249
'Spare Diet' 180
Speakman, Dr. (Bristol) 32, 53 (note)
specialisms, precursors of medical specialities 6
specialists, treated as quacks or of limited capacity 6
spiritualism 207
Sprengel, Kurt *History of Medicine* 49
Squire, Peter (1798-1884) 151
  Companion to the British Pharmacopoeia, A 151
  Pharmacopoeias of the London Hospitals, The 151
  Three Pharmacopoeias, The 151
Squire's Original Grand Elixir 112
Statute of Monopolies (1624) 79
Stead, William Thomas (1849-1912), defends Herbert Barker 166
Stevens, John 201, 220
  demystification of medicine 221
  Medical Reform 220
Stewart, Leonard 8
Stillé, Alfred 256 (note)
Stirling, regulars/irregulars in 124
Struve, Christian 186
strychnine 143
Suffolk, regulars/irregulars in 123
surgeon-apothecaires *see* apothecaries
surgeon(s)
  claim to travel by Act of Parliament 34
  split with barber-surgeons 31
Surgeon's Hall, public anatomy lectures in 31
Swift, Charles, publication on venereal disease 11
Sydenham, Thomas (1623-1688)
  on syphilis 9
  'regimen in the cure of fevers' 180
syphilis
  euphemisms 6

herbal remedies 17-18
mercury for 6, 15
surgical prerogative 9
virus 13, 17

Taylor, Dr. (itinerant irregular) 115
Taylor, James (bone-setter) 165
Taylor, John ('Chevalier') 30, 30-1, 40, 56-7
  shortness of stay in one place 41
  visits to West Country 53 (note)
Taylor, Thomas (1758-1835) 178
Taylor, Thomas (the Platonist) 194-5 (note)
T.C. (author of *The Charitable Surgeon*) 18
teetotalers (teetotalism) 174, 226
temperance, appeals to 184
temperance movement 226
Temperance Societies 186
temperatures, bodily 189
The People 208
Thiéry, François *Voeux d'un patriote sur la Médicine en France* 86-7
Thomas, Ann (bone-setter) 170
Thomas, Evan (bone-setter) 160-1
  prosecutions against 160-1
  sons 165
Thomas, Hugh Owen (1843-1891) 158, 167-8
Thomas, Josiah (botanical practitioner) 202-3
Thomas Morson & Son 150
Thompson, C.J.S. *Quacks of Old London* 5
Thomson, James (1700-1748) 178
Thomson, Samuel 220, 236
Thomson, William H. (Mississippi physician) 256 (note)
Thomsonian(s)
  American 236
  arrival in Bristol 46
Thomsonian herbalists 221, 222
Thornhill, Dr. Benjamin 30
Townsend (surgeon) 31
trade symbol of professional groups 31
transparency, in therapeutics 82
Travis, Henry (Owenite) 213 (note)
Trial by Jury Society 205
Trimmer, Mrs. Sarah (educationalist) 186
True Daffy's Elixir 113
Truth Seeker 208
Turner, Daniel (1667-1741) 19-21, 77

(note)
   medical degree of Yale University 21
   publications on venereal disease 11, 20
   Syphilis 20
   The Modern Quack 20
Turner, Robert *The Compleat Bonesetter* 180
Turner, William *A Booke of the Natures and Properties of Baths in England* 193 (note)
Tweed, J. 184
Tyron, Thomas (vegetarian) 177, 178

Underhill, John (Bristol) 32
Union for the Discouragement of Vicious Advertisements 218
universal suffrage, Chartist demand for 204
Universal Vegetable Medicine 184
University College Hospital Medical Committee 229
Upton, Robert (Clerk of the Society of Apothecaries) 120
urine-casting (uroscopy) 58, 115
'urinomania' 65
urology, origin as marginal specialism 6
uroscopy (urine-casting) 58, 115

vapour baths 189
Vaubaillon, secret remedies 96
vegetarianism 174, 205, 206, 211
   eighteenth-century 178
   seventeenth-century 177
venereal disease 5-28
   acquisition 13-15
   'cavalier's disease' 6
   herbal remedies 17
   medical division of labour 8-12
   publications on, in 18th century 10-11
   surgical prerogative 9
   treatment by quacks 114
Venette, Nicolas *Mysteries of Conjugal Love Reveal'd* 13
Venner, Tobias *Via Recta ad Vitam Longman* 193 (note)
Ventôse law on medicine (France) 90
veratrine 143
vernacular medical advice 175-7
Vicq d'Azyr, Félix *Nouveau plan de constitution pour la médecine en France* 87

Vincent, remedy for hernia 95
Vincent père, treatment of priapism 95
'Virtues' of remedies 82
vital energy, draining off 238
vital physiology 186
Voarino, Signor 185

Wakefield, attendance at druggists 118
Wakley, Thomas (editor of *The Lancet*) 46, 52
   on apothecaries 119
Wallace, Alfred Russel (1823-1913) 212 (note)
Ward, Dr., list of cheap medicines 43
Warmon, remedies proposed by 95
warm water/bath 189
Warren, John, publication on venereal disease 11
wart-charmers 117
water-casters *see* urine-casting
'Water from the Pool of Bethesda' 216
Waterton, Charles (1782-1865) 166
Webster, Joshua (vegetable drug-vendor) 179
Wesley, John (1703-1791) 186
   Primitive Physic (1747) 13, 47, 155
   cold water therapy 180
'whites' 13, 15
wholefood 205
Wholesale Druggists Club 131
Wilkes, Richard (1690-1760 — clergyman-physician) 125 (note)
Wilkinson, James J. Garth 205
   Medical Specialism 165
Will, H. (pupil of Liebig) 145
Willan, John (vindicator of Myersbach) 68
   letter to *Gazetteer* 68-9
William Allen, Hanburys & Barry 148
Willich, A.F.M. 182, 186
   macrobiotic diets 184
   sense impression of skin 187
Willows Francis Ltd 150
Wilson, James 225, 226
Winter, George (farmer-physician) 41, 53 (note), 107, 125 (note)
Wiseman, Richard (1622?-1676) 9
   on bone-setters 159
Working Men's College 207

Yorkshire, Greenland doctors in 124

Zimmerman, Johann Georg (quoted) 100